Current Status and Future Directions of Bone Trauma Surgery

Current Status and Future Directions of Bone Trauma Surgery

Editors

Ivo Dumić-Čule
Tomislav Čengić

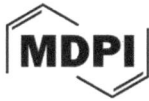

Basel • Beijing • Wuhan • Barcelona • Belgrade • Novi Sad • Cluj • Manchester

Editors
Ivo Dumić-Čule
University North
Varazdin
Croatia

Tomislav Čengić
University Hospital Centre
Sestre Milosrdnice
Zagreb
Croatia

Editorial Office
MDPI AG
Grosspeteranlage 5
4052 Basel, Switzerland

This is a reprint of articles from the Special Issue published online in the open access journal *Medicina* (ISSN 1648-9144) (available at: https://www.mdpi.com/journal/medicina/special_issues/3X08M7OQYA).

For citation purposes, cite each article independently as indicated on the article page online and as indicated below:

Lastname, A.A.; Lastname, B.B. Article Title. *Journal Name* **Year**, *Volume Number*, Page Range.

ISBN 978-3-7258-2249-2 (Hbk)
ISBN 978-3-7258-2250-8 (PDF)
doi.org/10.3390/books978-3-7258-2250-8

© 2024 by the authors. Articles in this book are Open Access and distributed under the Creative Commons Attribution (CC BY) license. The book as a whole is distributed by MDPI under the terms and conditions of the Creative Commons Attribution-NonCommercial-NoDerivs (CC BY-NC-ND) license.

Contents

About the Editors vii

Ivo Dumic-Cule
Current Status and Future Directions of Bone Trauma Surgery
Reprinted from: *Medicina* 2024, *60*, 1297, doi:10.3390/medicina60081297 1

Chi-Hsuan Tsai, Meng-Yu Wu, Da-Sen Chien, Po-Chen Lin, Jui-Yuan Chung, Chi-Yuan Liu, et al.
Association between Time to Emergent Surgery and Outcomes in Trauma Patients: A 10-Year Multicenter Study
Reprinted from: *Medicina* 2024, *60*, 960, doi:10.3390/medicina60060960 3

Po-Chen Lin, Meng-Yu Wu, Da-Sen Chien, Jui-Yuan Chung, Chi-Yuan Liu, I-Shiang Tzeng, et al.
Use of Reverse Shock Index Multiplied by Simplified Motor Score in a Five-Level Triage System: Identifying Trauma in Adult Patients at a High Risk of Mortality
Reprinted from: *Medicina* 2024, *60*, 647, doi:10.3390/medicina60040647 16

Shu-Jui Lee, Lin Jian, Chi-Yuan Liu, I-Shiang Tzeng, Da-Sen Chien, Yueh-Tseng Hou, et al.
A Ten-Year Retrospective Cohort Study on Neck Collar Immobilization in Trauma Patients with Head and Neck Injuries
Reprinted from: *Medicina* 2023, *59*, 1974, doi:10.3390/medicina59111974 28

Jui-Ting Mao, Hao-Wei Chang, Tsung-Li Lin, I-Hao Lin, Chia-Yu Lin and Chin-Jung Hsu
Clinical Outcomes of Single Versus Double Plating in Distal-Third Humeral Fractures Caused by Arm Wrestling: A Retrospective Analysis
Reprinted from: *Medicina* 2022, *58*, 1654, doi:10.3390/medicina58111654 40

Paulo Ottoni di Tullio, Vincenzo Giordano, William Dias Belangero, Robinson Esteves Pires, Felipe Serrão de Souza, Pedro José Labronici, et al.
Computed Tomography Does Not Improve Intra- and Interobserver Agreement of Hertel Radiographic Prognostic Criteria
Reprinted from: *Medicina* 2022, *58*, 1489, doi:10.3390/medicina58101489 50

Tomislav Madzar, Tonci Masina, Roko Zaja, Snjezana Kastelan, Jasna Pucarin Cvetkovic, Hana Brborovic, et al.
Overtraining Syndrome as a Risk Factor for Bone Stress Injuries among Paralympic Athletes
Reprinted from: *Medicina* 2024, *60*, 52, doi:10.3390/medicina60010052 62

Luka Dudaric, Ivo Dumic-Cule, Eugen Divjak, Tomislav Cengic, Boris Brkljacic and Gordana Ivanac
Bone Remodeling in Osteoarthritis—Biological and Radiological Aspects
Reprinted from: *Medicina* 2023, *59*, 1613, doi:10.3390/medicina59091613 73

Mislav Cavka, Domagoj Delimar, Robert Rezan, Tomislav Zigman, Kresimir Sasa Duric, Mislav Cimic, et al.
Complications of Percutaneous Vertebroplasty: A Pictorial Review
Reprinted from: *Medicina* 2023, *59*, 1536, doi:10.3390/medicina59091536 84

Danilo Leonetti, Giorgio Carmelo Basile, Gabriele Giuca, Elena Corso, Domenico Fenga and Ilaria Sanzarello
Total Talar Prosthesis, Learning from Experience, Two Reports of Total Talar Prosthesis after Talar Extrusion and Literature Review
Reprinted from: *Medicina* **2023**, *59*, 1498, doi:10.3390/medicina59081498 . . . . **94**

Chiedozie Kenneth Ugwoke, Domenico Albano, Nejc Umek, Ivo Dumić-Čule and Žiga Snoj
Application of Virtual Reality Systems in Bone Trauma Procedures
Reprinted from: *Medicina* **2023**, *59*, 562, doi:10.3390/medicina59030562 . . . . **107**

Stjepan Dokuzović, Sathish Muthu, Jure Pavešić, Mario Španić, Stjepan Ivandić, Gregor Eder, et al.
Conservative Treatment for Spontaneous Resolution of Postoperative Symptomatic Thoracic Spinal Epidural Hematoma—A Case Report
Reprinted from: *Medicina* **2023**, *59*, 1590, doi:10.3390/medicina59091590 . . . . **124**

Pan Hong, Yuhong Ding, Ruijing Xu, Saroj Rai, Ruikang Liu and Jin Li
A Combination of Ilizarov Frame, Externalized Locking Plate and Tibia Bridging for an Adult with Large Tibial Defect and Severe Varus Deformity Due to Chronic Osteomyelitis in Childhood: A Case Report
Reprinted from: *Medicina* **2023**, *59*, 262, doi:10.3390/medicina59020262 . . . . **132**

About the Editors

Ivo Dumić-Čule

Ivo Dumić-Čule graduated from the Zagreb School of Medicine in 2012 and received PhD in 2016 and MHA in 2021. In recognition of his work, he received the Dean's and Rector's Award. He is the youngest winner of the New Investigator Award, awarded by the European Calcified Tissue Society. He was the recipient of the Dean's Award for obtaining the highest scientific productivity in his PhD class. He is the author or co-author of more than 35 articles published in CC and SCI, international patents and five book chapters, which have been cited more than 1200 times. He was responsible for several research projects at the School of Medicine, the University of Zagreb, and was a Postdoctoral Fellow at the International Center for Genetic Engineering and Biotechnology in Trieste. He was the Chief Executive Officer at Children's Hospital in Croatia. Currently, he is Assistant Professor at University North and CEO of Polyclinic DaVinci. He is President of the Board of Senate of Economy in Croatia and a Member of the Advisory Board of M Plus Croatia.

Tomislav Čengić

Tomislav Čengić is a specialist in orthopedics and traumatology with an interest in minimally invasive and reconstructive surgery of the lower extremity. He has been attending a specialist internship since 2011 at the Traumatology Department of the Sestre Milosrdnice University Hospital Center in Zagreb and the Orthopedics Department of the University Hospital Center, Zagreb, after which he will take a specialist exam in orthopedics and traumatology. He defended his doctoral dissertation entitled "The effect of anteversion of the cementless femoral component of the "Zweymüller" hip endoprosthesis on primary stability and proneness to periprosthetic fracture—a biomechanical study on an artificial bone model". He graduated from the Faculty of Medicine of the University of Rijeka in 2009. While training abroad in 2021, he stayed at Center Orthopédique Santy, Lyon, France, under the mentorship of Dr. Mathieu Thaunat. In 2016, he stayed at the London Sarcoma Unit, Royal National Orthopedic Hospital, London, United Kingdom, under the mentorship of Prof. Will Aston. In 2014, he resided as a Clinical and Research Associate at the Clinic for Orthopedics and Traumatology, Universitätspital Basel, Switzerland, under the mentorship of Prof. Geert Pagenstert. He is the recipient of numerous scholarships and awards for innovations in medicine. In 2015, he was awarded the State Award of Technical Culture of the Republic of Croatia "Faust Vrančić" for a 3D reconstructive personalized pelvic implant. In 2021, he was awarded the American–Austrian Foundation (AAF) Bone&Joint Fellowship organized by AAF and Weil Cornell Medical School, New York, USA. In 2014, he received a Musculoskeletal Tumor Fellowship organized by the AAF and Memorial Sloan Kettering Cancer Center, New York, USA. In 2008, he won a scholarship from the Ministry of Science, Education and Sports for gifted students. In 2006, he was awarded the Rector's Award at the University of Rijeka and, in 2005, the Award of the Faculty of Medicine in Rijeka. He is an Assistant Professor at the Department of Orthopaedics, Zagreb School of Medicine and Department of Anatomy and Physiology at the University of Applied Health Sciences in Zagreb. He was a mentor for several graduate theses. He is the author of three university textbooks and over 20 scientific and professional papers.

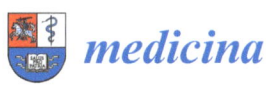 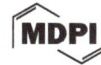

Editorial

Current Status and Future Directions of Bone Trauma Surgery

Ivo Dumic-Cule [1,2]

1. University North, 104 Brigade 3, 42000 Varazdin, Croatia; ivodc1@gmail.com; Tel.: +385-98-1655-686
2. Polyclinic Da Vinci, Petrovaradinska 110, 10000 Zagreb, Croatia

Citation: Dumic-Cule, I. Current Status and Future Directions of Bone Trauma Surgery. *Medicina* **2024**, *60*, 1297. https://doi.org/10.3390/medicina60081297

Received: 2 August 2024
Accepted: 7 August 2024
Published: 11 August 2024

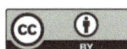

Copyright: © 2024 by the author. Licensee MDPI, Basel, Switzerland. This article is an open access article distributed under the terms and conditions of the Creative Commons Attribution (CC BY) license (https://creativecommons.org/licenses/by/4.0/).

The ever-evolving field of bone trauma surgery and bone regeneration is characterized by continuous transformation due to advancements in medical technology, enhancements in surgical techniques, and a deeper understanding of biological interactions underlying the processes of bone healing and regeneration. Therefore, this Special Issue of *Medicina*, "Current Status and Future Directions of Bone Trauma Surgery", is dedicated to presenting the latest knowledge and exploring future directions in bone trauma surgery. It comprises twelve articles focusing on all relevant aspects of bone trauma surgery and bone regeneration, including upgrades to the current techniques used for the management of bone trauma. Additionally, this Special Issue aimed to provide comprehensive reviews that can be useful and applicable to everyday traumatology practice.

Bone trauma surgery has made remarkable strides in recent decades. The integration of minimally invasive techniques, the development of sophisticated fixation devices, and the use of biologics for bone healing have revolutionized the field [1]. Currently, surgeons have a plethora of tools at their disposal, enabling them to tackle complex fractures with greater precision, resulting in improved outcomes. In this Special Issue, Mao and collaborators described less-invasive surgical techniques that yielded reduced rates of postoperative complications and faster recovery periods. In patients with distal-third humeral fractures resulting from arm wrestling, single plating has demonstrated a union rate and elbow range of motion comparable to that achieved using double plating. Moreover, significant advantages were described, including fewer complications, reduced surgical time, and lower blood loss. These benefits contribute to improved early functional outcomes, making single plating a more favorable option when treating these specific fractures [2].

Recent studies have underscored the importance of early intervention and individualized treatment plans, thereby ensuring functional recovery and, subsequently, increased quality of life for patients. Lee, S.J. and collaborators suggested that prehospital cervical and spinal immobilization should be more selectively applied to certain head and neck injury groups. This selective approach is particularly important for individuals older than 65, those with impaired consciousness (GCS 8), individuals suffering from severe traumatic injuries (ISS 16 or RTS 7), and patients experiencing shock. They emphasized a retrospective study design as well as its limitations and potential biases [3].

Although enhanced imaging technologies, such as 3D CT scans and MRI, play a crucial role in preoperative planning and intraoperative navigation, Tullio P.O.D. et al. demonstrated that there are certain conditions in which CT scans are no more useful than conventional X-rays. CT scans did not enhance the surgeons' primary interpretation of the Hertel prognostic criteria, nor did they provide additional value compared to radiographic examinations [4].

Emerging innovations in bone trauma surgery are also promising in terms of enhancing surgeon performance. The use of augmented reality (AR) in surgery is an exciting frontier, providing surgeons with augmented visualization and enhanced precision during procedures [5]. Over the past decade, the introduction of both high- and low-fidelity virtual reality systems for bone trauma procedures has resulted in significant benefits. These systems have enhanced procedural teaching and learning, improved preoperative planning, increased intraoperative precision and efficiency, and contributed to better postoperative outcomes. Despite these advancements, there is a need for further technical developments that meet industry benchmarks and metrics. Additionally, more standardized and rigorous clinical validation is required to fully realize the potential of these virtual reality systems in bone trauma procedures.

Percutaneous vertebroplasty is a minimally invasive technique employed to treat vertebral body compression fractures, offering significant relief and functional improvement. The most common complication is cement leakage, which can infiltrate the epidural, intradiscal, foraminal, paravertebral regions, and even the venous system. While many complications are asymptomatic, they pose the potential for severe consequences. A review published in this Special Issue is based on single-center experiences, comprised of various complications associated with vertebroplasty, and aimed to improve our understanding of the pathology and mitigate objective risks [6].

Despite the variability in terminology (hypertrophic arthritis, degenerative arthritis, arthritis deformans, etc.), our understanding of osteoarthritis has advanced due to extensive in vitro and in vivo research, elucidating the disease's pathophysiology and pathology at both histological and cellular levels. Nonetheless, the precise cause of osteoarthritis remains unknown. Therefore, a review written by Dudaric et al. consolidates the recent findings on the biological processes that occur in bone tissue during osteoarthritis, aiming to provide insights beneficial for clinical practice. Emphasizing the importance of selecting appropriate radiological techniques is crucial for the early diagnosis and effective management of this prevalent and debilitating chronic condition [7].

In summary, this Special Issue is dedicated to advancements in bone trauma surgery and bone regeneration that are transforming patient care and outcomes. Through comprehensive reviews and clinical studies, contributors have suggested modifications of surgical techniques, radiologic methods, and innovative technologies that enable better diagnostics, enhance healing, and reduce complications.

Funding: This research received no external funding.

Conflicts of Interest: The author declares no conflicts of interest.

References

1. Dumic-Cule, I.; Pecina, M.; Jelic, M.; Jankolija, M.; Popek, I.; Grgurevic, L.; Vukicevic, S. Biological aspects of segmental bone defects management. *Int. Orthop.* **2015**, *39*, 1005–1011. [CrossRef]
2. Mao, J.T.; Chang, H.W.; Lin, T.L.; Lin, I.H.; Lin, C.Y.; Hsu, C.J. Clinical Outcomes of Single Versus Double Plating in Distal-Third Humeral Fractures Caused by Arm Wrestling: A Retrospective Analysis. *Medicina* **2022**, *58*, 1654. [CrossRef] [PubMed]
3. Lee, S.J.; Jian, L.; Liu, C.Y.; Tzeng, I.S.; Chien, D.S.; Hou, Y.T.; Lin, P.C.; Chen, Y.L.; Wu, M.Y.; Yiang, G.T. A Ten-Year Retrospective Cohort Study on Neck Collar Immobilization in Trauma Patients with Head and Neck Injuries. *Medicina* **2023**, *59*, 1974. [CrossRef] [PubMed]
4. Tullio, P.O.D.; Giordano, V.; Belangero, W.D.; Pires, R.E.; de Souza, F.S.; Labronici, P.J.; Zamboni, C.; Malzac, F.; Belangero, P.S.; Ikemoto, R.Y.; et al. Computed Tomography Does Not Improve Intra- and Interobserver Agreement of Hertel Radiographic Prognostic Criteria. *Medicina* **2022**, *58*, 1489. [CrossRef] [PubMed]
5. Ugwoke, C.K.; Albano, D.; Umek, N.; Dumić-Čule, I.; Snoj, Ž. Application of Virtual Reality Systems in Bone Trauma Procedures. *Medicina* **2023**, *59*, 562. [CrossRef] [PubMed]
6. Cavka, M.; Delimar, D.; Rezan, R.; Zigman, T.; Duric, K.S.; Cimic, M.; Dumic-Cule, I.; Prutki, M. Complications of Percutaneous Vertebroplasty: A Pictorial Review. *Medicina* **2023**, *59*, 1536. [CrossRef] [PubMed]
7. Dudaric, L.; Dumic-Cule, I.; Divjak, E.; Cengic, T.; Brkljacic, B.; Ivanac, G. Bone Remodeling in Osteoarthritis-Biological and Radiological Aspects. *Medicina* **2023**, *59*, 1613. [CrossRef] [PubMed]

Disclaimer/Publisher's Note: The statements, opinions and data contained in all publications are solely those of the individual author(s) and contributor(s) and not of MDPI and/or the editor(s). MDPI and/or the editor(s) disclaim responsibility for any injury to people or property resulting from any ideas, methods, instructions or products referred to in the content.

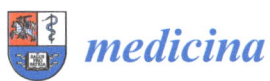

Article

Association between Time to Emergent Surgery and Outcomes in Trauma Patients: A 10-Year Multicenter Study

Chi-Hsuan Tsai [1,2], Meng-Yu Wu [1,2,3], Da-Sen Chien [1,2], Po-Chen Lin [1,2], Jui-Yuan Chung [3,4,5,6], Chi-Yuan Liu [7,8], I-Shiang Tzeng [9], Yueh-Tseng Hou [1,2], Yu-Long Chen [1,2] and Giou-Teng Yiang [1,2,*]

1. Department of Emergency Medicine, Taipei Tzu Chi Hospital, Buddhist Tzu Chi Medical Foundation, New Taipei 231, Taiwan
2. Department of Emergency Medicine, School of Medicine, Tzu Chi University, Hualien 970, Taiwan
3. Graduate Institute of Injury Prevention and Control, Taipei Medical University, Taipei 231, Taiwan
4. Department of Emergency Medicine, Cathay General Hospital, Taipei 106, Taiwan
5. School of Medicine, Fu Jen Catholic University, Taipei 242, Taiwan
6. School of Medicine, National Tsing Hua University, Hsinchu 300, Taiwan
7. Department of Orthopedic Surgery, Taipei Tzu Chi Hospital, Buddhist Tzu Chi Medical Foundation, New Taipei 231, Taiwan
8. Department of Orthopedics, School of Medicine, Tzu Chi University, Hualien 970, Taiwan
9. Department of Research, Taipei Tzu Chi Hospital, Buddhist Tzu Chi Medical Foundation, New Taipei 970, Taiwan
* Correspondence: gtyiang@gmail.com

Abstract: *Background*: Research on the impact of reduced time to emergent surgery in trauma patients has yielded inconsistent results. Therefore, this study investigated the relationship between waiting emergent surgery time (WEST) and outcomes in trauma patients. *Methods*: This retrospective, multi-center study used data from the Tzu Chi Hospital trauma database. The primary clinical outcomes were in-hospital mortality, intensive care unit (ICU) admission, and prolonged hospital length of stay (LOS) of $\geq$30 days. *Results*: A total of 15,164 patients were analyzed. The median WEST was 444 min, with an interquartile range (IQR) of 248–848 min for all patients. Patients who died in the hospital had a shorter median WEST than did those who survived (240 vs. 446 min, $p < 0.001$). Among the trauma patients with a WEST of <2 h, the median time was 79 min (IQR = 50–100 min). No significant difference in WEST was observed between the survival and mortality groups for patients with a WEST of <120 min (median WEST: 85 vs. 78 min, $p < 0.001$). Multivariable logistic regression analysis revealed that WEST was not associated with an increased risk of in-hospital mortality (adjusted odds ratio [aOR] = 1.05, 95% confidence interval [CI] = 0.17–6.35 for 30 min $\leq$ WEST < 60 min; aOR = 1.12, 95% CI = 0.22–5.70 for 60 min $\leq$ WEST < 90 min; and aOR = 0.60, 95% CI = 0.13–2.74 for WEST $\geq$ 90 min). *Conclusions*: Our findings do not support the "golden hour" concept because no association was identified between the time to definitive care and in-hospital mortality, ICU admission, and prolonged hospital stay of $\geq$30 days.

Keywords: golden hour; time to definitive care; mortality; trauma

1. Introduction

Traumatic injuries present a substantial global threat; they contribute considerably to global morbidity and mortality. Early definite care is crucial for high-risk trauma patients, with interventions for such patients including surgery [1–6]. According to the "golden hour" concept, the first hour following a traumatic injury is the most crucial [7].

The term "golden hour" is often attributed to R. Adams Cowley, the founder of Baltimore's Shock Trauma Institute. In a 1975 article, Cowley asserted that "the first hour after injury will largely determine a critically injured person's chances for survival". The golden hour concept emphasizes that critically injured patients must receive definitive care within 60 min of sustaining injuries. During this crucial period, immediate medical

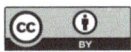

attention can profoundly influence a patient's prognosis. Swift and effective intervention within this timeframe often determines whether a patient will live or die or will experience full recovery or lasting disability. Prompt assessment, stabilization, and transport to appropriate medical facilities during this hour are essential to reduce complications and improve survival and recovery outcomes. Providing medical care within the golden hour is imperative because delays can lead to worsened outcomes and increased mortality rates. The golden hour concept was proposed in the 1970s; it has not been supported by empirical data or research but has gained widespread acceptance because of its clinical plausibility. Therefore, its validity remains unclear.

Trauma patients requiring emergent surgery may benefit from prompt surgical intervention, as suggested by the golden hour concept, with such intervention potentially improving their prognosis. However, research on the relationship between the waiting emergent surgery time (WEST) and trauma patient outcomes has produced inconsistent findings. Most studies investigating the impact of reduced surgical wait times have focused on patients with hip fracture, and they have obtained varying results. Additionally, research efforts have often been limited by small sample sizes or a primary emphasis on reducing time intervals rather than improving patient outcomes.

Gaining a comprehensive understanding of the golden hour concept is imperative. In Taiwan, level 1 trauma centers, which are accredited on the basis of their emergency capacity, have attending surgeons available 24/7 for all major trauma resuscitations. These centers also provide resuscitation interventions such as transcatheter arterial embolization or surgery, even on weekends and holidays [6,8]. Although studies have reported the optimal time to definitive care to be 2 h for procedures such as exploratory laparotomy and craniotomy at level 1 hospitals, in Taiwan, the time limit for emergent trauma surgeries is typically 30 min [9,10]. The current study investigated the relationship between the time to definitive care and trauma patient outcomes.

2. Methods

2.1. Study Design and Setting

This study was a retrospective cohort analysis of data from the Tzu Chi Hospital trauma registry, and the study protocol was approved by the Institutional Review Board of Taipei Tzu Chi Hospital (IRB number: 12-XD-077). The trauma database of Tzu Chi Hospital is a collaborative effort among four hospitals within the Tzu Chi Hospital system, with the hospitals located in Hualien, Taipei, Taichung, and Dalin. This database includes the data of patients admitted with trauma-related conditions identified by International Classification of Diseases, Ninth Revision, Clinical Modification codes 800–959 (excluding 905–909 and 930–939) or International Classification of Diseases, Tenth Revision, Clinical Modification codes S00–T98 (excluding T15–T19 and T90–T98) as well as those with major traumatic injuries. The database includes information regarding a comprehensive set of 152 variables associated with trauma, covering aspects such as demographics, injury mechanisms, injury types, injury severity, vital signs, surgical interventions, and in-hospital mortality. The current study adhered to the Strengthening the Reporting of Observational Studies in Epidemiology (STROBE) guidelines (Supplementary Table S1) [11].

2.2. Participant Selection

This study included patients listed on the Tzu Chi Hospital trauma database between January 2009 and December 2021. Initially, 48,524 patients were considered for analysis. However, patients who did not undergo surgery (n = 33,094), those without a recorded time to definitive care (n = 211), and those without data on mortality outcomes (n = 55) were excluded. Ultimately, 15,164 patients were included in the analysis. A detailed flow diagram of the participant selection process is presented in Figure 1.

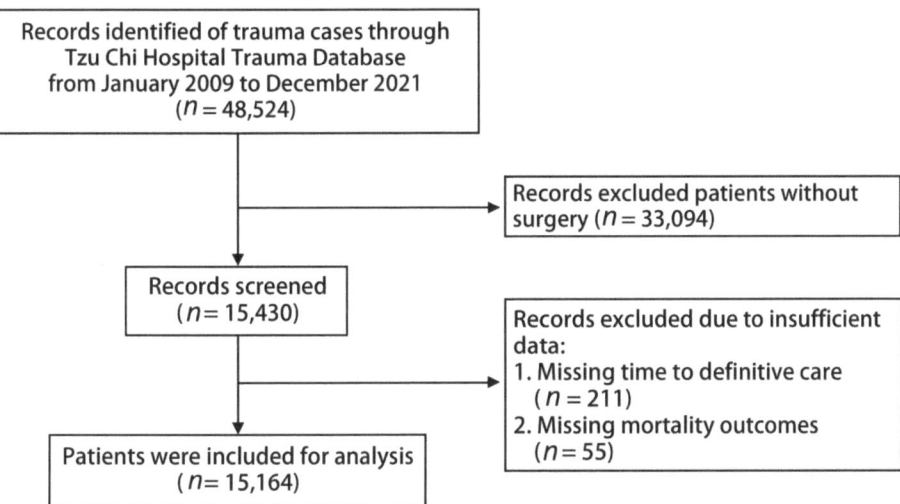

Figure 1. Flow diagram of participant selection.

2.3. *Variable Measurements*

The study analyzed the fundamental characteristics of the trauma cohort, including age, sex, pre-existing medical conditions, emergency triage classification, vital signs, injury etiology, and injury severity. Vital parameters, such as heart rate (HR), systolic blood pressure (SBP), diastolic blood pressure (DBP), and respiratory rate (RR), were documented. Trauma severity was assessed using the injury severity score (ISS) and the revised trauma score (RTS). The ISS is used to evaluate the severity of multiple injuries, with scores from various body regions (head, chest, abdomen, extremities, and other areas) combined into a single value ranging from 0 to 75, with higher scores indicating more severe trauma [12]. The RTS is used to assess trauma severity on the basis of a patient's physiological parameters, including SBP, RR, and level of consciousness [13]. These scoring systems are critical for the initial assessment and classification of trauma patients; they assist health-care providers in quickly assessing injury severity and developing appropriate treatment plans. Use of the ISS and RTS can help improve survival rates and patient outcomes as well as assist heal-care providers in effectively allocating emergency and medical resources. In the current study, patients with an ISS $\geq$ 16 or an RTS < 7 were defined as the major trauma population. The patients were categorized into two groups: those with traumatic brain injury (TBI, head Abbreviated Injury Score [AIS] $\geq$ 3) and those without TBI (head AIS score < 3). For the subgroup analysis, the geriatric population was defined as individuals aged $\geq$ 65 years. The mechanisms of injury included motor vehicle collision, low falls (falling from < 1 m), high falls (falling from $\geq$ 1 m), and others (such as drowning, burns, and cold injuries).

The primary variable in this study was each patient's time to definitive care, defined as the time to surgical intervention for acute trauma injury. Time to emergent surgery was calculated as the interval from the patient's arrival at the hospital to the start of surgical intervention. We categorized the WEST into 30 min intervals. Although emergency intervention is generally defined as that occurring within 1 h of injury, studies have indicated that the optimal time to definitive care for most emergent trauma interventions may extend up to 2 h, with this timeframe employed in some level 1 trauma centers [9,14]. To account for this, we conducted a sensitivity analysis focusing on patients who received emergent surgery within 2 h of injury.

2.4. Clinical Outcomes

We focused on three primary clinical outcomes: in-hospital mortality, admission to the intensive care unit (ICU), and extended hospitalization, defined as a length of stay (LOS) of ≥30 days. Additionally, we evaluated the frequency of ICU readmissions, the duration of ICU stays, extended ICU LOS (specified as an ICU stay exceeding 14 days), and the total duration of hospitalization for each patient.

2.5. Statistical Analysis

We conducted a comprehensive statistical analysis of all demographic information, injury details, and clinical outcomes by using SPSS software (version 20.0, SPSS, Chicago, IL, USA). The distribution patterns of continuous data were assessed using the Kolmogorov–Smirnov test. Continuous variables are presented as medians with interquartile ranges (IQRs), and categorical variables are presented as counts and percentages. Continuous data were analyzed using either nonparametric analysis of variance or the Mann–Whitney U test. Categorical and nominal data were evaluated using Pearson's chi-square test or Fisher's exact test. The relationship between the scoring systems and the three major trauma patient outcomes was determined using multivariable logistic regression. The factors considered in the regression analysis were variables with a p value < 0.10 in the chi-square or Mann–Whitney U tests or those of clinical significance, such as age, sex, injury type, and injury mechanism, by using a forced entry method. Sensitivity analyses were conducted to evaluate the associations across different groups, including categories of injury severity (minor injury: ISS < 16 or RTS ≥ 7 and major injury: ISS ≥ 16 or RTS < 7), age groups (nongeriatric: age < 65 years and geriatric: age ≥ 65 years), WEST durations (WEST < 30 min, 30 min ≤ WEST < 60 min, 60 min ≤ WEST < 90 min, and WEST ≥ 90 min), and major injury sites (head AIS ≥ 3, chest AIS ≥ 3, and abdominal AIS ≥ 3). All tests were two-sided, with significance set at $p < 0.05$.

3. Results

3.1. Characteristics of Study Participants

The in-hospital mortality rate, ICU admission rate, and rate of prolonged hospital LOS of ≥30 days were 1.0%, 12.0%, and 4.5%, respectively. Table 1 presents the demographic characteristics of all patients. The geriatric population (age ≥ 65 years) accounted for 41.4% and 63.4% of the mortality group. Patients in the in-hospital mortality group had higher triage levels, with 49.7% classified as triage level I. Penetrative injuries were present in only 5.3% of all patients. Cardiovascular disease was the most common chronic condition, accounting for 27.6% of the conditions, followed by diabetes (15.9%). Major injuries (ISS ≥ 16) were present in 7.4% of all patients and 67.6% of the in-hospital mortality group. Low falls were the most common injury mechanism, accounting for 39.9% of the injuries, followed by road traffic injuries, at 37.7%. TBI occurred in 6.7% of all patients and in 58.6% of the in-hospital mortality group.

Table 1. Comparison of demographic characteristics of included patients.

Characteristics	Total Patients	Survival	Mortality	*p*-Value
Patient number	15,164 (100%)	15,019 (99%)	145 (1%)	
Age (years)				<0.001
Age < 65 years old	8890 (58.6%)	8837 (58.8%)	53 (36.6%)	
Age ≥ 65 years old	6272 (41.4%)	6180 (41.2%)	92 (63.4%)	
Sex, n (%)				<0.001
Female	7520 (49.6%)	7479 (49.8%)	41 (28.3%)	
Male	7644 (50.4%)	7540 (50.2%)	104 (71.7%)	

Table 1. Cont.

Characteristics	Total Patients	Survival	Mortality	p-Value
Vital sign				
SBP	142 (124–161)	142 (124–161)	146 (109.5–174)	0.864
DBP	83 (73–94)	83 (73–94)	84 (66–99)	0.332
RR	18 (16–20)	18 (16–20)	18 (16–20)	0.094
HR	84 (73–96)	84 (73–96)	89 (74–101)	0.023
Triage				<0.001
1	667 (4.4%)	595 (4.0%)	72 (49.7%)	
2	5908 (39.0%)	5866 (39.1%)	42 (29.0%)	
3	8444 (55.8%)	8413 (56.1%)	31 (21.4%)	
4 and 5	125 (0.8%)	125 (0.8%)	0 (0.0%)	
Injury severity				
RTS	7.84 (7.84–7.84)	7.84 (7.84–7.84)	6.90 (5.00–7.84)	<0.001
RTS < 7	668 (4.4%)	594 (4.0%)	74 (51.4%)	<0.001
ISS	9 (4–9)	9 (4–9)	25 (9–29)	<0.001
ISS ≥ 16	1125 (7.4%)	1027 (6.8%)	98 (67.6%)	<0.001
Trauma team activation	495 (3.3%)	444 (3.0%)	51 (35.2%)	<0.001
Time for surgery	444 (248–848)	446 (251–850)	240 (116.5–473)	<0.001
Traumatic brain injury				<0.001
Non-TBI	14,151 (93.3%)	14,091 (93.8%)	60 (41.4%)	
TBI	1013 (6.7%)	928 (6.2%)	85 (58.6%)	
Injury type				0.080
Penetrating injury	807 (5.3%)	804 (5.4%)	3 (2.1%)	
Non-penetrating injury	14,357 (94.7%)	14,215 (94.6%)	142 (97.9%)	
Mechanism of injury				0.002
Traffic road injury	5112 (37.7%)	5045 (37.6%)	67 (51.5%)	
High fall	1370 (10.1%)	1353 (10.1%)	17 (13.1%)	
Low fall	5403 (39.9%)	5362 (39.9%)	41 (31.5%)	
Others	3279 (21.6%)	3259 (21.7%)	20 (13.8%)	
Comorbidity				
CNS diseases	672 (4.4%)	66 (4.4%)	6 (4.1%)	0.863
CVD	3965 (26.1%)	3925 (26.1%)	40 (27.6%)	0.692
CKD	351 (2.3%)	339 (2.3%)	12 (8.3%)	0.003
Diabetes mellitus	1676 (11.1%)	1653 (11.0%)	23 (15.9%)	0.250
Hospitalization				
Total LOS days	7 (4–10)	7 (4–10)	10 (4–22.5)	<0.001
Total LOS ≥ 30 days	687 (4.5%)	661 (4.4%)	26 (17.9%)	<0.001
ICU admission	1818 (12.0%)	1695 (11.3%)	123 (84.8%)	0.040
ICU LOS, days	5 (3–11)	5 (3–11)	6 (3–19)	<0.001
ICU LOS ≥ 14 days	369 (22.0%)	328 (21.1%)	41 (33.3%)	0.002
In-hospital mortality	145	---	145	----
Death within 24 h	10 (6.9%)	----	10 (6.9%)	----

Abbreviations: SBP, systolic blood pressure; DBP, diastolic blood pressure; RR, respiratory rate; HR, heart rate; CNS diseases, central nervous system diseases; CKD, chronic kidney disease; CVD, cardiovascular disease; ISS, injury severity score; RTS, revised trauma score; TBI, traumatic brain injury; LOS, length of stay; ICU, intensive care unit. The continuous variables are presented as median and interquartile range (IQR).

3.2. Time to Emergent Surgery in Subgroups

Table 2 presents the results of comparisons of the WEST among all patients across various subgroups. The median WEST for all patients was 444 min, with an IQR of 248–848 min. Patients who died in hospital had a notably shorter WEST than survivors did (median WEST: 240 vs. 446 min, $p < 0.001$). After stratification by other patient characteristics, a significantly shorter WEST was observed among patients younger than 65 years (median WEST: 419 vs. 478 min, $p < 0.001$), those with major injuries to the abdomen (median WEST in patients with abdominal AIS ≥ 3 vs. head AIS ≥ 3 vs. chest AIS ≥ 3: 353 vs. 413 vs. 492 min, $p < 0.001$), those with major injuries (ISS ≥ 16 or RTS < 7; median WEST in patients with RTS < 7 vs. RTS ≥ 7 and ISS ≥ 16 vs. ISS < 16:

301 vs. 450 min and 397 vs. 447 min, respectively, $p < 0.001$), and those with a hospital stay exceeding 30 days (median WEST: 446 vs. 406 min, $p < 0.001$).

Table 2. Comparison of waiting emergent surgery times (WESTs) among all patients across various subgroups.

Subgroup	Median (IQR)	p-Value
WEST per 30 min		
WEST < 30 min	16 (9–23)	
30 ≤ WEST < 60 min	48 (38–55)	<0.001
60 ≤ WEST < 90 min	76 (70–84)	
WEST ≥ 90 min	468 (275–873)	
Age		
Age < 65 years old	419 (231–802)	<0.001
Age ≥ 65 years old	478 (276–905)	
RTS		
RTS < 7	301 (136–760)	<0.001
RTS ≥ 7	450 (255–849)	
ISS		
ISS < 16	447 (256–840)	<0.001
ISS ≥ 16	397 (155–948)	
Major injury site		
Head AIS ≥ 3	413 (157–956)	
Chest AIS ≥ 3	492 (197–1077)	<0.001
Abdominal AIS ≥ 3	353 (156–946)	
Hospitalization		
Total LOS < 30 days	446 (252–847)	<0.001
Total LOS ≥ 30 days	406 (182–881)	
ICU admission		
Yes	432 (189–982)	0.273
No	445 (256–830)	
In-hospital mortality		
Yes	240 (116–473)	<0.001
No	446 (251–850)	

Abbreviations: WEST, waiting emergent surgery time; SBP, systolic blood pressure; DBP, diastolic blood pressure; RR, respiratory rate; HR, heart rate; ISS, injury severity score; AIS, abbreviated injury scale; RTS, revised trauma score; TBI, traumatic brain injury; LOS, length of stay; ICU, intensive care unit.

3.3. Trauma Patients with WEST Less than 2 h

According to previous studies, many level 1 trauma centers have implemented the optimal time interval of 2 h for emergent trauma interventions [9,14]. Table 3 presents the results of sensitivity analyses for trauma patients who received emergent surgery within 2 h. Among the trauma patients with a WEST of <2 h, the median time was 79 min, with an IQR of 50–100 min. No significant difference in WEST was noted between the survival and mortality groups of patients with a WEST of <120 min (median WEST: 85 vs. 78 min, $p < 0.001$). The patients aged ≥ 65 years (median WEST: 81 vs. 72 min, $p < 0.001$), those with minor injuries (ISS < 16 or RTS ≥ 7; median WEST in patients with RTS ≥ 7 vs. RTS < 7 and ISS < 16 vs. ISS ≥ 16: 76 vs. 56 min and 88 vs. 76 min, respectively, $p < 0.001$), those with major injuries to the chest (median WEST in patients with chest AIS ≥ 3 vs. head AIS ≥ 3 vs. abdominal AIS ≥ 3: 77 vs. 91 vs. 81 min, $p < 0.001$), and those without ICU admission (median WEST: 76 vs. 87 min, $p < 0.001$) had a shorter WEST.

Table 3. Comparison of waiting emergent surgery time (WEST) among trauma patients receiving emergent surgery within 2 h across various subgroups.

Subgroup	Median (IQR)	p-Value
Age		
Age < 65 years old	81 (56–99.75)	<0.001
Age ≥ 65 years old	72 (40–99)	
RTS		
RTS < 7	89 (70.5–102)	<0.001
RTS ≥ 7	76 (48–99)	
ISS		
ISS < 16	76 (47–99)	<0.001
ISS ≥ 16	88 (64–103)	
Major injury site		
Head AIS ≥ 3	91 (72–105)	
Chest AIS ≥ 3	77 (53–93)	<0.001
Abdominal AIS ≥ 3	81 (60.5–96)	
Hospitalization		
Total LOS < 30 days	78 (49–99)	0.174
Total LOS ≥ 30 days	87 (60–99)	
ICU admission		
Yes	87 (58.75–100)	<0.001
No	76 (48–99)	
In-hospital mortality		
Yes	85 (62–98)	0.463
No	78 (50–99)	

Abbreviations: WEST, waiting emergent surgery time; SBP, systolic blood pressure; DBP, diastolic blood pressure; RR, respiratory rate; HR, heart rate; ISS, injury severity score; AIS, abbreviated injury scale; RTS, revised trauma score; TBI, traumatic brain injury; LOS, length of stay; ICU, intensive care unit.

3.4. Association between WEST and Clinical Outcomes

The results of the multivariable logistic regression in Table 4, which included all patient data, revealed several variables to be significantly associated with increased odds of mortality. These variables included age ≥ 65 years (adjusted odds ratio [aOR] = 3.62), male sex (aOR = 2.12), RTS < 7 (aOR = 5.15), and ISS ≥ 16 (aOR = 8.29). Notably, WEST was not correlated with an elevated risk of in-hospital mortality. Additionally, no significant association was noted between WEST and ICU admission or prolonged hospital stay of ≥30 days. The results of the subgroup analysis (Figure 2) indicated that a longer WEST was associated with a reduced risk of in-hospital mortality in patients with WEST ≥ 90 min (aOR = 0.994, 95% confidence interval [CI] = 0.991–0.997) in those aged < 65 years (aOR = 0.990, 95% CI = 0.984–0.995) and ≥65 years (aOR = 0.996, 95% CI = 0.992–0.999), as well as in those with minor injuries (RTS ≥ 7: aOR = 0.995, 95% CI = 0.992–0.998; ISS < 16: aOR = 0.995, 95% CI = 0.991–1.000) or major injuries (RTS < 7: aOR = 0.992, 95% CI = 0.988–0.997; ISS ≥ 16: aOR = 0.993, 95% CI = 0.989–0.996), and those with head AIS ≥ 3 (aOR = 0.992, 95% CI = 0.988–0.996).

Table 4. Results of multivariable logistic regression analysis of in-hospital mortality, ICU admission, and prolonged hospital stay (≥30 days).

Variables	In-Hospital Mortality		ICU Admission		Prolonged Hospital Stay ≥ 30 Days	
	Adjusted OR (95% CI)	p-Value	Adjusted OR (95% CI)	p-Value	Adjusted OR (95% CI)	p-Value
WEST per 30 min						
WEST < 30 min	Reference	---	Reference	---	Reference	---
30 ≤ WEST < 60 min	1.05 (0.17–6.35)	0.955	0.85 (0.41–1.80)	0.678	2.93 (0.92–9.33)	0.068
60 ≤ WEST < 90 min	1.12 (0.22–5.70)	0.890	0.62 (0.30–1.28)	0.199	1.80 (0.58–5.53)	0.307
WEST ≥ 90 min	0.60 (0.13–2.74)	0.510	0.70 (0.40–1.24)	0.225	1.69 (0.59–4.83)	0.324

Table 4. Cont.

Variables	In-Hospital Mortality		ICU Admission		Prolonged Hospital Stay ≥ 30 Days	
	Adjusted OR (95% CI)	p-Value	Adjusted OR (95% CI)	p-Value	Adjusted OR (95% CI)	p-Value
Age						
Age < 65 years old	Reference	---	Reference	---	Reference	---
Age ≥ 65 years old	3.62 (2.44–5.35)	<0.001	1.84 (1.59–2.13)	<0.001	1.22 (1.01–1.46)	0.038
Sex						
Male	Reference	Ref	Reference	---	Reference	Ref
Female	0.47 (0.31–0.70)	<0.001	0.67 (0.58–0.77)	<0.001	0.83 (0.70–0.99)	0.042
Major injury or not						
RTS score						
RTS < 7	5.15 (3.32–7.99)	<0.001	5.97 (4.58–7.78)	<0.001	2.75 (2.16–3.51)	<0.001
RTS ≥ 7	Reference	---	Reference	---	Reference	---
ISS score						
ISS < 16	Reference	---	Reference	---	Reference	---
ISS ≥ 16	8.29 (4.54–15.1)	<0.001	20.3 (16.5–25.0)	<0.001	5.74 (4.39–7.50)	<0.001
TBI status						
No TBI	Reference	---	Reference	---	Reference	---
TBI	1.59 (0.91–2.81)	0.106	9.63 (7.66–12.1)	<0.001	1.90 (1.43–2.52)	<0.001
Injury type						
Blunt injury	Reference	---	Reference	---	Reference	---
Penetrating injury	1.36 (0.38–4.90)	0.636	0.48 (0.34–0.67)	<0.001	1.28 (0.86–1.90)	0.223
Mechanism						
Road traffic injury	Reference	---	Reference	---	Reference	---
High fall	1.09 (0.61–1.93)	0.776	0.77 (0.60–0.98)	0.033	1.25 (0.95–1.63)	0.106
Low fall	0.98 (0.61–1.55)	0.920	0.55 (0.46–0.66)	<0.001	0.66 (0.52–0.84)	0.001
Others	0.70 (0.39–1.26)	0.234	1.78 (1.49–2.12)	<0.001	1.13 (0.89–1.44)	0.304

Abbreviations: OR: odds ratio; CI: confidence interval; RTS: revised trauma score; ISS: injury severity score; TBI: traumatic brain injury.

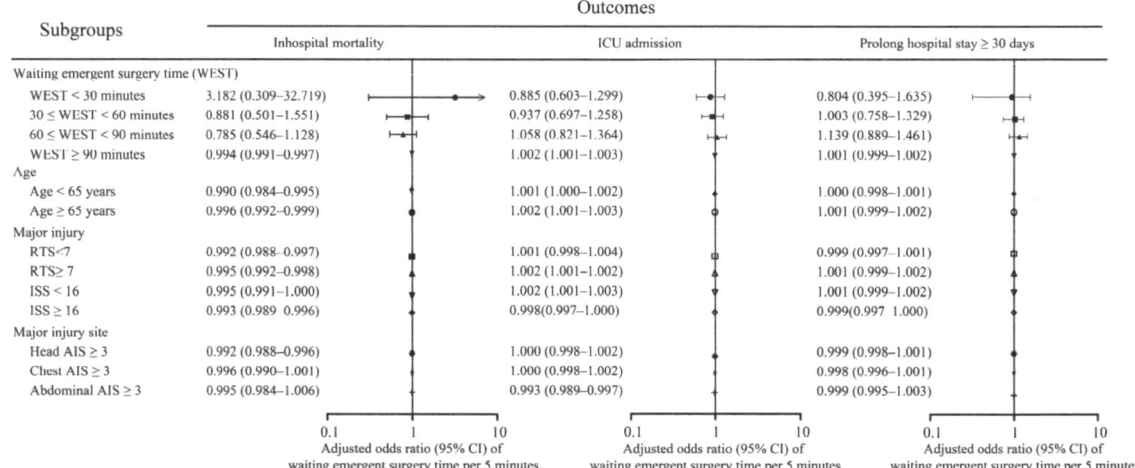

Figure 2. Subgroup analysis illustrating association between a 5 min increase in waiting emergent surgery time (WEST) and in-hospital mortality, ICU admission, and prolonged hospital stay (≥30 days) across various subgroups.

4. Discussion

Our findings revealed no association between WEST and in-hospital mortality, ICU admission, and prolonged hospital stay (≥30 days). However, the subgroup analysis indicated that a longer WEST (per 5 min) was associated with increased survival in patients with a WEST ≥ 90 min, those aged < 65 years, those aged ≥ 65 years, those with minor injuries (RTS ≥ 7 and ISS < 16), those with major injuries (RTS < 7 or ISS ≥ 16), and those with major injuries to the head (head AIS ≥ 3). Additionally, a longer WEST was associated with an increased risk of ICU admission in patients with a WEST ≥ 90 min, those aged ≥ 65 years, those with minor injuries, and those with major injuries in the abdomen.

Previous studies investigating the relationship between waiting time for surgery and mortality and functional outcomes have predominantly focused on fracture surgeries. For example, the TRON Study, a propensity score–matched multicenter investigation involving 779 patients who underwent ankle fracture surgery, revealed significantly longer operative times and higher infection rates in their delayed operation group compared with their early operation group [15]. Pincus et al. [16] analyzed 42,230 patients with hip fractures and revealed that prolonged wait times were associated with an increased risk of 30-day mortality and other complications. The time window for waiting for surgery is considerably narrower for complex fractures and major traumatic injuries than it is for simple fractures. Several studies have provided support for the golden hour concept with respect to emergent surgery. Hsieh et al. analyzed the data of 963 trauma patients from the Pan-Asian Trauma Outcome Study registry and revealed a positive association between a shorter time to definitive care within 2 h and patient survival and functional outcomes [14]. Another observational study that used data from the Trauma and Audit Research Network revealed that trauma patients who underwent secondary transfer experienced a prolonged time to urgent surgery and increased crude mortality rates [17]. However, our study did not obtain evidence supporting these associations, even among the subgroups with major trauma, TBI, major chest injuries, and torso injuries. The relationship between WEST and trauma outcomes might be influenced by presurgical treatments, which can attenuate the effect of WEST and render the effect nonsignificant. This underscores the importance of actively promoting recovery during the waiting period for surgery through interventions such as proactive blood and fluid transfusions, administration of hemostatic medications, maintenance of body temperature, and ensuring adequate ventilation to prevent acidosis [18,19]. Furthermore, the number and type of presurgical treatments can influence the time to emergent surgery. Surgeons and anesthesiologists generally consider stable baseline blood pressure and HR to be necessary for effective surgery. Conservative trauma practitioners may even advocate for ensuring acceptable blood pressure levels before surgery to avoid potential complications associated with operating on hemodynamically unstable patients. Therefore, patients with major trauma might experience a slightly higher WEST than those with minor injuries do; this extended WEST may be partially attributable to implementation of preoperative stabilization treatments and may reflect the greater complexity of injuries requiring more interventions. Nevertheless, studies investigating WEST and patient outcomes have failed to account for the potential confounding effect of presurgical treatments, which may have introduced bias into their results [14,17].

In our study, a subgroup analysis focusing on patients with major head, chest, and abdominal injuries revealed that longer intervals prior to surgical intervention did not increase the risk of mortality in the TBI population, nor did it have any association with the outcomes of patients with major chest or abdominal injuries. This finding contrasts with those of previous research primarily focused on TBIs [20,21]. A key reason for this inconsistency is that the location and severity of head trauma exert a more substantial influence on clinical outcomes than the timing of surgical procedures does. In clinical practice, neurosurgeons typically evaluate the prognoses of patients with head trauma and recommend surgery accordingly. For patients with severe injuries, surgical intervention may not significantly influence outcomes, whereas for those with less severe injuries, immediate surgery may not be required. Instead, the patient may be observed to determine whether surgical intervention is necessary as the condition evolves. Therefore, the inclusion of observation time in calculations of WEST for patients with TBI may introduce bias. Considering patients who are under observation before surgery in combination with those who require immediate surgery, such as those with epidural hematomas, may lead to findings indicating lower in-hospital mortality rates and longer intervals to definitive care. This underscores the influence of patient heterogeneity on outcomes and indicates that certain types of TBI may not require immediate intervention. Consistent with our findings, a meta-analysis of 16 studies revealed that patient outcomes were not significantly influenced by the timing of surgery in 68.7% of the included studies. Moreover, the effect of time to surgery on outcomes was not significant in the majority (75%) of studies focusing on patients with severe TBI [22]. In the current study, we considered different TBI severities (mild, moderate, and severe). The results indicated that shorter intervals to emergent surgery did not reduce in-hospital mortality in mild or severe TBI populations (mild TBI: aOR = 0.993, 95% CI = 0.987–0.999; moderate TBI: aOR = 0.997, 95% CI = 0.988–1.006; severe TBI: aOR = 0.992, 95% CI = 0.985–0.999). Future studies should conduct in-depth analyses of various traumatic intracranial hemorrhage types and include parameters such as the bleeding volume and brain herniation to minimize bias.

This study has several strengths. First, it validated the golden hour concept for surgical intervention in trauma patients. This finding holds clinical importance because it underscores the importance of timely stabilization of injury conditions and adequate resuscitation. Second, we conducted many subgroup analyses to investigate the association between WEST and clinical outcomes. These analyses confirmed that a shorter WEST did not significantly reduce the risk of mortality in trauma patients, even in those with major trauma injuries. This indicates that adequate resuscitation may be more crucial than shortening the WEST is.

This study has some limitations that should be considered. First, because this was a retrospective study, data may be missing, which may have introduced bias. The unmeasured variables in this study may also have influenced the study results. Moreover, our exclusion of unreasonable data points and outliers may have introduced selection bias into the final dataset. Although a randomized controlled trial could address these limitations, ethical considerations might render such a trial infeasible. The majority of the excluded patients lacked documentation for critical variables such as time to definitive care and mortality outcomes, which are crucial aspects of our analysis. Furthermore, imputing missing data for time to definitive care and mortality outcome data would be inappropriate because of the considerable variability in these measures related to factors such as hospital capacity, injury severity, and personalized treatment plans. Imputation under these circumstances could lead to inaccurate estimations. Additionally, imputing missing data for other variables would not notably improve the accuracy of the analysis. To mitigate these limitations, we compared the baseline characteristics between the included patients and patients excluded because of missing data (refer to Supplementary Table S2). Significant differences were noted between the two groups, particularly for outcome variables such as in-hospital mortality, ICU admission, and prolonged hospitalization. However, the in-hospital mortality rates were not statistically different between the included and excluded samples. Moreover, some missing data for time to definitive care may be considered "missing at random" because case managers may not have accurately predicted patient outcomes when documenting this variable. Second, emergency medical system dispatch times can considerably influence a patient's WEST and clinical outcomes. However, because prehospital transport times in Taiwan are generally < 20 min, we excluded this variable from the analysis; in Taipei, the median transport interval is 7 min, and the median prehospital interval is 23 min, which are significantly shorter than those in other countries [23]. Third, our study excluded patients who did not receive surgical intervention. However, we were unable to determine the reasons for these patients ultimately not undergoing surgery. Possible reasons include 'Do not resuscitate' orders and poor prognosis leading to palliative care. Fourth, although the severity of injury is a major determinant of mortality among trauma patients, surgeons employing a proactive approach may also influence patient outcomes. Currently, no objective assessment method is available for this surgeon-specific factor. Fifth, missing data on resuscitation interventions for trauma patients, such as fluid resuscitation volume, blood transfusion, transcatheter arterial embolization, and emergent thoracotomy, may have influenced the study outcomes. These interventions can prolong the WEST, and accounting for them is crucial to accurately evaluating the effect of time to surgery. However, current studies supporting the golden hour concept often lack adjustment for these variables [14,24]. Finally, our findings may not be applicable to the general population. Major injuries were uncommon in our data (7.4%), with blunt injuries being the most prevalent (5.3%). Falls were the leading cause of injury (50%), with high falls accounting for 10.1% and lower falls accounting for 39.9% of the injuries. Further research involving broader populations and robustly controlling for confounding factors is required to validate our findings.

5. Conclusions

Our findings revealed no significant association between time to emergent surgery and in-hospital mortality, ICU admission, or prolonged hospital stays of ≥ 30 days, which contradicts the golden hour concept. Furthermore, our subgroup analysis revealed that a longer WEST (per 5 min) was associated with increased survival for patients with a WEST of ≥ 90 min, regardless of age group (<65 and ≥ 65 years), injury severity (minor injury with RTS ≥ 7 and ISS < 16 and major injury with RTS < 7 or ISS ≥ 16), and injury site (major injuries to the head, with head AIS ≥ 3).

Supplementary Materials: The following supporting information can be downloaded at: https://www.mdpi.com/article/10.3390/medicina60060960/s1, Table S1: STROBE Statement of current cohort study; Table S2: Comparison of demographic characteristics of included patients and patients with missing values.

Author Contributions: Study design: C.-H.T., M.-Y.W., D.-S.C., J.-Y.C. and P.-C.L.; data collection and analysis: C.-Y.L., I.-S.T. and Y.-T.H.; manuscript preparation: C.-H.T., M.-Y.W., Y.-L.C. and G.-T.Y.; writing—original draft preparation: C.-H.T., M.-Y.W., D.-S.C., J.-Y.C. and G.-T.Y. All authors have read and agreed to the published version of the manuscript.

Funding: This research was supported by grants from Taipei Tzu Chi Hospital (TCRD-TPE-113-RT-4, TCRD-TPE-113-48).

Institutional Review Board Statement: This retrospective cohort study was approved by Taipei Tzu Chi Hospital's Institutional Review Board (number: 12-XD-077, approved date: 20 September 2023). The ethics committee waived the requirement for participant consent because of the retrospective nature of the study and the use of anonymized data.

Informed Consent Statement: Patient consent was waived due to retrospective nature of the study and the use of anonymized data by Taipei Tzu Chi Hospital's Institutional Review Board.

Data Availability Statement: The data that support the findings of this study are available from the corresponding author upon reasonable request.

Conflicts of Interest: The authors declare that they have no conflicts of interest with respect to the publication of this article.

Abbreviations

WEST	Waiting emergent surgery time
ICU	Intensive care unit
LOS	Length of stay
IQR	Interquartile range
aOR	Adjusted odds ratio
CI	Confidence interval
HR	Heart rate
SBP	Systolic blood pressure
DBP	Diastolic blood pressure
RR	Respiratory rate
ISS	Injury severity score
RTS	Revised trauma score

	TBI	Traumatic brain injury
	AIS	Abbreviated injury score
	CNS diseases	Central nervous system diseases
	CKD	Chronic kidney disease
	CVD	Cardiovascular disease

References

1. Lin, P.-C.; Wu, M.-Y.; Chien, D.-S.; Chung, J.-Y.; Liu, C.-Y.; Tzeng, I.-S.; Hou, Y.-T.; Chen, Y.-L.; Yiang, G.-T. Use of Reverse Shock Index Multiplied by Simplified Motor Score in a Five-Level Triage System: Identifying Trauma in Adult Patients at a High Risk of Mortality. *Medicina* **2024**, *60*, 647. [CrossRef] [PubMed]
2. Chen, T.-H.; Wu, M.-Y.; Shin, S.D.; Jamaluddin, S.F.; Son, D.N.; Hong, K.J.; Jen-Tang, S.; Tanaka, H.; Hsiao, C.-H.; Hsieh, S.-L.; et al. Discriminant ability of the shock index, modified shock index, and reverse shock index multiplied by the Glasgow coma scale on mortality in adult trauma patients: A PATOS retrospective cohort study. *Int. J. Surg.* **2023**, *109*, 1231–1238. [CrossRef] [PubMed]
3. Yang, Y.-C.; Lin, P.-C.; Liu, C.-Y.; Tzeng, I.-S.; Lee, S.-J.; Hou, Y.-T.; Chen, Y.-L.; Chien, D.-S.; Yiang, G.-T.; Wu, M.-Y. Prehospital shock index multiplied by AVPU scale as a predictor of clinical outcomes in traumatic injury. *Shock* **2022**, *58*, 524–533. [CrossRef] [PubMed]
4. Lin, P.-C.; Liu, C.-Y.; Tzeng, I.-S.; Hsieh, T.-H.; Chang, C.-Y.; Hou, Y.-T.; Chen, Y.-L.; Chien, D.-S.; Yiang, G.-T.; Wu, M.-Y. Shock index, modified shock index, age shock index score, and reverse shock index multiplied by Glasgow Coma Scale predicting clinical outcomes in traumatic brain injury: Evidence from a 10-year analysis in a single center. *Front. Med.* **2022**, *9*, 3478. [CrossRef] [PubMed]
5. Huang, H.-K.; Liu, C.-Y.; Tzeng, I.-S.; Hsieh, T.-H.; Chang, C.-Y.; Hou, Y.-T.; Lin, P.-C.; Chen, Y.-L.; Chien, D.-S.; Yiang, G.-T.; et al. The association between blood pressure and in-hospital mortality in traumatic brain injury: Evidence from a 10-year analysis in a single-center. *Am. J. Emerg. Med.* **2022**, *58*, 265–274. [CrossRef] [PubMed]
6. Chien, D.-S.; Yiang, G.-T.; Liu, C.-Y.; Tzeng, I.-S.; Chang, C.-Y.; Hou, Y.-T.; Chen, Y.-L.; Lin, P.-C.; Wu, M.-Y. Association of In-Hospital Mortality and Trauma Team Activation: A 10-Year Study. *Diagnostics* **2022**, *12*, 2334. [CrossRef]
7. Forrester, J.D.; August, A.; Cai, L.Z.; Kushner, A.L.; Wren, S.M. The Golden Hour After Injury Among Civilians Caught in Conflict Zones. *Disaster Med. Public Health Prep.* **2019**, *13*, 1074–1082. [CrossRef]
8. Wu, M.-Y.; Lin, P.-C.; Liu, C.-Y.; Tzeng, I.-S.; Hsieh, T.-H.; Chang, C.-Y.; Hou, Y.-T.; Chen, Y.-L.; Chien, D.-S.; Yiang, G.-T. The impact of holiday season and weekend effect on traumatic injury mortality: Evidence from a 10-year analysis. *Tzu-Chi Med. J.* **2023**, *35*, 69. [CrossRef]
9. McIsaac, D.I.; Abdulla, K.; Yang, H.; Sundaresan, S.; Doering, P.; Vaswani, S.G.; Thavorn, K.; Forster, A.J. Association of delay of urgent or emergency surgery with mortality and use of health care resources: A propensity score–matched observational cohort study. *Can. Med. Assoc. J.* **2017**, *189*, E905–E912. [CrossRef]
10. Ahmed, K.; Zygourakis, C.; Kalb, S.; Pennington, Z.; Molina, C.; Emerson, T.; Theodore, N. Protocol for Urgent and Emergent Cases at a Large Academic Level 1 Trauma Center. *Cureus* **2019**, *11*, e3973. [CrossRef]
11. von Elm, E.; Altman, D.G.; Egger, M.; Pocock, S.J.; Gøtzsche, P.C.; Vandenbroucke, J.P. The Strengthening the Reporting of Observational Studies in Epidemiology (STROBE) statement: Guidelines for reporting observational studies. *J. Clin. Epidemiol.* **2008**, *61*, 344–349. [CrossRef]
12. Baker, S.P.; O'Neill, B.; Haddon, W., Jr. Long, W.B. The injury severity score: A method for describing patients with multiple injuries and evaluating emergency care. *J. Trauma* **1974**, *14*, 187–196. [CrossRef] [PubMed]
13. Champion, H.R.; Sacco, W.J.; Copes, W.S.; Gann, D.S.; Gennarelli, T.A.; Flanagan, M.E. A revision of the Trauma Score. *J. Trauma* **1989**, *29*, 623–629. [CrossRef] [PubMed]
14. Hsieh, S.-L.; Hsiao, C.-H.; Chiang, W.-C.; Shin, S.D.; Jamaluddin, S.F.; Son, D.N.; Hong, K.J.; Jen-Tang, S.; Tsai, W.; Chien, D.-K.; et al. Association between the time to definitive care and trauma patient outcomes: Every minute in the golden hour matters. *Eur. J. Trauma Emerg. Surg.* **2022**, *48*, 2709–2716. [CrossRef] [PubMed]
15. Sugino, T.; Takegami, Y.; Bando, K.; Sato, T.; Fujita, T.; Oka, Y.; Imagama, S. The Wait Time for Surgery Following Injury Affects Functional Outcomes and Complications After an Ankle Fracture: A Propensity Score–Matched Multicenter Study, the TRON Study. *Foot Ankle Spec.* **2023**. [CrossRef]
16. Pincus, D.; Ravi, B.; Wasserstein, D.; Huang, A.; Paterson, J.M.; Nathens, A.B.; Kreder, H.J.; Jenkinson, R.J.; Wodchis, W.P. Association Between Wait Time and 30-Day Mortality in Adults Undergoing Hip Fracture Surgery. *JAMA* **2017**, *318*, 1994–2003. [CrossRef]
17. Haslam, N.R.; Bouamra, O.; Lawrence, T.; Moran, C.G.; Lockey, D.J. Time to definitive care within major trauma networks in England. *BJS Open* **2020**, *4*, 963–969. [CrossRef]
18. Galbraith, C.M.; Wagener, B.M.; Chalkias, A.; Siddiqui, S.; Douin, D.J. Massive Trauma and Resuscitation Strategies. *Anesthesiol. Clin.* **2023**, *41*, 283–301. [CrossRef]
19. Cantle, P.M.; Cotton, B.A. Balanced Resuscitation in Trauma Management. *Surg. Clin. N. Am.* **2017**, *97*, 999–1014. [CrossRef]
20. Chockalingam, K.; A Rahman, N.A.; Idris, Z.; Theophilus, S.C.; Abdullah, J.M.; Ghani, A.R.I.; Ali, A. Door-to-Skin Time in Patient Undergoing Emergency Trauma Craniotomy. *Malays. J. Med. Sci.* **2023**, *30*, 71–84. [CrossRef]

21. Kim, Y.J. The Impact of Time from ED Arrival to Surgery on Mortality and Hospital Length of Stay in Patients with Traumatic Brain Injury. *J. Emerg. Nurs.* **2011**, *37*, 328–333. [CrossRef] [PubMed]
22. Kim, Y.-J. The impact of time to surgery on outcomes in patients with traumatic brain injury: A literature review. *Int. Emerg. Nurs.* **2014**, *22*, 214–219. [CrossRef] [PubMed]
23. Shih, J.Y.M.; Shih, J.J.M. Pre-Hospital Time Intervals among Trauma Patients in Northern Taiwan. *Taiwan Crit. Care Med.* **2011**, *12*, 166–174.
24. Mader, M.M.-D.; Rotermund, R.; Lefering, R.; Westphal, M.; Maegele, M.; Czorlich, P.; DGU. The faster the better? Time to first CT scan after admission in moderate-to-severe traumatic brain injury and its association with mortality. *Neurosurg. Rev.* **2021**, *44*, 2697–2706. [CrossRef] [PubMed]

Disclaimer/Publisher's Note: The statements, opinions and data contained in all publications are solely those of the individual author(s) and contributor(s) and not of MDPI and/or the editor(s). MDPI and/or the editor(s) disclaim responsibility for any injury to people or property resulting from any ideas, methods, instructions or products referred to in the content.

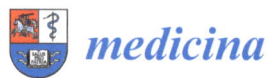 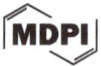

Article

Use of Reverse Shock Index Multiplied by Simplified Motor Score in a Five-Level Triage System: Identifying Trauma in Adult Patients at a High Risk of Mortality

Po-Chen Lin [1,2], Meng-Yu Wu [1,2,3], Da-Sen Chien [1,2], Jui-Yuan Chung [3,4,5,6], Chi-Yuan Liu [7,8], I-Shiang Tzeng [9], Yueh-Tseng Hou [1,2], Yu-Long Chen [1,2] and Giou-Teng Yiang [1,2,*]

1. Department of Emergency Medicine, Taipei Tzu Chi Hospital, Buddhist Tzu Chi Medical Foundation, New Taipei 231, Taiwan; taipeitzuchier@gmail.com (P.-C.L.); skyshangrila@gmail.com (M.-Y.W.); sam.jan1978@msa.hinet.net (D.-S.C.); briann75@gmail.com (Y.-T.H.); yulong0129@gmail.com (Y.-L.C.)
2. Department of Emergency Medicine, School of Medicine, Tzu Chi University, Hualien 970, Taiwan
3. Graduate Institute of Injury Prevention and Control, Taipei Medical University, Taipei 110, Taiwan; bybarian@gmail.com
4. Department of Emergency Medicine, Cathay General Hospital, Taipei 106, Taiwan
5. School of Medicine, Fu Jen Catholic University, Taipei 242, Taiwan
6. School of Medicine, National Tsing Hua University, Hsinchu 300, Taiwan
7. Department of Orthopedic Surgery, Taipei Tzu Chi Hospital, Buddhist Tzu Chi Medical Foundation, New Taipei 231, Taiwan
8. Department of Orthopedics, School of Medicine, Tzu Chi University, Hualien 970, Taiwan
9. Department of Research, Taipei Tzu Chi Hospital, Buddhist Tzu Chi Medical Foundation, New Taipei 970, Taiwan; istzeng@gmail.com
* Correspondence: gtyiang@gmail.com

Abstract: *Background and Objectives*: The Taiwan Triage and Acuity Scale (TTAS) is reliable for triaging patients in emergency departments in Taiwan; however, most triage decisions are still based on chief complaints. The reverse-shock index (SI) multiplied by the simplified motor score (rSI-sMS) is a more comprehensive approach to triage that combines the SI and a modified consciousness assessment. We investigated the combination of the TTAS and rSI-sMS for triage compared with either parameter alone as well as the SI and modified SI. *Materials and Methods*: We analyzed 13,144 patients with trauma from the Taipei Tzu Chi Trauma Database. We investigated the prioritization performance of the TTAS, rSI-sMS, and their combination. A subgroup analysis was performed to evaluate the trends in all clinical outcomes for different rSI-sMS values. The sensitivity and specificity of rSI-sMS were investigated at a cutoff value of 4 (based on previous study and the highest score of the Youden Index) in predicting injury severity clinical outcomes under the TTAS system were also investigated. *Results*: Compared with patients in triage level III, those in triage levels I and II had higher odds ratios for major injury (as indicated by revised trauma score < 7 and injury severity score [ISS] ≥ 16), intensive care unit (ICU) admission, prolonged ICU stay (≥14 days), prolonged hospital stay (≥30 days), and mortality. In all three triage levels, the rSI-sMS < 4 group had severe injury and worse outcomes than the rSI-sMS ≥ 4 group. The TTAS and rSI-sMS had higher area under the receiver operating characteristic curves (AUROCs) for mortality, ICU admission, prolonged ICU stay, and prolonged hospital stay than the SI and modified SI. The combination of the TTAS and rSI-sMS had the highest AUROC for all clinical outcomes. The prediction performance of rSI-sMS < 4 for major injury (ISS ≥ 16) exhibited 81.49% specificity in triage levels I and II and 87.6% specificity in triage level III. The specificity for mortality was 79.2% in triage levels I and II and 87.4% in triage level III. *Conclusions*: The combination of rSI-sMS and the TTAS yielded superior prioritization performance to TTAS alone. The integration of rSI-sMS and TTAS effectively enhances the efficiency and accuracy of identifying trauma patients at a high risk of mortality.

Keywords: trauma; reverse-shock index multiplied by simplified motor score; Taiwan Triage and Acuity Scale; triage

Citation: Lin, P.-C.; Wu, M.-Y.; Chien, D.-S.; Chung, J.-Y.; Liu, C.-Y.; Tzeng, I.-S.; Hou, Y.-T.; Chen, Y.-L.; Yiang, G.-T. Use of Reverse Shock Index Multiplied by Simplified Motor Score in a Five-Level Triage System: Identifying Trauma in Adult Patients at a High Risk of Mortality. *Medicina* **2024**, *60*, 647. https://doi.org/10.3390/medicina60040647

Academic Editors: Ivo Dumić-Čule and Tomislav Čengić

Received: 29 March 2024
Revised: 12 April 2024
Accepted: 14 April 2024
Published: 18 April 2024

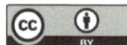

Copyright: © 2024 by the authors. Licensee MDPI, Basel, Switzerland. This article is an open access article distributed under the terms and conditions of the Creative Commons Attribution (CC BY) license (https://creativecommons.org/licenses/by/4.0/).

1. Introduction

Traumatic injury is a major global health problem, contributing to both mortality and disability and placing a substantial burden on healthcare systems [1]. Several triage tools have been developed for use in both prehospital and hospital settings, including the Canadian Triage and Acuity Scale (CTAS) [2], the Emergency Severity Index (ESI) [3], the Manchester Triage Scale [4], the Taiwan Triage and Acuity Scale (TTAS) [5,6], and the Australasian Triage Scale [7]. The ESI is a five-level triage scale based on physical signs and expected resource use, which focuses on quickly categorizing patients in settings with limited resources. One advantage of the ESI is the rapid identification of patients needing immediate attention [8]. However, multiple studies have highlighted an overrepresentation of ESI III assignments and a lack of accurate differentiation in patient acuity levels. This trend has been linked to emergency department (ED) overcrowding and poorer patient outcomes. Addressing these issues is crucial for enhancing ED efficiency and ensuring optimal patient care [9,10]. The ATS is based on adult physiological predictors (airway, breathing, circulation, and disability). A meta-analysis included six studies showed that the pooled coefficient for the ATS was substantial at 0.428 (95%CI 0.340–0.509) and the mis-triage rate was less than fifty percent. Compared to ESI, which has a strong tendency towards categorizing patients as level 2, ATS can appropriately distribute patients in triage levels [11,12]. In addition, the Manchester Triage Scale is a five-level triage algorithm that consists of 52 flowcharts, covering patients' chief signs and symptoms. Each flowchart in turn consists of additional signs and symptoms, named discriminators, which are ranked by priority [13]. Compared to ESI in the ED triage, the mean length of stay by using MTS triage was significantly lower [14]. CTAS and TTSA are based on presenting signs and symptoms, which provides more information regarding early treatment than the ESI (which is a triage tool that predicts ED resource allocation). In the study by Joany M Zachariasse et al. [15], the authors included 66 eligible studies and evaluated 33 different triage systems, revealing numerous different triage systems are being used; they found that many lack a rigorous evaluation. The most commonly used and evaluated triage systems, CTAS, ESI, and MTS, show a moderate–good validity in identifying high- and low-urgency patients. In the results, there is no strong evidence supporting differences between CTAS, ESI, and MTS; therefore, none of them should be preferred over the other.

Accurate triage is essential in ensuring that patients with trauma receive the appropriate level of care, given that undertriage or overtriage can lead to poor outcomes and waste valuable resources [16]. The TTAS is reliable for triaging patients in emergency departments (EDs) in Taiwan [5,6]. TTAS can vary based on regional healthcare systems. Different regions or countries may use different three-tier emergency classification systems, or they may be customized based on local medical needs and resources. Therefore, the specific implementation of TTAS systems may vary by region. The TTAS was adapted from the CTAS and maintains most of the key features of the CTAS. In addition, it uses a patient classification system that prioritizes treatment on the basis of five levels of acuity—level I (most urgent) to level V (least urgent) [17]—and is based on chief complaints and first-order modifiers (such as vital signs (including respiration, hemodynamics, consciousness level, and body temperature), pain severity, and injury mechanism (for patients with trauma) to determine triage severity. Although the TTAS system uses explicit threshold levels for hemodynamic stability (e.g., tachycardia [140 bpm]/bradycardia [50 bpm], with or without symptoms of shock or blood pressure < 70 mm Hg) as order modifiers, most triage decisions are still based on chief complaints. According to an analysis of 36,395 major patients with trauma from the Nationwide Emergency Department Sample of the United States, nearly one in three patients who experienced major trauma were undertriaged [18]. Similarly, relying solely on the TTAS system for trauma triage may result in patients being undertriaged or overtriaged. Triage systems must be frequently evaluated to assess their efficacy in identifying patients at high risk of severe injury in order to ensure high patient safety and appropriate and timely utilization of ED resources.

The 2021 National Guidelines for the Field Triage of Injured Patients (field triage guideline) updated and added new criteria for field triage [19]. The two major concepts were the application of the shock index (SI) and simplified consciousness assessment. These two components can be combined in a novel tool known as the reverse SI (rSI) multiplied by simplified motor score (sMS), as rSI-sMS, which aims to provide a relatively user-friendly, easily applicable, and comprehensive approach to triage. The decision to utilize rSI multiplied by sMS rather than SI multiplied by sMS is grounded in the correlation of lower values of rSI or sMS with poorer outcomes. Conversely, higher values of SI would suggest a worse outcome. This reasoning remains consistent when employing rSI multiplied by GCS as well [20]. This novel tool incorporates the rSI and the 3-point sMS to assess both hypovolemic shock status and neurological condition in patients with trauma.

In this study, we evaluated the effectiveness of incorporating rSI-sMS to identify patients with severe injury at high risk of mortality within a level category of the TTAS system. We hypothesized that the addition of rSI-sMS would decrease the proportion of undertriage and overtriage among patients with trauma.

2. Methods

2.1. Study Design and Cohort

The present retrospective cohort analysis used data from the Taipei Tzu Chi Hospital registry and was approved by the Institutional Review Board of Taipei Tzu Chi Hospital (IRB number: 11-XD-148 and 12-XD-079). This hospital's trauma database includes hospitalized patients with ICD-9-CM codes 800–959 (excluding 905–909 and 930–939) or ICD-10-CM codes S00–T98 (excluding T15–T19 and T90–T98). The ICD-9-CM codes 905–909 (ICD-10-CM codes T90–T98) pertain to the late effects of injury, poisoning, toxic effects, and other external causes, rather than the immediate effects associated with acute trauma. As they are not directly related to acute trauma, they were excluded from this study. Furthermore, the ICD-9-CM codes 930–939 (ICD-10-CM codes T15–T19) represent the effects of foreign bodies entering the body through natural orifices, which are also unrelated to trauma. Consequently, they were also excluded from our analysis. In addition, the database records 152 variables associated with trauma injury, including demographics, injury mechanism, injury types, injury severity, vital signs, surgical intervention, and in-hospital mortality. We included all patients with major traumatic injuries from January 2009 to June 2019; we excluded those under the age of 20 years because of differences in normal vital sign ranges for pediatric patients.

2.2. TTAS System

The TTAS is a computerized decision support system used in EDs in Taiwan and was adapted from the CTAS [5,21,22]. The TTAS classifies patients into three domains: trauma (14 categories and 41 chief complaints), nontrauma (13 categories and 125 chief complaints), and environmental injuries (11 chief complaints). Triage severity is assessed on the basis of chief complaints and first-order modifiers, including vital signs, consciousness level, and pain severity. When first-order modifiers are insufficient in determining the appropriate triage acuity level, second-order modifiers—such as visual disturbance for eye trauma or neurologic deficit for head, neck, and back trauma—are applied. Patients are prioritized on the basis of their acuity level as follows: level 1, resuscitation; level 2, emergency; level 3, urgent; level 4, less urgent; and level 5, nonurgent.

In Taipei Tzu Chi Hospital, to qualify as a candidate for the role of triage nurse in the ED, a nurse must meet the following requirements: (1) completion of 3 years of basic nursing training, including general nursing, observation nursing, emergency and critical care nursing, pediatric nursing, trauma nursing, and care for toxic and environmental injuries; (2) recognition by the Taiwan Nurses Association based on the Clinical Ladder System for the nurses program in a hospital; and (3) completion of triage classification education courses. The candidates are led by senior triage nurses to perform triage classification for a minimum of 100 patients for 5 days. After passing the evaluation, a nurse is qualified as a formal triage nurse. Currently, Taipei Tzu Chi Hospital has 25 emergency triage nurses.

One designated triage nurse who has undergone specific training regarding the application of the five-level TTAS protocol and the computer-assisted system generates the TTAS level for each patient in real time. Studies have demonstrated that the TTAS is a reliable triage system that accurately prioritizes treatment, avoids overtriage, and efficiently allocates appropriate resources to ED patients.

2.3. Variable Measurements

We retrieved data regarding the analyzed patients' clinicodemographic characteristics, including age, sex, chronic diseases, triage level, vital signs, and injury mechanism and severity. Vital sign data—including those related to heart rate, systolic blood pressure (SBP), diastolic blood pressure (DBP), respiratory rate, Glasgow Coma Scale (GCS) score, and sMS—were recorded upon arrival at the hospital and employed to calculate rSI-sMS. The sMS assesses the GCS motor response, with a score of 2 indicating that the patient can follow commands (equivalent to a GCS motor subscale score of 6), a score of 1 indicating that the patient can localize to pain (equivalent to a GCS motor subscale score of 5), and a score of 0 indicating that the patient has a GCS motor subscale score of ≤ 4. However, the rSI-sMS was calculated as $1/SI \times sMS$. We cannot use a score of 0 of sMS to calculate rSI-sMS. Therefore, we modified the sMS by changing the highest score to 3 and the lowest score to 1. We also included the SI and mSI for analysis. The SI was calculated as heart rate (HR)/SBP; the mSI was calculated as HR/mean arterial pressure. Based on a previous study [23], we used 4 as the cutoff value of rSI-sMS for predicting trauma patients with high risk of mortality.

We used the injury severity score (ISS) to determine trauma severity. Major trauma was defined as an ISS score of ≥ 16. Patients with traumatic brain injury (TBI) were stratified into mixed TBI (head abbreviated injury scale (AIS) score > 3 and any other AIS score ≥ 0) and isolated TBI (head AIS score > 3 and any other AIS score = 0) groups. We defined the geriatric population as age ≥ 65 years for subgroup analysis.

2.4. Outcomes

The primary outcome was in-hospital mortality. The secondary outcomes were admission to the intensive care unit (ICU), readmission to the ICU, ICU length of stay (LOS), prolonged ICU stay (>14 days), total hospital stay, and prolonged hospital stay (>30 days).

2.5. Statistical Analysis

Demographic data, injury data, and clinical outcomes were analyzed using SPSS (Version 20.0, SPSS, Chicago, IL, USA). In this paper, we assessed the normality of continuous data using the Kolmogorov–Smirnov test. Each continuous variable is reported as the mean ± standard deviation for normally distributed data and the median with interquartile range for nonnormally distributed data. Categorical variables are reported as numbers and percentages. Independent-samples t-tests were conducted for normally distributed continuous variables, whereas Mann-Whitney U tests were performed for nonnormally distributed continuous variables. Pearson's chi-squared test or Fisher's exact test was used for categorical variables. Multivariable logistic regression was performed to predict the primary and secondary outcomes in patients with trauma, with significant variables or variables deemed important included in the analysis. The area under the receiver operating characteristic curve (AUROC) was calculated to assess the discrimination of the logistic regression model for each outcome. A p value of <0.05 was considered statistically significant, and all tests were two-sided.

3. Results

3.1. Patient Characteristics

Of the 13,144 eligible patients, 1384 were excluded owing to their age being <20 years (n = 1198), death upon arrival (n = 151), or insufficient data for calculating rSI-sMS (n = 35). Ultimately, we included the data of 11,760 patients for analysis; these patients' clinicodemographic characteristics are presented in Table 1. Triage level II had the largest proportion of patients (51.7%), followed by level III (41.8%) and then level I (6%). Compared with triage levels II and III, the level I population had higher proportions of men (63.9%) and older adults (age $\geq$ 65 years; 38.4%); lower SBP, DBP, and GCS scores; a higher HR and respiratory rate; and a higher proportion of isolated brain injury (39.5%). Nonpenetrating injuries were the primary cause of trauma in this study, with traffic accidents and falls being the most common mechanisms. Among all the triage levels, level I had the highest incidence of road transport injuries (46.8%), whereas level III had the highest incidence of low falls (46.1%). Cardiovascular disease was the most common underlying condition across all the triage levels. The triage level III population had higher proportions of cardiovascular disease and diabetes mellitus than the level I and II populations.

Table 1. Clinicodemographic characteristics of the included patients, stratified by triage level.

Characteristics	Triage I	Triage II	Triage III	Triage IV/V	p-Value
Patient number	711 (6.0%)	6080 (51.7%)	4914 (41.8%)	55 (0.5%)	
Age (years)	56 (39–74)	59 (43–77)	63 (47–77)	52 (36–62)	<0.001
Age < 65 ys	438 (61.6%)	3562 (58.6%)	2642 (53.8%)	43 (78.2%)	<0.001
Age $\geq$ 65 ys	273 (38.4%)	2518 (41.4%)	2272 (46.2%)	12 (21.8%)	
Sex, n (%)					<0.001
Female	257 (36.1%)	2772 (45.6%)	2577 (52.4%)	25 (45.5%)	
Male	454 (63.9%)	3308 (54.4%)	2337 (47.6%)	30 (54.5%)	
Vital sign					
SBP	143 (115–170)	147 (127–169)	148 (129–165)	141 (122–154)	<0.001
DBP	81.5 (68–96)	85 (74–97)	85 (76–95)	81 (73–93)	<0.001
HR	88 (76–105)	84 (74–96)	82 (72–93)	85 (72–97)	<0.001
RR	19 (18–20)	18 (18–20)	18 (18–20)	18 (18–20)	<0.001
GCS score	14 (7–15)	15 (15–15)	15 (15–15)	15 (15–15)	
Injury score systems					
rSIsms	3.5 (2.0–5.0)	5.2 (4.3–6.3)	5.4 (4.5–6.3)	4.8 (4.1–5.8)	<0.001
rSIsms < 4	425 (59.8%)	1069 (17.6%)	625 (12.7%)	13 (23.6%)	<0.001
rSIsms $\geq$ 4	286 (40.2%)	5011 (82.4%)	4289 (87.3%)	42 (76.4%)	
Injury severity					
RTS	7.1 (6.0–7.8)	7.8 (7.8–7.8)	7.8 (7.8–7.8)	7.8 (7.8–7.8)	<0.001
RTS < 7	353 (49.6%)	211 (3.5%)	62 (1.3%)	0 (0.0%)	<0.001
ISS	11 (9–20)	9 (4–9)	9 (4–9)	4 (4–9)	<0.001
ISS $\geq$ 16	300 (42.2%)	444 (7.3%)	201 (4.1%)	2 (3.6%)	<0.001
Isolated head injury *	281 (39.5%)	1080 (17.8%)	500 (10.2%)	10 (18.2%)	<0.001
Injury type					<0.001
Penetration	57 (8.0%)	366 (6.0%)	142 (2.9%)	1 (1.8%)	
Non-penetration	654 (92.0%)	5714 (94.0%)	4772 (97.1%)	54 (98.2%)	
Mechanism of injury					<0.001
Road transport	333 (46.8%)	2255 (37.1%)	1691 (34.4%)	20 (36.4%)	
Low fall	142 (20.0%)	2298 (37.8%)	2264 (46.1%)	19 (34.5%)	
High fall	129 (18.1%)	789 (13.0%)	556 (11.3%)	5 (9.1%)	
Others	107 (15.0%)	738 (12.1%)	403 (8.2%)	11 (20.0%)	
Comorbidity					
CNS diseases	48 (6.8%)	405 (6.7%)	283 (5.8%)	0 (0.0%)	0.052
CVD	142 (20.0%)	1791 (29.5%)	1626 (33.1%)	9 (16.4%)	<0.001
Respiratory diseases	13 (1.8%)	155 (2.5%)	109 (2.2%)	1 (1.8%)	0.510
CKD	19 (2.7%)	206 (3.4%)	150 (3.1%)	1 (1.8%)	0.568
Diabetes mellitus	63 (8.9%)	770 (12.7%)	683 (13.9%)	3 (5.5%)	0.001

Table 1. Cont.

Characteristics	Triage I	Triage II	Triage III	Triage IV/V	p-Value
ICU care					
ICU admission	491 (69.1%)	1052 (17.3%)	343 (7.0%)	5 (9.1%)	<0.001
Re-admission ICU	8 (1.1%)	27 (0.4%)	9 (0.2%)	0 (0.0%)	0.001
ICU LOS, days	6 (3–13)	4 (3–6)	4 (3–6)	2 (2–3)	<0.001
LOS < 14 days	372 (75.8%)	928 (88.2%)	315 (91.8%)	5 (100.0%)	<0.001
LOS ≥ 14 days	119 (24.2%)	124 (11.8%)	28 (8.2%)	0 (0.0%)	
Surgical intervention					
Operation	327 (46.0%)	3748 (61.6%)	3544 (72.1%)	29 (52.7%)	<0.001
Re-operation	75 (10.5%)	188 (3.1%)	81 (1.6%)	0 (0.0%)	<0.001
Complications	176 (24.8%)	830 (13.7%)	165 (3.4%)	2 (3.6%)	<0.001
Total LOS	11 (5–25)	6 (4–10)	6 (4–8)	5 (3–7)	<0.001
<30 days	570 (80.2%)	5279 (94.2%)	4811 (97.9%)	54 (98.2%)	<0.001
≥30 days	141 (19.8%)	351 (5.8%)	103 (2.1%)	1 (1.8%)	

CKD: chronic kidney disease; CVD: cardiovascular diseases; ISS: injury severity score; RTS: revised trauma score; LOS: length of stay; ICU: intensive care unit. * Isolated head injury: patients with an AIS code limited to the head and no AIS-coded injury in any other region.

The level I group had a higher ISS than the other groups, with 42.2% of patients presenting with an ISS of ≥16. The revised trauma score (RTS) was lowest for triage level I, with 49.6% of the triage level I patients with RTS < 7. The level I group had a higher proportion of patients requiring admission to the ICU, readmission, and prolonged ICU stay. The triage level III group had the highest operation rate (72.1%), whereas the level I group had the highest reoperation rate (10.5%), the highest complication rate (24.8%), the longest total LOS (19.8%), and the highest in-hospital mortality rate (15.0%).

3.2. Prioritization Performance of Patients Using the TTAS System

We observed that the TTAS system was effective in prioritizing patients with major trauma, with significant differences observed between the triage level groups related to RTS < 7, ISS ≥ 16, hospital stay, ICU stay, the proportion of patients admitted to the ICU, prolonged ICU stay (≥14 days), prolonged hospital stay (≥30 days), and mortality. Specifically, the level I and II triage groups had higher odds ratios for major injury (as indicated by RTS < 7 and ISS ≥ 16), ICU admission, prolonged ICU stay, prolonged hospital stay, and mortality and lower odds ratios for operation than the level III group (Figure 1).

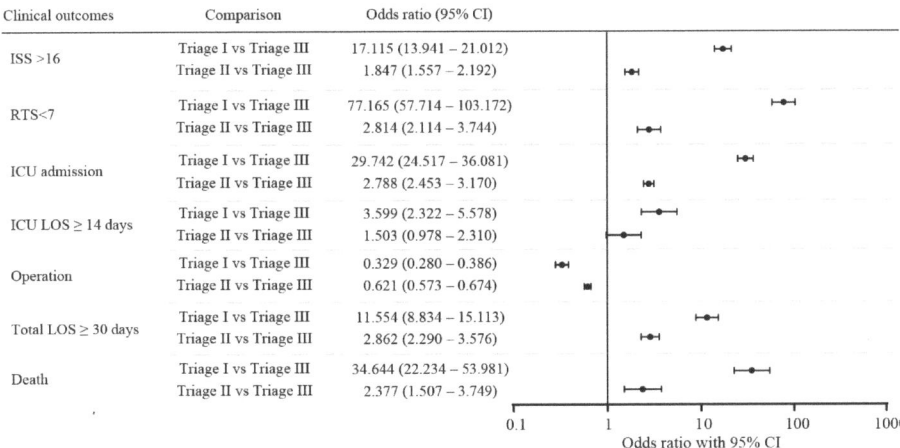

Figure 1. Odds ratios for logistic regression analysis for injury severity and clinical outcomes between different triage levels in the TTAS.

3.3. Risk Stratification Based on rSI-sMS < 4 in the TTAS

The results of risk stratification based on rSI-sMS < 4 in the TTAS are presented in Table 2. The triage level I group had the highest percentage of patients (59.8%) with rSI-sMS < 4, followed by the level II group (17.6%) and then the level III (12.7%) group. In all three triage levels, a significant difference regarding injury severity (ISS $\geq$ 16 and RTS < 7) was noted between patients with rSI-sMS < 4 and those with rSI-sMS $\geq$ 4. The rSI-sMS < 4 group had a higher RTS and ISS, a higher proportion of ISS $\geq$ 16 and RTS < 7 patients, and less favorable outcomes related to ICU admission, reoperation, complications, prolonged hospitalization, and mortality than the rSI-sMS $\geq$ 4 group. Notably, no significant differences in clinical outcomes were observed between the two groups in triage levels IV and V.

Table 2. Risk stratification between patients with rSI-sMS < 4 and $\geq$ 4 in different triage levels.

Outcomes	Triage I		Triage II		Triage III		Triage IV/V	
	rSI-sMS < 4	rSI-sMS $\geq$ 4	rSI-sMS < 4	rSI-sMS $\geq$ 4	rSI-sMS < 4	rSI-sMS $\geq$ 4	rSI-sMS < 4	rSI-sMS $\geq$ 4
Patient number	425 (59.8%)	286 (40.2%)	1069 (17.6%)	5011 (82.4%)	625 (12.7%)	4289 (87.3%)	13 (23.6%)	42 (76.4%)
Injury severity								
ISS $\geq$ 16	241 (56.7%) ***	59 (20.6%) ***	134 (12.5%) ***	310 (6.2%) ***	40 (6.4%) **	161 (3.8%) **	0 (0.0%)	2 (4.8%)
RTS < 7	315 (74.1%) ***	38 (13.3%) ***	147 (13.8%) ***	64 (1.3%) ***	39 (6.2%) ***	23 (0.5%) ***	0 (0.0%)	0 (0.0%)
ICU care								
ICU admission	334 (78.6%) ***	157 (54.9%) ***	267 (25.0%) ***	785 (15.7%) ***	70 (11.2%) ***	273 (6.4%) ***	1 (7.7%)	4 (9.5%)
Re-admission ICU	7 (1.6%)	1 (0.3%)	9 (0.8%) *	18 (0.4%) *	3 (0.5%)	6 (0.1%)	0 (0.0%)	0 (0.0%)
ICU LOS $\geq$ 14 days	98 (29.3%) ***	21 (13.4%) ***	39 (14.6%)	85 (10.8%)	5 (7.1%)	23 (8.4%)	0 (0.0%)	0 (0.0%)
Surgical intervention								
Operation	211 (49.6%) *	116 (40.6%) *	640 (59.9%)	3108 (62.0%)	425 (68.0%) *	3119 (72.7%) *	6 (46.2%)	23 (54.8%)
Re-operation	57 (13.4%) **	18 (6.3%) **	54 (5.1%) ***	134 (2.7%) ***	18 (2.9%) **	63 (1.5%) **	0 (0.0%)	0 (0.0%)
Complications	121 (28.5%) **	55 (19.2%) **	197 (18.4%) ***	633 (12.6%) ***	40 (6.4%) ***	125 (2.9%) ***	0 (0.0%)	2 (4.8%)
Total LOS $\geq$ 30 days	106 (24.9%) ***	35 (12.2%) ***	89 (8.3%) ***	262 (5.2%) ***	24 (3.8%) ***	79 (1.8%) ***	0 (0.0%)	1 (2.4%)
Death	91 (21.4%) ***	16 (5.6%) ***	25 (2.3%) ***	48 (1.0%) ***	9 (1.4%) ***	16 (0.4%) ***	0 (0.0%)	0 (0.0%)

* $p < 0.05$, ** $p < 0.01$, *** $p < 0.001$.

Table 3 compares the results of the SI, mSI, and rSI-sMS AUROCs for predicting trauma outcomes. The TTAS and rSI-sMS had higher AUROCs for mortality, ICU admission, prolonged ICU stay, and prolonged hospital stay than the SI and mSI. The combination of the TTAS and rSI-sMS had a higher AUROC for all clinical outcomes than that of the TTAS and the SI or mSI. The subgroup analysis of the rSI-sMS < 4 group across multiple triage levels is presented in Figure 2. In triage levels I–III, patients with rSI-sMS < 4 had higher odds ratios of ICU admission, prolonged hospital stay, and mortality than those with rSI-sMS $\geq$ 4. Additionally, in triage levels I and II, patients with rSI-sMS < 4 had a higher risk of prolonged ICU stay than those with rSI-sMS $\geq$ 4. The mortality rates of the rSI-sMS < 4 group across the various triage levels are presented in Figure 3A. The overall mortality rates were 3% in triage levels I and II and 1% in triage level III. Patients with rSI-sMS < 4 had a significantly higher mortality rate than those with rSI-sMS $\geq$ 4 in triage levels I and II (16.07% vs. 1.52%, respectively) and level III (3.28% vs. 0.47%, respectively).

The trends for all clinical outcomes for the various rSI-sMS values are presented in Figure 3B. A cutoff value of 4 for rSI-sMS facilitated effective discrimination between all the clinical outcomes (Table 4). The trend of the mortality rate, prolonged hospitalization rate, ICU admission rate, ICU prolonged hospitalization rate, and major injury rate (ISS $\geq$ 16) remained relatively flat after the application of the cutoff value. The predictive performance of rSI-sMS < 4 for major injury was 81.49% specificity in triage levels I and II and 87.6% specificity in triage level III. The sensitivity and specificity for mortality were 64.4% and 79.2%, respectively, in triage levels I and II and 36% and 87.4%, respectively, in triage level III.

Table 3. Comparison of SI, mSI, and rSI-sMS AUROC curves for predicting mortality, ICU admission, prolonged ICU stay (≥14 days), and prolonged hospital stay (≥30 days).

Scoring Systems	Mortality		ICU Admission		Prolong ICU Stay		Prolong Total Hospital Stay	
	AUROC (95% CI)	p-Value	AUROC (95% CI)	p-Value	AUROC (95% CI)	p-Value	AUROC (95% CI)	p-Value
SI	0.505 (0.458–0.552)	0.819	0.522 (0.506–0.537)	0.003	0.527 (0.488–0.567)	0.147	0.547 (0.522–0.573)	<0.001
mSI	0.541 (0.495–0.587)	0.046	0.535 (0.519–0.550)	<0.001	0.545 (0.506–0.584)	0.018	0.559 (0.534–0.584)	<0.001
rSI-sMS	0.733 (0.688–0.778)	<0.001	0.605 (0.590–0.621)	<0.001	0.623 (0.584–0.662)	<0.001	0.616 (0.591–0.642)	<0.001
Triage	0.780 (0.743–0.816)	<0.001	0.702 (0.689–0.715)	<0.001	0.621 (0.584–0.657)	<0.001	0.676 (0.654–0.699)	<0.001
Triage + SI	0.770 (0.733–0.807)	<0.001	0.699 (0.686–0.713)	<0.001	0.617 (0.579–0.655)	<0.001	0.689 (0.667–0.711)	<0.001
Triage + mSI	0.780 (0.744–0.816)	<0.001	0.703 (0.690–0.717)	<0.001	0.623 (0.585–0.660)	<0.001	0.692 (0.670–0.713)	<0.001
Triage + rSI-sMS	0.797 (0.759–0.835)	<0.001	0.714 (0.701–0.728)	<0.001	0.641 (0.603–0.679)	<0.001	0.699 (0.677–0.721)	<0.001

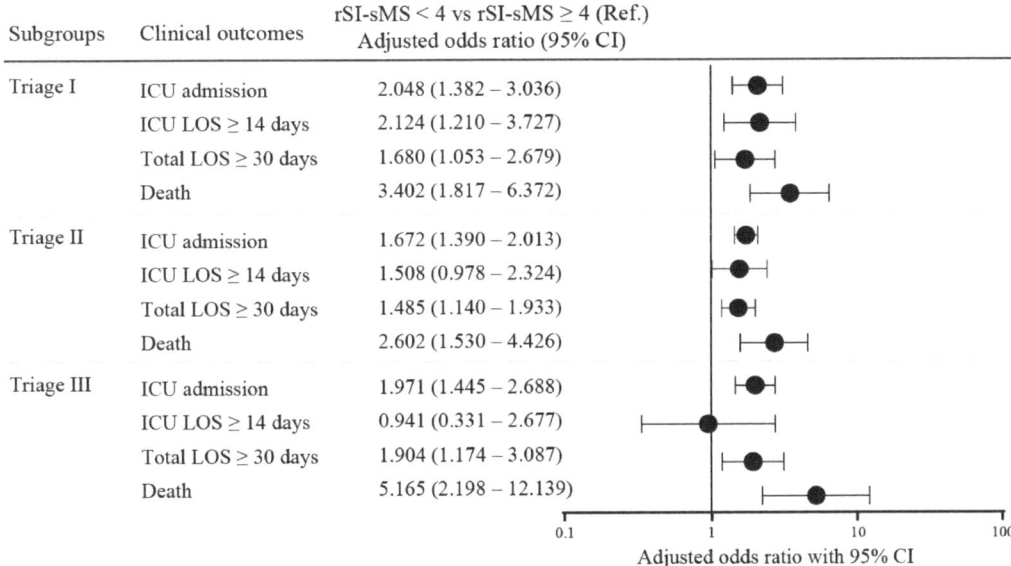

Figure 2. Odds ratios for logistic regression analysis for clinical outcomes of the rSI-sMS < 4 group at different triage levels.

Table 4. Performance of the rSI-sMS score for clinical outcomes at different triage levels.

Outcomes.	Triage I/II				Triage III				Triage IV/V			
	Sens.	Spec.	PLR	NLR	Sens.	Spec.	PLR	NLR	Sens.	Spec.	PLR	NLR
ISS ≥ 16	50.40%	81.49%	2.72	0.61	19.9%	87.6%	1.60	0.91	----	----	----	----
ICU admission	39.0%	83.0%	2.29	0.73	20.4%	87.9%	1.68	0.91	20.0%	76.0%	0.83	1.05
ICU LOS ≥ 14 days	56.4%	64.3%	1.58	0.68	17.9%	79.4%	0.86	1.03	----	----	----	----
Operation	20.9%	76.3%	0.88	1.04	12.0%	85.4%	0.82	1.03	20.7%	73.1%	0.77	1.08
Total LOS ≥ 30 days	39.6%	79.4%	1.92	0.76	23.3%	87.5%	1.86	0.88	----	----	----	----
Death	64.4%	79.2%	3.10	0.45	36.0%	87.4%	2.86	0.73	----	----	----	----

Sens., sensitivity; Spec., specificity; PLR, positive likelihood ratio; NLR, negative likelihood ratio.

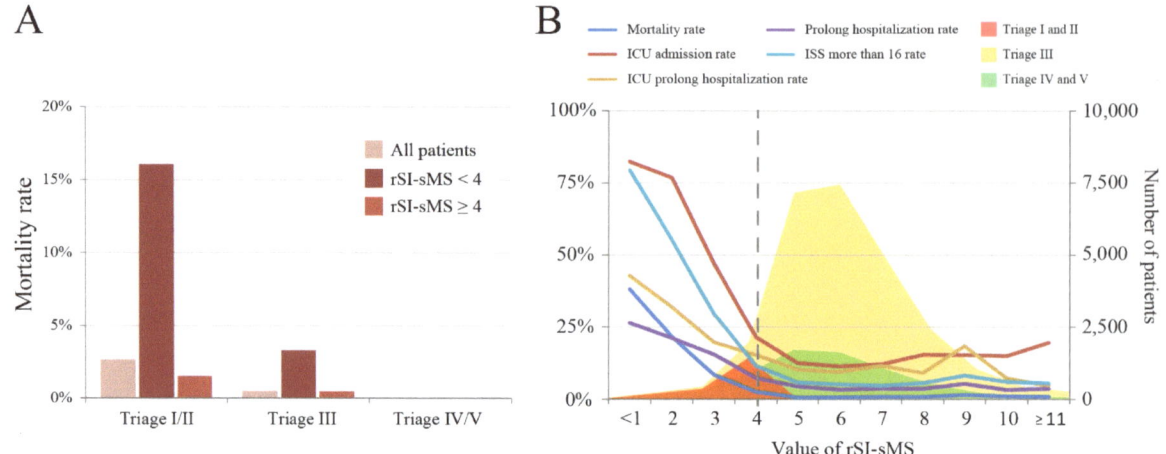

Figure 3. (**A**) Mortality rate of the rSI-sMS < 4 group in different triage levels. (**B**) Trends in all clinical outcomes for different rSI-sMS values.

4. Discussion

Triage is an essential element of the trauma care system used to determine the extent of injuries and treatment priorities to facilitate appropriate resource allocation to patients with trauma. However, accurately identifying patients who require trauma care can be challenging given that prehospital providers and emergency physicians often have limited data to inform such identification. The rSI-sMS method was promoted based on the current concept of the Field Triage Guidelines in 2021 [19]. The rSI-sMS method has two major advantages: use of the SI to reflect patients' hemodynamic status, and use of the sMS instead of the GCS to simplify consciousness assessment in order to reflect neurological status. The present study demonstrated that rSI-sMS is effective in identifying high-risk populations, including those with major injury (ISS $\geq$ 16), high mortality and ICU admission rates, and prolonged hospitalization and ICU stays. Although the five-level TTAS can effectively prioritize patients with major trauma, patients with rSI-sMS < 4 had less favorable outcomes than those with rSI-sMS $\geq$ 4 within the same triage level. This finding implies that rSI-sMS should be included in the triage system for better identification of patients who require trauma care and more accurate prediction of their outcomes to enhance the quality of care and improve trauma outcomes.

The TTAS system mainly categorizes and determines triage levels on the basis of patients' chief complaints, which are subdivided into 163 categories. Although vital signs are included as modifiers in the primary adjusting variables, chief complaints still play a major role in determining triage levels. Therefore, the determination of chief complaints during triage is crucial. In cases of a lack of triage nurses or triage training resources, inaccuracies may arise in the determination of triage levels. In addition, nurses may develop their own personalized usage of the TTAS through years of practice, which could lead to variations in the interpretation and integration of the tool, resulting in lower interrater reliability. A study that analyzed 100 patients arriving by ambulance assessed by five experienced ED nurses reported that the overall interrater agreement of the CTAS was moderate (global Kappa coefficient: 0.44) [24], suggesting a need for further research to verify the reliability of the CTAS. The use of an objective scoring tool can mitigate the limitations of the TTAS and reduce differences among triage personnel. The rSI-sMS method is suitable for quick use by emergency medical workers upon patient arrival without any additional equipment or cost. The core variables used in the calculation of rSI-sMS are those that are commonly collected in clinical practice, and this calculation is based on a simple algorithm. An rSI-sMS score of <4 can be used as a primary trigger for action in an ED. In addition, using rSI-sMS < 4 as a risk stratification tool in the TTAS can facilitate the identification of high-risk patients. In the current study, we observed that even after risk stratification using the TTAS, patients with rSI-sMS < 4 in triage levels I–III had greater injury severity and less favorable clinical outcomes, as reflected by their relatively high odds ratios for mortality, ICU admission, prolonged total LOS, and prolonged ICU stay. Overall, implementing rSI-sMS < 4 as a risk stratification tool in the TTAS can improve patient outcomes and help to optimize resource utilization. In addition, we expect that morbidity and mortality can decrease with the addition of rSI-sMS to the TTAS system; however, further prospective studies are necessary to verify this assumption.

In the present study, rSI-sMS was significantly associated with trauma outcomes and enhanced the ability of the TTAS to predict mortality, ICU admission, prolonged total LOS, and ICU stay in patients with trauma. These findings are in line with those of other studies that have suggested that incorporating vital sign prediction scoring systems into the triage process can help reduce delays in evaluating and treating undertriaged patients and can decrease the associated morbidity [25]. Jung-Fang Chuang et al. [25] used the rSI as an additional criterion under the TTAS had better classification performance in triage levels I and II. In addition, patients with a severe SI of <1 also had worse outcomes. Furthermore, the subgroup analysis revealed that the combination of rSI-sMS and triage had better predictive performance than the combination of SI and mSI [16]. Another concern is inaccurate prioritization in levels II and III of the TTAS system when patients have an rSI of <1. In the present study, the prioritization performance of rSI-sMS in levels II and III of the TTAS system did not yield the same results as Chuang et al. [25]. This difference may have been partially due to our cohort having higher severe injury and higher mortality rates: 51.7% of all the analyzed patients were classified as level II and 41.8% were classified as level III. Although the TTAS exhibited strong prioritization performance, using rSI-sMS as an additional criterion may increase physicians' attention to high-risk patients with trauma.

This study had several strengths. First, we investigated a novel prediction scoring system that had better predictive performance than the SI and mSI. We applied an objective scoring system, namely rSI-sMS, in the TTAS for the reclassification of high-risk patients with trauma to mitigate the limitations of the TTAS. Second, we analyzed an Asian triage system, namely the TTAS, which has not been widely evaluated. The TTAS is typically designed to screen all patients evenly on the basis of chief complaints. Although the main description-based injury assessment in the TTAS is quick and easy, it overlooks the risk of misalignment due to ignorance of personal reactions, such as those related to age and comorbidities. Therefore, the incorporation of an objective additional criterion is useful for increasing predictive performance. Finally, the present large cohort was adjusted for many confounders to eliminate the possibility of any potential influence and thus reflect real-world conditions.

Notably, this study also had some limitations. First, the retrospective design precluded the collection of data related to vital signs; consequently, we excluded patients with missing records for vital signs of interest. However, patients with missing records for age, sex, and other physiological variables were not excluded. The number of cases with missing values was found to be negligible (<0.3%); thus, imputation was deemed unnecessary. Imputing data from vital sign records would have been inappropriate and could have introduced inaccuracies into the findings. Second, detailed triage information was not included in the database. We recognize that such information could further validate the performance of TTAS prioritization and further our understanding of the heterogeneity of triage determination. Accordingly, future studies are recommended to include such data to enhance the accuracy and comprehensiveness of their findings. Third, we did not include injured patients who died before arrival at the hospital, and this omission may have introduced bias. Moreover, this study lacked access to long-term outcome data after discharge and follow-up information from other hospitals, both of which could have facilitated more comprehensive understanding of the performance of the TTAS with rSI-sMS prioritization. Finally, although the Tzu Chi Trauma Database includes data related to a large number of patients over the preceding decade, this study was conducted at a single center; thus, the findings may have limited generalizability. Accordingly, further prospective multicenter studies are warranted to validate our results.

5. Conclusions

In this study, patients with rSI-sMS < 4 had more severe injuries (ISS $\geq$ 16) and experienced worse outcomes—including prolonged hospital and ICU stay, a higher proportion of ICU admission, and increased in-hospital mortality—compared with patients with rSI-sMS $\geq$ 4. Although the five-level TTAS system was effective in prioritizing patients with major trauma, patients with rSI-sMS < 4 had less favorable outcomes than those with rSI-sMS $\geq$ 4 within the same triage level (I–III). The combination of rSI-sMS and the TTAS yielded superior prioritization performance to rSI-sMS, the TTAS alone, the SI, or the mSI. Thus, our findings indicate that incorporating rSI-sMS into the TTAS system can help identify patients with serious injuries who may require reclassification to a higher triage level.

Author Contributions: Conceptualization, P.-C.L. and M.-Y.W.; methodology, I.-S.T.; software, I.-S.T.; validation, D.-S.C., J.-Y.C. and C.-Y.L.; investigation, I.-S.T. and Y.-T.H.; data curation, Y.-L.C. and G.-T.Y.; writing—original draft preparation, P.-C.L., M.-Y.W., D.-S.C., J.-Y.C., C.-Y.L. and G.-T.Y.; writing—review and editing, P.-C.L., M.-Y.W., D.-S.C., J.-Y.C., C.-Y.L. and G.-T.Y.; visualization, M.-Y.W.; project administration, P.-C.L. and G.-T.Y.; funding acquisition, P.-C.L. All authors have read and agreed to the published version of the manuscript.

Funding: This study was supported by the grant of Taipei Tzu Chi Hospital and Buddhist Tzu Chi Medical Foundation. (TCMF-A 113-02, TCRD-TPE-112-33, and TCRD-TPE-113-34).

Institutional Review Board Statement: This study was approved by the Institutional Review Board of Taipei Tzu Chi Hospital (IRB number: 11-XD-148 and 12-XD-079).

Informed Consent Statement: Patient consent was waived from IRB due to retrospective study design.

Data Availability Statement: The data is unavailable due to privacy andor ethical restrictions.

Acknowledgments: This study was supported by Buddhist Tzu Chi Medical Foundation (TCMF-A 113-02).

Conflicts of Interest: The authors declare no conflict of interest.

References

1. Wu, M.-Y.; Lin, P.-C.; Liu, C.-Y.; Tzeng, I.-S.; Hsieh, T.-H.; Chang, C.-Y.; Hou, Y.-T.; Chen, Y.-L.; Chien, D.-S.; Yiang, G.-T. The impact of holiday season and weekend effect on traumatic injury mortality: Evidence from a 10-year analysis. *Tzu Chi Med. J.* **2023**, *35*, 69–77. [CrossRef]
2. Dong, S.L.; Bullard, M.J.; Meurer, D.P.; Colman, I.; Blitz, S.; Holroyd, B.R.; Rowe, B.H. Emergency triage: Comparing a novel computer triage program with standard triage. *Acad. Emerg. Med.* **2005**, *12*, 502–507. [CrossRef]
3. Wuerz, R.C.; Milne, L.W.; Eitel, D.R.; Travers, D.; Gilboy, N. Reliability and validity of a new five-level triage instrument. *Acad. Emerg. Med.* **2000**, *7*, 236–242. [CrossRef]
4. Cronin, J. The introduction of the Manchester triage scale to an emergency department in the Republic of Ireland. *Accid. Emerg. Nurs.* **2003**, *11*, 121–125. [CrossRef]
5. Ng, C.-J.; Yen, Z.-S.; Tsai, J.C.-H.; Chen, L.C.; Lin, S.J.; Sang, Y.Y.; Chen, J.-C. TTAS national working group Validation of the Taiwan triage and acuity scale: A new computerised five-level triage system. *Emerg. Med. J.* **2010**, *28*, 1026–1031. [CrossRef]
6. Chang, Y.-C.; Ng, C.-J.; Wu, C.-T.; Chen, L.-C.; Chen, J.-C.; Hsu, K.-H. Effectiveness of a five-level Paediatric Triage System: An analysis of resource utilisation in the emergency department in Taiwan. *Emerg. Med. J.* **2012**, *30*, 735–739. [CrossRef]
7. Jelinek, G.A.; Little, M. Inter-rater reliability of the National Triage Scale over 11,500 simulated occasions of triage. *Emerg. Med.* **1996**, *8*, 226–230. [CrossRef]
8. Shelton, R. The emergency severity index 5-level triage system. *Dimens. Crit. Care Nurs.* **2009**, *28*, 9–12. [CrossRef]
9. Levin, S.; Toerper, M.; Hamrock, E.; Hinson, J.S.; Barnes, S.; Gardner, H.; Dugas, A.; Linton, B.; Kirsch, T.; Kelen, G. Machine-Learning-Based Electronic Triage More Accurately Differentiates Patients with Respect to Clinical Outcomes Compared With the Emergency Severity Index. *Ann. Emerg. Med.* **2018**, *71*, 565–574.e2. [CrossRef]
10. Chmielewski, N.D.; Moretz, J.M. ESI Triage Distribution in U.S. Emergency Departments. *Adv. Emerg. Nurs. J.* **2022**, *44*, 46–53. [CrossRef]

11. Mirhaghi, A.; Heydari, A.; Mazlom, R.; Hasanzadeh, F. Reliability of the Emergency Severity Index: Meta-analysis. *Sultan Qaboos Univ. Med. J.* **2015**, *15*, e71–e77. [PubMed]
12. Ebrahimi, M.; Heydari, A.; Mazlom, R.; Mirhaghi, A. The reliability of the Australasian Triage Scale: A meta-analysis. *World J. Emerg. Med.* **2015**, *6*, 94–99. [CrossRef]
13. Zachariasse, J.M.; Seiger, N.; Rood, P.P.M.; Alves, C.F.; Freitas, P.; Smit, F.J.; Roukema, G.R.; Moll, H.A. Validity of the Manchester Triage System in emergency care: A prospective observational study. *PLoS ONE* **2017**, *12*, e0170811. [CrossRef]
14. Zakeri, H.; Saleh, L.A.; Niroumand, S.; Ziadi-Lotfabadi, M. Comparison the Emergency Severity Index and Manchester Triage System in Trauma Patients. *Bull. Emerg. Trauma* **2022**, *10*, 65–70. [CrossRef]
15. Zachariasse, J.M.; van der Hagen, V.; Seiger, N.; Mackway-Jones, K.; van Veen, M.; Moll, H.A. Performance of triage systems in emergency care: A systematic review and meta-analysis. *BMJ Open* **2019**, *9*, e026471. [CrossRef]
16. Chien, D.-S.; Yiang, G.-T.; Liu, C.-Y.; Tzeng, I.-S.; Chang, C.-Y.; Hou, Y.-T.; Chen, Y.-L.; Lin, P.-C.; Wu, M.-Y. Association of In-Hospital Mortality and Trauma Team Activation: A 10-Year Study. *Diagnostics* **2022**, *12*, 2334. [CrossRef]
17. Ng, C.-J.; Hsu, K.-H.; Kuan, J.-T.; Chiu, T.-F.; Chen, W.-K.; Lin, H.-J.; Bullard, M.J.; Chen, J.-C. Comparison Between Canadian Triage and Acuity Scale and Taiwan Triage System in Emergency Departments. *J. Formos. Med. Assoc.* **2010**, *109*, 828–837. [CrossRef]
18. Xiang, H.; Wheeler, K.K.; Groner, J.I.; Shi, J.; Haley, K.J. Undertriage of major trauma patients in the US emergency departments. *Am. J. Emerg. Med.* **2014**, *32*, 997–1004. [CrossRef]
19. Newgard, C.D.M.; Fischer, P.E.; Gestring, M.; Michaels, H.N.; Jurkovich, G.J.M.; Lerner, E.B.P.; Fallat, M.E.; Delbridge, T.R.; Brown, J.B.M.; Bulger, E.M.; et al. National guideline for the field triage of injured patients: Recommendations of the National Expert Panel on Field Triage, 2021. *J. Trauma Acute Care Surg.* **2022**, *93*, e49–e60. [CrossRef]
20. Kuo, S.C.H.; Kuo, P.-J.; Hsu, S.-Y.; Rau, C.-S.; Chen, Y.-C.; Hsieh, H.-Y.; Hsieh, C.-H. The use of the reverse shock index to identify high-risk trauma patients in addition to the criteria for trauma team activation: A cross-sectional study based on a trauma registry system. *BMJ Open* **2016**, *6*, e011072. [CrossRef]
21. Chang, W.; Liu, H.-E.; Goopy, S.; Chen, L.-C.; Chen, H.-J.; Han, C.-Y. Using the Five-Level Taiwan Triage and Acuity Scale Computerized System: Factors in Decision Making by Emergency Department Triage Nurses. *Clin. Nurs. Res.* **2016**, *26*, 651–666. [CrossRef] [PubMed]
22. Lin, Y.-K.; Niu, K.-Y.; Seak, C.-J.; Weng, Y.-M.; Wang, J.-H.; Lai, P.-F. Comparison between simple triage and rapid treatment and Taiwan Triage and Acuity Scale for the emergency department triage of victims following an earthquake-related mass casualty incident: A retrospective cohort study. *World J. Emerg. Surg.* **2020**, *15*, 20. [CrossRef] [PubMed]
23. Wu, M.-Y.; Hou, Y.-T.; Chung, J.-Y.; Yiang, G.-T. Reverse shock index multiplied by simplified motor score as a predictor of clinical outcomes for patients with COVID-19. *BMC Emerg. Med.* **2024**, *24*, 26. [CrossRef] [PubMed]
24. Dallaire, C.; Poitras, J.; Aubin, K.; Lavoie, A.; Moore, L. Emergency department triage: Do experienced nurses agree on triage scores? *J. Emerg. Med.* **2012**, *42*, 736–740. [CrossRef]
25. Chuang, J.-F.; Rau, C.-S.; Wu, S.-C.; Liu, H.-T.; Hsu, S.-Y.; Hsieh, H.-Y.; Chen, Y.-C.; Hsieh, C.-H. Use of the reverse shock index for identifying high-risk patients in a five-level triage system. *Scand. J. Trauma Resusc. Emerg. Med.* **2016**, *24*, 12. [CrossRef]

Disclaimer/Publisher's Note: The statements, opinions and data contained in all publications are solely those of the individual author(s) and contributor(s) and not of MDPI and/or the editor(s). MDPI and/or the editor(s) disclaim responsibility for any injury to people or property resulting from any ideas, methods, instructions or products referred to in the content.

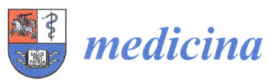
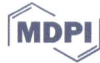

Article

A Ten-Year Retrospective Cohort Study on Neck Collar Immobilization in Trauma Patients with Head and Neck Injuries

Shu-Jui Lee [1,2,†], Lin Jian [3,4,†], Chi-Yuan Liu [5,6], I-Shiang Tzeng [7], Da-Sen Chien [1,2], Yueh-Tseng Hou [1,2], Po-Chen Lin [1,2], Yu-Long Chen [1,2], Meng-Yu Wu [1,2] and Giou-Teng Yiang [1,2,*]

1. Department of Emergency Medicine, Taipei Tzu Chi Hospital, Buddhist Tzu Chi Medical Foundation, New Taipei 231, Taiwan
2. Department of Emergency Medicine, School of Medicine, Tzu Chi University, Hualien 970, Taiwan
3. Department of Medical Education, Changhua Christian Hospital, Changhua 500, Taiwan
4. Department of Medicine, College of Medicine, Tzu Chi University, Hualien 970, Taiwan
5. Department of Orthopedic Surgery, Taipei Tzu Chi Hospital, Buddhist Tzu Chi Medical Foundation, New Taipei 231, Taiwan
6. Department of Orthopedics, School of Medicine, Tzu Chi University, Hualien 970, Taiwan
7. Department of Research, Taipei Tzu Chi Hospital, Buddhist Tzu Chi Medical Foundation, New Taipei 231, Taiwan
* Correspondence: gtyiang@gmail.com; Tel.: +886-2-6628-9779; Fax: +886-2-6628-9009
† These authors contributed equally to this work.

Citation: Lee, S.-J.; Jian, L.; Liu, C.-Y.; Tzeng, I.-S.; Chien, D.-S.; Hou, Y.-T.; Lin, P.-C.; Chen, Y.-L.; Wu, M.-Y.; Yiang, G.-T. A Ten-Year Retrospective Cohort Study on Neck Collar Immobilization in Trauma Patients with Head and Neck Injuries. *Medicina* **2023**, *59*, 1974. https://doi.org/10.3390/medicina59111974

Academic Editors: Salvatore Chibbaro, Ivo Dumić-Čule and Tomislav Čengić

Received: 15 September 2023
Revised: 23 October 2023
Accepted: 7 November 2023
Published: 9 November 2023

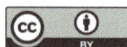

Copyright: © 2023 by the authors. Licensee MDPI, Basel, Switzerland. This article is an open access article distributed under the terms and conditions of the Creative Commons Attribution (CC BY) license (https://creativecommons.org/licenses/by/4.0/).

Abstract: *Background and Objectives*: In the context of prehospital care, spinal immobilization is commonly employed to maintain cervical stability in head and neck injury patients. However, its use in cases of unclear consciousness or major trauma patients is often precautionary, pending the exclusion of unstable spinal injuries through appropriate diagnostic imaging. The impact of prehospital C-spinal immobilization in these specific patient populations remains uncertain. *Materials and Methods*: We conducted a retrospective cohort study at Taipei Tzu Chi Hospital from January 2009 to May 2019, focusing on trauma patients suspected of head and neck injuries. The primary outcome assessed was in-hospital mortality. We employed multivariable logistic regression to investigate the relationship between prehospital C-spine immobilization and outcomes, while adjusting for various factors such as age, gender, type of traumatic brain injury, Injury Severity Score (ISS), Revised Trauma Score (RTS), and activation of trauma team. *Results*: Our analysis encompassed 2733 patients. Among these, patients in the unclear consciousness group (GCS ≤ 8) who underwent C-spine immobilization exhibited a higher mortality rate than those without immobilization. However, there was no statistically significant difference in mortality among patients with alert consciousness (GCS > 8). Multivariable logistic regression analysis revealed that advanced age (age ≥ 65), unclear consciousness (GCS ≤ 8), major traumatic injuries (ISS ≥ 16 and RTS ≤ 7), and the use of neck collars for immobilization (adjusted OR: 1.850, 95% CI: 1.240–2.760, $p = 0.003$) were significantly associated with an increased risk of mortality. Subgroup analysis indicated that C-spine immobilization was significantly linked to an elevated risk of mortality in older adults (age ≥ 65), patients with unclear consciousness (GCS ≤ 8), those with major traumatic injuries (ISS ≥ 16 and RTS ≤ 7), and individuals in shock (shock index > 1). *Conclusions*: While our findings do not advocate for the complete abandonment of neck collars in all suspected head and neck injury patients, our study suggests that prehospital cervical and spinal immobilization should be applied more selectively in certain head and neck injury populations. This approach is particularly relevant for older individuals (age ≥ 65), those with unclear consciousness (GCS ≤ 8), individuals experiencing major traumatic injuries (ISS ≥ 16 or RTS ≤ 7), and patients in a state of shock (shock index ≥ 1). Our study employs a retrospective cohort design, which may introduce selection bias. Therefore, in the future, there is a need for confirmation of our results through a two-arm randomized controlled trial (RCT) arises, as this design is considered ideal for addressing this issue.

Keywords: head and neck injury; c-spinal immobilization; neck collar; mortality

1. Introduction

Over 50 million patients visit emergency departments for trauma-related reasons each year, which increases burden of health care costs [1,2]. Head and neck injuries (HNI) account for 39% of all injury casualties [3]. Injury severity can range from soft tissue lacerations to traumatic neurological injury. The mechanism may be broad from minor falls to severe motor vehicle accidents [4]. Although the prevalence of concomitant cervical spinal injury in patients with TBI was 6.5%, prehospital spinal immobilization is widely used for cervical in-line stabilization in highly suspect C-spinal injury patients [5]. Current practices are based on the assumption that head and neck injury may cause neurological injury due to an unstable spinal column without immobilization. However, C-spinal immobilization entails its own risks of complications and possible adverse effects, including increased risk of respiratory compromise [6], back and neck pain [7–9], pressure sores [10], and increased intracranial pressure [11]. C-spinal immobilization may also prolong rescue airway management and on-scene time to delay transport [12–14]. In addition, airway compromise and elevation of intracranial pressure may also trigger hypoxemia, intracranial hypertension, and hypoperfusion in severe TBI. More and more studies recommend that the HNI population with clear consciousness should early receive spinal clearance at the scene based on National Emergency X-Radiography Utilization Study (NEXUS) criteria or clinical symptoms.

In the consciousness-unclear population or severe injury mechanism, especially in the setting of a motor vehicle collision, fall, or sports-related injury, prophylactic spinal immobilization in the traumatic injury group is usually used due to difficult evaluation until exclusion of unstable spinal injury or appropriate diagnostic imaging. But the effect of prehospital C-spinal immobilization in these populations remains unclear. In Wesley B. Vanderlan et al. [15], the authors revealed that penetrating neck trauma with C-spine immobilization was associated with a high risk of mortality and an increased risk of cardiopulmonary resuscitation (CPR). In Elliott R. Haut et al. [16], the authors showed similar result in spine-immobilized penetrating trauma patients. Therefore, the benefit of prehospital C-spine immobilization has been called into question, because clinical benefit may not be worth delaying definitive care [17]. In the blunt HNI population and shock condition, there is a lack of high-level evidence on the effect of prehospital cervical spine immobilization on head and neck injury patient outcomes [18]. In our study, we aim to determine the impact of prehospital c-spinal immobilization in suspected HNI patient outcomes, whether removing a neck collar can provide benefit in suspected HNI, and which subgroups have less benefit from C-spine immobilization. Additionally, we also tried to investigate potential factors that may influence the benefit of C-spine immobilization. We believed prehospital c-spinal immobilization should be more specific and selective in population.

2. Methods

2.1. Study Setting and Patients Data Source

We conducted a retrospective cohort study of trauma patients in Taipei Tzu Chi Hospital from January 2009 to May 2019 by Taipei Tzu Chi Hospital, Buddhist Tzu Chi Medical Foundation, New Taipei City. The Institutional Review Board of Taipei Tzu Chi Hospital gave approval for this study (IRB number: 11-XD-148). Patient data were retrospectively reviewed from the Taipei Tzu Chi Hospital Trauma Database. Patients were included if they visited Taipei Tzu Chi Hospital and had hospitalization history from January 2009 to May 2019. These patients received outpatient department following up. The exclusion criteria for this study cohort were missing data on important parameters including in-hospital data and clinical outcome.

The detailed demographic, overall survival and clinical outcome data were collected from the trauma database, computerized records, and charts. The basic characteristics of the patients included age and sex, comorbid conditions, injury location, types of injuries, and EMT treatment. The in-hospital parameters included triage, activation of trauma team, in-hospital vital sign, and clinical outcome. Patients were divided into non-geriatric patients and geriatric patients by a cut-off value of 65 in age for the subgroup analysis [19]. In prehospital management, rescue airway included supraglottic airway or endotracheal tube intubation. Oxygen support included nasal cannula, oxygen mask, and non-rebreathing oxygen mask. Injury severity was analyzed by Injury Severity Score (ISS), Revised Trauma Score (RTS), New Trauma and Injury Severity Score (TRISS) and New Injury Severity Score (NISS). We adopted two major score, ISS and RTS, as the indices of trauma severity. ISS was calculated by summing the square of the 3 highest Abbreviated Injury Scale scores of different injury body regions. RTS was calculated by the following formula: RTS = (GCS score coded $\times$ 0.9368) + (SBP coded $\times$ 0.7326) + (RR coded $\times$ 0.2908). We dichotomized major trauma by ISS with cut-off value of 16 and RTS with a cut-off value of 7 [20,21]. We also used the shock index, defined as the heart rate (HR) divided by systolic blood pressure (SBP), to dichotomize shock status by a cut-off value of 1 [22]. The clinical outcome was analyzed via hospitalization time, ICU admission, re-admission ICU, ICU admission time, operation, re-operation and mortality.

2.2. Statistical Analysis

All continuous data were analyzed as normally distributed by the Kolmogorov–Smirnov test. Dichotomous and categorical variables are reported as sample numbers (percentages). Continuous variables are reported as the median (interquartile range or Q1–Q3). Non-parametric ANOVA or the Mann–Whitney U test was used for comparison of continuous variables. The Pearson chi-squared test or Fisher's exact test was used for comparison of categorical and nominal variables. Multivariable logistic regression was used to determine the association between parameters and clinical outcomes in the head and neck injury population. Variables that had $p < 0.10$ on the chi-squared test or the Mann–Whitney U test were selected for multivariable logistic regression analysis using the forced entry method. Variance inflation factors were used to recognized multicollinearity among a set of explanatory variables. The VIFs are less than 10, indicating that the multicollinearity does not pose a serious problem for those models, and the VIFs exceeding 10 are signs of serious multicollinearity requiring correction. We drop the variables with VIFs exceeding 10 to eliminate the extreme multicollinearity. The model fit was assessed using the Hosmer–Lemeshow goodness-of-fit test. The discrimination of the multivariable regression model was tested using the area under the receiver operating characteristic curve (AUROC) for mortality outcome. In the subgroup analysis, multivariable logistic regression was used via SPSS software (Version 13.0 SPSS Inc., Chicago, IL, USA) for statistical analysis. Statistically significance was defined as p-value < 0.05.

3. Results

Patient Characteristics and Prehospital Analysis

A total of 13,144 patients were eligible for review in the Taipei Tzu Chi Hospital Trauma Database. After exclusion of patients without head and neck injury (n = 9942), 3202 patients remained. Among them, 469 patients were excluded for missing data or age below 20 years. The remaining 2733 patients were included in this study (Figure 1). The characteristics of the total included patients were shown in Table 1. There were 2733 patients included with median age (IQR): 62 (45–77) and 1632 (59.7%) patients were male. In total, 1245 (45.6%) patients were age $\geq$65 and 1488 (54.4%) patients were age < 65. The Glasgow coma scale (GCS) at triage in the C-spine immobilization group (CSI) is lower than in the non-C-spine immobilization group (nCSI); and in the CSI group, there are up to 227 (29.6%) patients with GCS $\leq$ 8. In the CSI group, triage level I accounted for approximately 42.8%, which was more than in the nCSI group (14.0%) and the proportion who required activation of trauma team is higher in the CSI group [259 (33.8%) vs. 66 (3.4%), $p < 0.001$]. Isolated TBI accounted for approximately 65.3% in all patients and more in the CSI group [1396 (71.0%) vs. 388 (50.6%), $p < 0.001$]. The proportion requiring EMT management was higher in the CSI than in the nCSI population, including stopping bleeding and banding, spinal board immobilization, splint immobilization, oxygen support, rescue airway management, and cardiopulmonary resuscitation (CPR). In the analysis of where accidents occurred, most occurred on the street, 52.8%, with a higher percentage, 69.8%, in the CSI group. Motor vehicle collision is the major injury type in the total head and neck injury population (34.1%), followed by contusion (34.1%). In the nCSI group, contusion is the major injury type. The injury severity analysis revealed that the CSI group had more severe injuries than the nCSI group, from RTS, ISS, NISS, and TRISS. There was also a higher major traumatic population in the CSI group than in the nCSI group based on ISS $\geq$ 16 [445 (22.6%) vs. 379 (49.4%), $p < 0.001$] and RTS $\leq$ 7 [273 (13.9%) vs. 328 (42.8%), $p < 0.001$]. In the clinical outcome analysis, the CSI group had a higher proportion of ICU admissions, re-ICU admissions, operations, re-operations, complications, and death. Length of stay (LOS) in ICU was also longer in the CSI population but total LOS was not significantly different between the two groups.

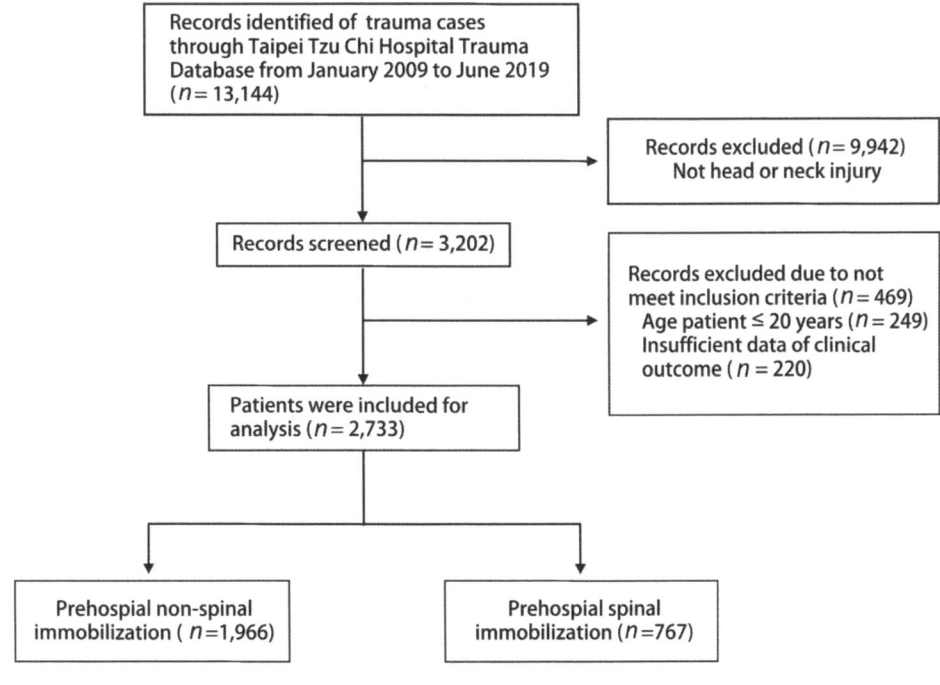

Figure 1. Flow diagram of included patients.

Table 1. Comparison of demographic characteristics of patients included in the study of in-hospital mortality.

Characteristics	Total Patient	Non-C-Spine Immobilization	C-Spine Immobilization	p-Value
Patient number	2733 (100.0%)	1966 (%)	767 (%)	
Age (years)	62 (45–77)	65 (48–79)	54 (37–68)	<0.001
Age < 65	1488 (54.4%)	964 (49.0%)	524 (68.3%)	<0.001
Age ≥ 65	1245 (45.6%)	1002 (51.0%)	243 (31.7%)	
Gender				0.046
Female	1101 (40.3%)	815 (41.5%)	286 (37.3%)	
Male	1632 (59.7%)	1151 (58.5%)	481 (62.7%)	
In-hospital vital sign				
SBP	149 (125–173)	150.5 (128–174)	142 (113–168)	<0.001
DBP	85 (73–98)	86 (75–98)	84 (68–98)	<0.001
RR	18 (18–20)	18 (18–20)	18 (18–20)	<0.001
HR	84 (72–96)	84 (74–96)	82 (68–96)	<0.001
Triage GCS	15 (14–15)	15 (15–15)	14 (7–15)	<0.001
Triage GCS ≤ 8	361 (13.2%)	134 (6.8%)	227 (29.6%)	<0.001
Triage				<0.001
1	604 (22.1%)	276 (14.0%)	328 (42.8%)	
2	1499 (54.8%)	1138 (57.9%)	361 (47.1%)	
3	620 (22.7%)	542 (27.6%)	78 (10.2%)	
4 and 5	10 (0.4%)	10 (0.5%)	0 (0%)	
Call trauma team	325 (11.9%)	66 (3.4%)	259 (33.8%)	<0.001
Injury severity				
RTS	7.84 (7.84–7.84)	7.84 (7.84–7.84)	7.84 (5.97–7.84)	<0.001
ISS	9 (8–16)	9 (6–13)	14 (9–25)	<0.001
NISS	10 (8–16)	9 (6–16)	16 (9–27)	<0.001
TRISS	0.97 (0.94–0.99)	0.97 (0.96–0.99)	0.96 (0.67–0.99)	<0.001
ISS ≥ 16	824 (30.2%)	445 (22.6%)	379 (49.4%)	<0.001
RTS ≤ 7	601 (22.0%)	273 (13.9%)	328 (42.8%)	<0.001
TBI				<0.001
Mixed TBI	949 (34.7%)	570 (29.0%)	379 (49.4%)	
Isolated TBI	1784 (65.3%)	1396 (71.0%)	388 (50.6%)	
Prehospital treatment				
Stopping bleeding and banding	869 (31.8%)	441 (22.4%)	428 (55.8%)	<0.001
Spinal board immobilization	537 (19.6%)	53 (2.7%)	484 (63.1%)	<0.001
Splint immobilization	106 (3.9%)	35 (1.8%)	71 (9.3%)	<0.001
Oxygen support	217 (7.9%)	51 (2.6%)	166 (21.6%)	<0.001
Rescue airway [†]	60 (2.2%)	6 (0.3%)	54 (7.0%)	<0.001
CPR	103 (3.8%)	16 (0.8%)	87 (11.3%)	<0.001
Injury place				<0.001
Home	869 (31.8%)	771 (39.2%)	98 (12.8%)	
Street	1442 (52.8%)	907 (46.1%)	535 (69.8%)	
Work	29 (1.1%)	24 (1.2%)	5 (0.7%)	
Public site	207 (7.6%)	120 (6.1%)	87 (11.3%)	
Others	186 (6.8%)	144 (7.3%)	42 (5.5%)	
Injury type				<0.001
Contusion	931 (34.1%)	845 (43.0%)	86 (11.2%)	
Motor vehicle collision	1153 (42.2%)	683 (34.7%)	470 (61.3%)	
Falling down	457 (16.7%)	295 (15.0%)	162 (21.1%)	
Penetration	22 (0.8%)	20 (1.0%)	2 (0.3%)	
Others	170 (6.2%)	123 (6.3%)	47 (6.1%)	
Past history				<0.001
CNS diseases	226 (8.3%)	191 (9.7%)	35 (4.6%)	
Cardiovascular diseases	825 (30.2%)	694 (35.3%)	131 (17.1%)	

Table 1. Cont.

Characteristics	Total Patient	Non-C-Spine Immobilization	C-Spine Immobilization	p-Value
Respiratory diseases	53 (1.9%)	42 (2.1%)	11 (1.4%)	
Gastrointestinal diseases	68 (2.5%)	54 (2.7%)	14 (1.8%)	
Chronic kidney disease	97 (3.5%)	86 (4.4%)	11 (1.4%)	
Diabetes mellitus	350 (12.8%)	296 (15.1%)	54 (7.0%)	
ICU admission	1440 (52.7%)	999 (50.8%)	441 (57.5%)	0.002
Re-admission ICU	29 (1.1%)	19 (1.0%)	10 (1.3%)	0.439
LOS in ICU	4 (3–7)	4 (3–6)	5 (3–9)	<0.001
Operation	651 (23.8%)	430 (21.9%)	221 (28.8%)	<0.001
Re-opertation	103 (3.8%)	59 (3.0%)	44 (5.7%)	0.001
Complications	400 (14.6%)	268 (13.6%)	132 (17.2%)	0.017
Total LOS	7 (4–14)	7 (4–13)	8 (3–17)	0.107
Death	315 (11.5%)	126 (6.4%)	189 (24.6%)	<0.001

Dichotomous and categorical variables are reported as the absolute sample size (percentage); continuous variables are reported as the median (IQR). CPR: cardiopulmonary resuscitation; SBP: systolic blood pressure; DBP: diastolic blood pressure; RR: respiration rate; HR: heart rate; ISS: Injury Severity Score; RTS: Revised Trauma Score; NISS: National Industrial Security System; TRISS: New Trauma and Injury Severity Score; LOS: length of stay; and ICU: intensive care unit. [†] Rescue airway includes prehospital supraglottic airway and endotracheal tube insertion.

The subgroup analysis of consciousness-alert (GCS > 8) and -unclear population (GCS ≤ 8) was shown in Table 2. Age < 65 and isolated TBI populations were the major populations in the CSI group with GCS > 8 or GCS ≤ 8. Based on injury severity of ISS and RTS, the major traumatic population was also higher in the CSI group than in the nCSI group in both the consciousness-alert (GCS > 8) and -unclear population (GCS ≤ 8) groups.

Table 2. Subgroup analysis of spinal immobilization in the consciousness-alert (GCS > 8) and -unclear populations (GCS ≤ 8).

Characteristics	GCS ≤ 8			GCS > 8		
	nCSI	CSI	p-Value	nCSI	CSI	p-Value
Patient	134	227		1832	540	
Age (years)			0.052			<0.001
Age < 65	79 (59.0%)	157 (69.2%)		885 (48.3%)	367 (68.0%)	
Age ≥ 65	55 (41.0%)	70 (30.8%)		947 (51.7%)	173 (32.0%)	
Gender			1.000			0.101
Female	47 (35.1%)	81 (35.7%)		1064 (58.1%)	335 (62.0%)	
Male	87 (64.9%)	146 (64.3%)		768 (41.9%)	205 (38.0%)	
TBI			<0.001			<0.001
Mixed TBI	47 (35.1%)	130 (57.3%)		523 (28.5%)	249 (46.1%)	
Isolated TBI	87 (64.9%)	97 (42.7%)		1309 (71.5%)	291 (53.9%)	
Injury severity						
ISS ≥ 16	94 (70.1%)	207 (91.2%)	<0.001	351 (19.2%)	172 (31.9%)	<0.001
RTS ≤ 7	134 (100.0%)	227 (100.0%)	-----	139 (7.6%)	101 (18.7%)	<0.001
Call trauma team	29 (21.6%)	167 (73.6%)	<0.001	37 (2.0%)	92 (17.0%)	<0.001
Death	63 (47.0%)	161 (70.9%)	<0.001	63 (3.4%)	28 (5.2%)	0.063

Dichotomous and categorical variables are reported as the absolute sample size (percentage); continuous variables are reported as the median (IQR). nCSI: non-C-spine immobilization; CSI: C-spine immobilization; ISS: Injury Severity Score; RTS: Revised Trauma Score; GCS: Glasgow coma scale; TBI: traumatic brain injury.

The unclear population (GCS ≤ 8) with the C-spine immobilization group had higher mortality rates than the nCSI group but there was no significant result in the consciousness-alert group (GCS > 8). In the isolated TBI population with or without consciousness-clear, the mortality rate is not significantly different between nCSI and CSI (Table 3). However, interestingly, a mixed TBI population with consciousness-unclear (GCS ≤ 8) had higher mortality rates in the C-spine immobilization group than the non-immobilization group [nCSI: 19 (40.4%) vs. CSI: 102 (78.5%), $p < 0.001$].

Table 3. Subgroup analysis of spinal immobilization in isolated TBI and mixed TBI with different consciousness status.

Characteristics	Isolated TBI with GCS ≤ 8			Isolated TBI with GCS > 8		
	nCSI	CSI	p-Value	nCSI	CSI	p-Value
Patient	87	97		1309	291	
Age (years)			<0.001			<0.001
Age < 65	39 (44.8%)	68 (70.1%)		567 (43.3%)	175 (60.1%)	
Age ≥ 65	48 (55.2%)	29 (29.9%)		742 (56.7%)	116 (39.9%)	
Gender			0.772			0.553
Female	35 (40.2%)	37 (38.1%)		536 (40.9%)	113 (38.8%)	
Male	52 (59.8%)	60 (61.9%)		773 (59.1%)	178 (61.2%)	
Injury severity						
ISS ≥ 16	59 (67.8%)	83 (85.6%)	0.005	253 (19.3%)	79 (27.1%)	0.004
RTS ≤ 7	87 (100.0%)	97 (100.0%)	-----	95 (7.3%)	58 (19.9%)	<0.001
Call trauma team	14 (16.1%)	67 (69.1%)	<0.001	11 (0.8%)	27 (9.3%)	<0.001
Death	44 (50.6%)	59 (60.8%)	0.182	52 (4.0%)	19 (6.5%)	0.060
Characteristics	Mixed TBI with GCS ≤ 8			Mixed TBI with GCS > 8		
	nCSI	CSI	p-Value	nCSI	CSI	p-Value
Patient	47	130		523	249	
Age (years)			0.035			<0.001
Age < 65	40 (85.1%)	89 (68.5%)		318 (60.8%)	192 (77.1)	
Age ≥ 65	7 (14.9%)	41 (31.5%)		205 (39.2%)	57 (22.9%)	
Gender			0.294			0.051
Female	12 (25.5%)	44 (33.8%)		232 (44.4%)	92 (36.9%)	
Male	35 (74.5%)	86 (66.2%)		291 (55.6%)	157 (63.1%)	
Injury severity						
ISS ≥ 16	35 (74.5%)	124 (95.4%)	<0.001	98 (18.7%)	93 (37.3%)	<0.001
RTS ≤ 7	47 (100.0%)	130 (100.0%)	-----	44 (8.4%)	43 (17.3%)	<0.001
Call trauma team	15 (31.9%)	100 (76.9%)	<0.001	26 (5.0%)	65 (26.1%)	<0.001
Death	19 (40.4%)	102 (78.5%)	<0.001	11 (2.1%)	9 (3.6%)	0.231

Dichotomous and categorical variables are reported as the absolute sample size (percentage); continuous variables are reported as the median (IQR). nCSI: non-C-spine immobilization; CSI: C-spine immobilization; ISS: Injury Severity Score; RTS: Revised Trauma Score; GCS: Glasgow coma scale.

Multivariable logistic regression of in-hospital mortality revealed that old age (age ≥ 65), consciousness-unclear (GCS ≤ 8), and major traumatic injury (ISS ≥ 16 and RTS ≤ 7) were significantly associated with an increased risk of mortality. Male, TBI type, injury type and activation of trauma team were not at a statistically significant level. Neck collar immobilization in the head and neck injury population was significantly associated with an increased odds of mortality (adjusted OR: 1.850, 95% CI: 1.240–2.760, p = 0.003) (Table 4). The Hosmer–Lemeshow test showed adequate fit (χ^2 = 10.60, p = 0.226) and the AUROC of the multiple logistic regression model for association of neck collar immobilization and mortality was 0.921 with 95% CI: 0.905–0.937. In the subgroup analysis (Table 5), compared to the nCSI group, the c-spine immobilization group had a higher odds ratio of mortality in old age (age ≥ 65), consciousness-unclear (GCS ≤ 8), major traumatic injury (ISS ≥ 16 and RTS ≤ 7), mixed TBI, isolated TBI, and shock population.

Table 4. Multivariable logistic regression of in-hospital mortality.

Variable	Adjusted OR (95% CI)	p-Value
Age (years)		
Age < 65	Reference	
Age ≥ 65	2.757 (1.886–4.029)	<0.001
Gender		
Female	Reference	
Male	1.018 (0.0.730–1.419)	0.918
Triage GCS ≤ 8	8.862 (5.425–14.476)	<0.001
ISS ≥ 16	5.380 (3.685–7.853)	<0.001
RTS ≤ 7	2.813 (1.703–4.645)	<0.001
TBI		
Mixed TBI	Reference	
Isolated TBI	0.977 (0.679–1.405)	0.899
Injury type		
Contusion	Reference	
Motor vehicle collision	0.671 (0.418–1.078)	0.099
Falling down	0.907 (0.551–1.493)	0.700
Penetration	0.833 (0.114–6.091)	0.857
Others	1.543 (0.800–2.976)	0.196
Call trauma team	1.168 (0.753–1.810)	0.488
Neck collar immobilization	1.850 (1.240–2.760)	0.003

Table 5. Multivariable logistic regression of in-hospital mortality in subgroups.

Subgroups	Non-C-Spine Immobilization Adjusted OR (95% CI)	C-Spine Immobilization Adjusted OR (95% CI)	p-Value
Age			
Age < 65	Reference	1.708 (0.981–2.976)	0.059
Age ≥ 65	Reference	2.035 (1.108–3.736)	0.022
GCS			
GCS ≤ 8	Reference	2.495 (1.342–4.640)	0.004
GCS > 8	Reference	1.434 (0.788–2.610)	0.238
ISS			
ISS < 16	Reference	1.084 (0.457–2.572)	0.855
ISS ≥ 16	Reference	2.248 (1.388–3.642)	0.001
RTS			
RTS ≤ 7	Reference	2.273 (1.383–3.733)	0.001
RTS > 7	Reference	1.250 (0.576–2.715)	0.573
TBI type			
Mixed TBI	Reference	2.181 (1.079–4.407)	0.030
Isolated TBI	Reference	1.685 (1.019–2.785)	0.042
Activation of trauma team			
Call trauma team	Reference	2.135 (0.854–5.338)	0.105
Non-call trauma team	Reference	1.942 (1.230–3.067)	0.004
Shock status			
Shock index ≥ 1	Reference	10.103 (1.673–61.008)	0.012
Shock index < 1	Reference	1.469 (0.897–2.407)	0.126

Co-variables used in multivariable logistic regression included age, sex, mechanism of injury, type of traumatic brain injury, Injury Severity Score, and Revised Trauma Score, except the variable of the subgroup. ISS: Injury Severity Score; RTS: Revised Trauma Score; GCS: Glasgow coma scale; TBI: traumatic brain injury.

4. Discussion

The present study explored the association between prehospital c-spinal immobilization and mortality in the HNI population and observed that the C-spinal immobilization group has a higher risk of mortality than the non-C-spinal immobilization group (aOR: 1.850, 95% CI: 1.240–2.760, p = 0.003). In the HNI population with old age (age ≥ 65), consciousness-unclear (GCS ≤ 8), major traumatic injury (ISS ≥ 16 or RTS ≤ 7), and shock status (shock index < 1), the C-spinal immobilization group has a higher adjusted OR of mortality than the non-C-spinal immobilization group.

This study has some strengths. First, our study involved the Asian population, which has not been widely investigated in previous studies on the association of prehospital c-spinal immobilization and mortality in the HNI population. Second, our study included many confounders in the multivariable logistic regressions, such as injury mechanism and TBI type, and different injury severity indices, and prehospital management. Previous studies did not include these clinical variables due to limitations of the database. Third, our study used the head and neck injury population to investigate neck collar effects instead of the definite diagnosis, as a prehospital setting for EMS and useful guide for emergency physicians. Finally, our results showed the association between prehospital C-spinal immobilization and mortality in the HNI population. In addition, we highlighted that the benefits of prehospital C-spinal immobilization may be less in HNI patients with old age (age $\geq$ 65), consciousness-unclear (GCS $\leq$ 8), major traumatic injury (ISS $\geq$ 16 or RTS $\leq$ 7), and shock status (shock index < 1).

Prehospital C-spinal immobilization is usually used to prevent neurologic complication in HNI. Overimmobilization may occur in difficult-to-manage patients, such as the old age, consciousness-unclear, shock and severe injury mechanism populations. However, in Mark Hauswald et al. [23], a 5-year retrospective chart review study, the authors found that prehospital immobilization in blunt spinal injuries has little or no effect on neurologic outcome, with an adjusted OR of 2.03 of disability under 95% CI 1.03–3.99. In terms of physical and biomechanical reasons, energy deposition during an injury is a complex process and spinal injury at the scene is usually caused by ejection from vehicles contacting the vehicle structure or the ground. Compared to a direct event, the energy of the spine's normal motion due to no immobilization is low, which may explain why immobilization immediately after injury has little effect [23]. Another study, conducted in Taiwan, with lightweight motorcycle injuries showed that 63/8633 (0.73%) patients had cervical spine injury and only 16 patients received surgical intervention [24]. There was no significant correlation between cervical spine injury and neck collar whether applied or not [24]. In addition, the authors have reported that there was a significant correlation of supraclavicular lesion, neck pain and neurologic deficit in patients with c-collars. Some studies also mentioned that c-spinal immobilization carries the risk of concealing neck injuries and increased scene time [12]. The practice of prehospital spinal immobilization in HNI may be an overly conservative and overprotective practice for neurological outcomes. More and more studies have focused on this issue and analyzed the subgroup population, such as penetrating HNI, to confirm the hypothesis.

In Wesley B. Vanderlan et al. [15], the authors included penetrating neck trauma, 94% of gunshot injuries, in a level 1 trauma center to evaluate the effect of spinal immobilization on mortality. The result showed that C-spine immobilization in this study was associated with an increased risk of death with an odds ratio of 2.77 (95% CI 1.18–6.49) and an increased risk of cardiopulmonary resuscitation (CPR) with an odds ratio 3.53 (95% CI, 1.06–12.95). In Elliott R. Haut et al. [16], the authors included 45,284 penetrating trauma patients and concluded that spine-immobilized penetrating trauma patients had a higher risk of mortality with an adjusted odds ratio of 2.06 under 95% CI 1.35–3.13 than those who did not undergo prehospital spine immobilization. In both studies, the authors highlighted that the factors that delay c-spinal immobilization in transport may be critically detrimental. In current concepts, the benefit of any prehospital procedure in traumatic injury has been called into question, because their clinical benefit may not be worth delaying definitive care. Moishe Liberman et al. [25] reported that trauma patients who received Advanced Life Support (ALS) did not have better survival rate than whose received Basic Life Support (BLS). In the severe traumatic brain injury population, ALS programs did not improve outcomes and worsened clinical outcomes [26]. A longer prehospital time in traumatic injury may also be associated with an increased risk of poor functional outcomes [27]. Therefore, more studies agree that prehospital cervical and spinal immobilization should be more selective. Our result showed similar data in the HNI population. In the severe injury population, such as consciousness-unclear (GCS $\leq$ 8), major traumatic injury (ISS $\geq$ 16 or RTS $\leq$ 7), and shock status (shock index < 1), the CSI population showed increases in the adjusted OR of mortality greater than that of the nCSI groups, especially in patients with shock status (aOR: 10.103 with 95% CI: 1.673–61.008, p = 0.012). We believed that time spent on dealing with significant clinical conditions may provide better clinical outcomes than time spent on spinal immobilization.

There are several limitations to our study. First, our study only reported in-hospital mortality. There was a lack of a functional outcome for C-spinal immobilization. Several studies have also focused on neurological outcomes in trauma patients. A recent PATOS study [28] found that prehospital spinal immobilization was not associated with favorable functional outcomes in trauma patients with spinal injuries, consistent with prior research, such as the work of Mark Hauswald et al. [23], which suggested that prehospital immobilization in cases of blunt spinal injuries has little or no impact on neurological outcomes. Although we believe that the identification of secondary injuries in cases of unstable cervical spine injuries is an ideal endpoint but not a final functional outcome, it is often difficult to distinguish whether sequential neurological deficits represent the progression of the initial traumatic spinal injury or secondary injury resulting from an unstable cervical spine without immobilization, particularly in prehospital care settings. In Taiwan, prehospital transport times are typically under 20 min, with a median transport interval of 7 min and a median prehospital interval of 23 min in Taipei—significantly shorter than in many other countries [29]. Consequently, the identification of secondary injuries related to unstable cervical spine injuries during these brief prehospital periods can be challenging. Patients suspected of head and neck injuries typically receive spinal injury assessments as quickly as possible on arrival in hospitals. Additionally, our hospital's brain CT scans routinely cover the C1–C2 regions, which are common sites for C-spinal injuries, even when physicians do not explicitly request a C-spinal CT scan. As a result, C-spinal injuries can be promptly identified to minimize the risk of secondary injuries. Therefore, we focused on mortality instead of secondary C-spinal injuries and we believe the incidence of secondary C-spinal injuries is unsignificant.

Second, this study has a retrospective cohort design. The baseline characteristics of the two groups were different, especially in injury severity, which may cause confounding issues through an indication bias. Although a two-arm randomized controlled trial (RCT) is the ideal study design on this issue, the study design may be against research ethics and current practice guidelines. Further, the incidence of secondary injury is low. The included sample number will be large. In 2001, a meta-analysis study focused on this issue and included randomized controlled trials comparing spinal immobilization strategies in trauma patients with suspected spinal cord injuries as selection criteria [30]. The research group showed no randomized controlled trials of spinal immobilization strategies in trauma patients. Up until 2023, there are still no randomized controlled trials on the current issue. Therefore, to minimize the influence of selection bias, we adjusted the differences using univariable, multivariable logistic regression, and subgroup analyses to make our results robust.

Third, in this database, there is a lack of information regarding neck collar types, such as rigid versus soft collars, the duration of collar wear, rescue airway time, resuscitation time, and the time when spinal injury was definitively excluded. We also did not measure intracranial pressure through parameters like optic nerve sheath diameter or increases in the internal jugular vein. Such data could offer a clearer understanding of the pathophysiological impact of neck collars on mortality.

Furthermore, our study did not distinctly categorize HNI into groups, differentiating between traumatic brain injury, spinal injury, and the combination of traumatic brain injury with spinal injury. In the prehospital setting, emergency medical technicians often make decisions regarding cervical spine immobilization based on the mechanism of injury and the patient's chief complaints. The definite diagnosis of TBI and spinal cord injury relies on imaging findings, which may not be readily available in the prehospital care context. Lastly, the sample size in our study was small. To obtain more conclusive results, it is essential to conduct large-sample randomized clinical trials in the future.

5. Conclusions

Although our results do not support removing a neck collar in all suspected HNI patients, prehospital cervical and spinal immobilization should be more selective in some HNI populations, especially in old age (age ≥ 65), consciousness-unclear (GCS ≤ 8), major traumatic injury (ISS ≥ 16 or RTS ≤ 7), and shock status (shock index ≥ 1). In these populations, the benefit of prehospital C-spinal immobilization may be less. Our study employs a retrospective cohort design, which may introduce selection bias. Therefore, in the future, there is a need for confirmation of our results through a two-arm RCT, as this design is considered ideal for addressing this issue.

Author Contributions: Methodology, S.-J.L., P.-C.L., Y.-L.C. and M.-Y.W.; Software, I.-S.T.; Validation, I.-S.T.; Formal analysis, Y.-T.H.; Investigation, I.-S.T.; Writing—original draft, S.-J.L., L.J., C.-Y.L., P.-C.L., M.-Y.W. and G.-T.Y.; Writing—review & editing, S.-J.L., L.J., C.-Y.L., D.-S.C., M.-Y.W. and G.-T.Y.; Visualization, Y.-T.H., Y.-L.C. and M.-Y.W.; Project administration, C.-Y.L. All authors have read and agreed to the published version of the manuscript.

Funding: This study was funded by grants of Taipei Tzu Chi Hospital (TCRD-TPE-112-09 TCRD-TPE-112-39).

Institutional Review Board Statement: The Institutional Review Board of Taipei Tzu Chi Hospital gave approval for this study (IRB number: 11-XD-148, 21 April 2023).

Informed Consent Statement: The Institutional Review Board of Taipei Tzu Chi Hospital gave approval for this study and patient consent was waived.

Data Availability Statement: Data are contained within the article.

Conflicts of Interest: The authors declare no conflict of interest.

References

1. Corso, P.; Finkelstein, E.; Miller, T.; Fiebelkorn, I.; Zaloshnja, E. Incidence and lifetime costs of injuries in the United States. *Inj. Prev.* **2006**, *12*, 212–218. [CrossRef] [PubMed]
2. MacKenzie, E.J.; Rivara, F.P.; Jurkovich, G.J.; Nathens, A.B.; Frey, K.P.; Egleston, B.L.; Salkever, D.S.; Weir, S.; Scharfstein, D.O. The National Study on Costs and Outcomes of Trauma. *J. Trauma Inj. Infect. Crit. Care* **2007**, *63*, S54–S67, discussion S81–S86. [CrossRef] [PubMed]
3. Wade, A.L.; Dye, J.L.; Mohrle, C.R.; Galarneau, M.R. Head, Face, and Neck Injuries During Operation Iraqi Freedom Ii: Results from the Us Navy-Marine Corps Combat Trauma Registry. *J. Trauma Acute Care Surg.* **2007**, *63*, 836–840. [CrossRef] [PubMed]
4. Sethi, R.K.V.; Kozin, E.D.; Fagenholz, P.J.; Lee, D.J.; Shrime, M.G.; Gray, S.T. Epidemiological Survey of Head and Neck Injuries and Trauma in the United States. *Otolaryngol. Neck Surg.* **2014**, *151*, 776–784. [CrossRef] [PubMed]
5. Pandrich, M.J.; Demetriades, A.K. Prevalence of concomitant traumatic cranio-spinal injury: A systematic review and meta-analysis. *Neurosurg. Rev.* **2018**, *43*, 69–77. [CrossRef] [PubMed]
6. Hankins, D.G.; Rivera-Rivera, E.J.; Ornato, J.P.; Swor, R.A.; Blackwell, T.; Domeier, R.M. Spinal Immobilization in the Field: Clinical Clearance Criteria and Implementation. *Prehospital Emerg. Care* **2001**, *5*, 88–93. [CrossRef] [PubMed]
7. Stroh, G.; Braude, D. Can an out-of-hospital cervical spine clearance protocol identify all patients with injuries? An argument for selective immobilization. *Ann. Emerg. Med.* **2001**, *37*, 609–615. [CrossRef]
8. Belanger, E.; Levi, A.D. The acute and chronic management of spinal cord injury. *J. Am. Coll. Surg.* **2000**, *190*, 603–618. [CrossRef]
9. Kang, D.G.; Lehman, R.A. Spine immobilization: Prehospitalization to final destination. *J. Surg. Orthop. Adv.* **2011**, *20*, 2–7.
10. Benger, J.; Blackham, J. Why Do We Put Cervical Collars on Conscious Trauma Patients? *Scand. J. Trauma Resusc. Emerg. Med.* **2009**, *17*, 44. [CrossRef]
11. Davies, G.; Deakin, C.; Wilson, A. The effect of a rigid collar on intracranial pressure. *Injury* **1996**, *27*, 647–649. [CrossRef] [PubMed]
12. Brown, J.B.; Bankey, P.E.; Sangosanya, A.T.; Cheng, J.D.; Stassen, N.A.; Gestring, M.L. Prehospital Spinal Immobilization Does Not Appear to Be Beneficial and May Complicate Care Following Gunshot Injury to the Torso. *J. Trauma Inj. Infect. Crit. Care* **2009**, *67*, 774–778. [CrossRef] [PubMed]

13. Brimacombe, J.; Keller, C.; Künzel, K.H.; Gaber, O.; Boehler, M.; Pühringer, F. Cervical Spine Motion During Airway Management: A Cinefluoroscopic Study of the Posteriorly Destabilized Third Cervical Vertebrae in Human Cadavers. *Anesth. Analg.* **2000**, *91*, 1274–1278. [CrossRef] [PubMed]
14. Donaldson, W.F., III; Heil, B.V.; Donaldson, V.P.; Silvaggio, V.J. The Effect of Airway Maneuvers on the Unstable C1-C2 Segment. A Cadaver Study. *Spine* **1997**, *22*, 1215–1218. [CrossRef]
15. Vanderlan, W.B.; Tew, B.E.; McSwain, N.E. Increased risk of death with cervical spine immobilisation in penetrating cervical trauma. *Injury* **2009**, *40*, 880–883. [CrossRef]
16. Haut, E.R.; Kalish, B.T.; Efron, D.T.; Haider, A.H.; Stevens, K.A.; Kieninger, A.N.; Cornwell, E.E., 3rd; Chang, D.C. Spine Immobilization in Penetrating Trauma: More Harm Than Good? *J. Trauma Acute Care Surg.* **2010**, *68*, 115–121, discussion 20–21. [CrossRef]
17. Stuke, L.E.; Pons, P.T.; Guy, J.S.; Chapleau, W.P.; Butler, F.K.; McSwain, N.E. Prehospital Spine Immobilization for Penetrating Trauma—Review and Recommendations From the Prehospital Trauma Life Support Executive Committee. *J. Trauma Inj. Infect. Crit. Care* **2011**, *71*, 763–770, discussion 69–70. [CrossRef]
18. Oteir, A.O.; Smith, K.; Stoelwinder, J.U.; Middleton, J.; Jennings, P.A. Should suspected cervical spinal cord injury be immobilised?: A systematic review. *Injury* **2015**, *46*, 528–535. [CrossRef]
19. Bischoff, H.A.; Stähelin, H.B.; Monsch, A.U.; Iversen, M.D.; Weyh, A.; von Dechend, M.; Akos, R.; Conzelmann, M.; Dick, W.; Theiler, R. Identifying a cut-off point for normal mobility: A comparison of the timed 'up and go' test in community-dwelling and institutionalised elderly women. *Age Ageing* **2003**, *32*, 315–320. [CrossRef]
20. Jeong, J.H.; Park, Y.J.; Kim, D.H.; Kim, T.Y.; Kang, C.; Lee, S.H.; Lee, S.B.; Kim, S.C.; Lim, D. The new trauma score (NTS): A modification of the revised trauma score for better trauma mortality prediction. *BMC Surg.* **2017**, *17*, 77. [CrossRef]
21. Boyd, C.R.; Tolson, M.A.; Copes, W.S. Evaluating trauma care: The TRISS method. Trauma Score and the Injury Severity Score. *J. Trauma* **1987**, *27*, 370–378. [CrossRef]
22. Koch, E.; Lovett, S.; Nghiem, T.; Riggs, R.; Rech, M.A. Shock index in the emergency department: Utility and limitations. *Open Access Emerg. Med.* **2019**, *11*, 179–199. [CrossRef] [PubMed]
23. Hauswald, M.; Ong, G.; Tandberg, D.; Omar, Z. Out-of-Hospital Spinal Immobilization: Its Effect on Neurologic Injury. *Acad. Emerg. Med.* **1998**, *5*, 214–219. [CrossRef] [PubMed]
24. Lin, H.L.; Lee, W.C.; Chen, C.W.; Lin, T.Y.; Cheng, Y.C.; Yeh, Y.S.; Lin, Y.K.; Kuo, L.C. Neck Collar Used in Treatment of Victims of Urban Motorcycle Accidents: Over- or Underprotection? *Am. J. Emerg. Med.* **2011**, *29*, 1028–1033. [CrossRef]
25. Liberman, M.; Mulder, D.; Lavoie, A.; Denis, R.; Sampalis, J.S. Multicenter Canadian Study of Prehospital Trauma Care. *Ann. Surg.* **2003**, *237*, 153–160. [CrossRef]
26. Stiell, I.G.; Nesbitt, L.P.; Pickett, W.; Munkley, D.; Spaite, D.W.; Banek, J.; Field, B.; Luinstra-Toohey, L.; Maloney, J.; Dreyer, J.; et al. The OPALS Major Trauma Study: Impact of advanced life-support on survival and morbidity. *Can. Med Assoc. J.* **2008**, *178*, 1141–1152. [CrossRef] [PubMed]
27. Chen, C.H.; Shin, S.D.; Sun, J.T.; Jamaluddin, S.F.; Tanaka, H.; Song, K.J.; Kajino, K.; Kimura, A.; Huang, E.P.; Hsieh, M.J.; et al. Association between Prehospital Time and Outcome of Trauma Patients in 4 Asian Countries: A Cross-National, Multicenter Cohort Study. *PLoS Med.* **2020**, *17*, e1003360. [CrossRef]
28. Chen, H.A.; Hsu, S.T.; Shin, S.D.; Jamaluddin, S.F.; Son, D.N.; Hong, K.J.; Tanaka, H.; Sun, J.T.; Chiang, W.C.; Ramakrishnan, T.V.; et al. A multicenter cohort study on the association between prehospital immobilization and functional outcome of patients following spinal injury in Asia. *Sci. Rep.* **2022**, *12*, 3492. [CrossRef]
29. Shih, J.Y.M.; Shih, J.J.M. Pre-Hospital Time Intervals among Trauma Patients in Northern Taiwan. *Taiwan Crit. Care Med.* **2011**, *12*, 166–174.
30. Kwan, I.; Bunn, F.; Roberts, I.G. Spinal immobilisation for trauma patients. *Cochrane Database Syst. Rev.* **2001**, *2001*, CD002803. [CrossRef] [PubMed]

Disclaimer/Publisher's Note: The statements, opinions and data contained in all publications are solely those of the individual author(s) and contributor(s) and not of MDPI and/or the editor(s). MDPI and/or the editor(s) disclaim responsibility for any injury to people or property resulting from any ideas, methods, instructions or products referred to in the content.

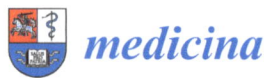

Article

Clinical Outcomes of Single Versus Double Plating in Distal-Third Humeral Fractures Caused by Arm Wrestling: A Retrospective Analysis

Jui-Ting Mao [1,†], Hao-Wei Chang [1,†], Tsung-Li Lin [1,2,3], I-Hao Lin [1], Chia-Yu Lin [1,4,*] and Chin-Jung Hsu [1,5,*]

1. Department of Orthopaedics, China Medical University Hospital, China Medical University, Taichung 40447, Taiwan
2. Department of Sports Medicine, College of Health Care, China Medical University, Taichung 40447, Taiwan
3. Graduate Institute of Biomedical Sciences, China Medical University, Taichung 40447, Taiwan
4. Spine Center, China Medical University Hospital, China Medical University, Taichung 40447, Taiwan
5. School of Chinese Medicine, China Medical University, Taichung 40447, Taiwan
* Correspondence: chiayulin1213@gmail.com (C.-Y.L.); jeffrey59835983@gmail.com (C.-J.H.)
† These authors contributed equally to the study.

Abstract: *Background and Objectives:* Arm wrestling is a simple and popular activity among young people that causes distal-third humeral fractures. However, injury to the young population may cause economic loss; therefore, they need to return to work as soon as possible. Accordingly, we aimed to compare radiological and functional outcomes of distal-third humeral fractures caused by arm wrestling treated with double and single plating. *Materials and Methods:* Thirty-four patients with distal-third humeral fractures caused by arm wrestling were treated between January 2015 and January 2021. They were separated into double- and single-plating groups and treated using a triceps-sparing approach. Regular follow-up was performed to evaluate elbow functionality, range of motion, bone union, and complications; the American Shoulder and Elbow Surgeons score was used for functional assessment. *Results:* Patients treated with single plating exhibited union rate, union time, and elbow range of motion similar to those of patients treated with double plating; however, they exhibited better pain and functional outcomes (American Shoulder and Elbow Surgeons score) at 2 weeks, 1 month, and 3 months postoperatively (84.50 ± 5.01 vs. 61.70 ± 12.53 at 2 weeks, 96.20 ± 2.63 vs. 84.25 ± 14.56 at 1 month, and 100.00 vs. 94.76 ± 9.71 at 3 months, $p < 0.05$). The two groups exhibited no significant differences after 1 year (100.00 vs. 98.54 ± 3.99, $p < 0.13$). The overall complication rate was significantly higher in patients treated with double plating than in those treated with single plating (18.75% vs. 5.56%). Radial nerve palsy was observed in patients in both groups. *Conclusions:* In patients with distal-third humeral fractures caused by arm wrestling, single plating provides a union rate and elbow range of motion similar to those of double plating, with significantly fewer complications and lower surgical time and blood loss with improved early functional outcomes.

Keywords: single plate; double plate; humerus; fracture; arm wrestling

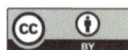

1. Introduction

The incidence of humeral fractures is 60%, 25.1%, and 10.7% in the middle, proximal, and distal third of the humeral diaphysis, respectively [1]. Arm wrestling is a cause of distal-third humeral fractures. It is a simple and popular activity among young people [2]. During the competition, torsional and axial forces in the humeral shaft may cause significant torque. When the defensive wrestler cannot resist the force, soft tissue damage may occur in the shoulder, elbow, or wrist, as well as fractures [3]. The most common fracture pattern observed after arm wrestling is the extra-articular spiral fracture of the distal third of the humerus [4]. Although the humeral shaft can efficiently tolerate coronal or sagittal plane angulation, non-operative treatment of distal humeral shaft fractures requires more union time, particularly when comparing arm wrestling fractures to other injury mechanisms [5]. Sirbu et al. showed that single plating is an effective treatment option for fractures caused by arm wrestling, with good union rates and functional outcomes [6]. However, some authors have reported superior biomechanical stability with double plating [7,8]. Therefore, the standard management of distal-third humeral fracture remains controversial. We hypothesised that double plating provides more stability in torsional and axial force-induced injuries and has a better functional outcome.

This study aimed to use our data to compare radiological and functional outcomes of distal-third humeral fractures caused by arm wrestling, which were treated with double or single plating.

2. Materials and Methods

2.1. Patient Population

Overall, 268 patients who experienced distal-third humeral fractures were treated at a level-1 trauma centre from January 2015 to January 2021. The inclusion criteria for the study were fractures that resulted from arm wrestling and those treated using open reduction and internal fixation with double or single plating by two experienced surgeons. The decision to use single or double plating was based on the surgeon's preference. The exclusion criteria were age <18 years, fractures involving the articular surface or humeral condyle, presence of multiple fracture sites, follow-up of <1 year, cancer history, ligament injury, and preoperative radial palsy. In total, we included 34 patients and categorised them into two groups as follows: single (Group S) and double plating (Group D) (Figure 1).

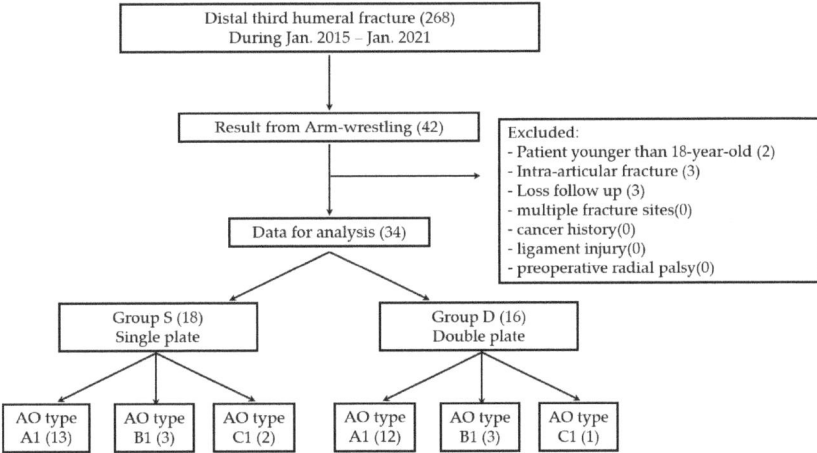

Figure 1. Participants flow. AO = Arbeitsgemeinschaftfür Osteosynthesefragen.

2.2. Surgical Technique

We used a triceps-sparing approach in both groups. First, patients were placed in the decubitus position. Next, a straight skin incision was made, beginning at the centre of the middle to the distal third of the humeral shaft and ending over the ulnar diaphysis. Subsequently, the incision was curved to avoid crossing over the tip of the olecranon. No drainage placements were observed, and we did not perform ulnar nerve transposition in both groups.

2.3. Double Plating

We initiated double plating from the ulnar window and subsequently switched to the radial window. In the ulnar window, the ulnar nerve was identified and superficially released through the cubital tunnel while preserving the perineural vessels. In contrast, the triceps fascia was split and mobilised from the lateral intermuscular septum and humerus towards the ulnar side in the radial window. The anconeus was elevated from the posterolateral distal humerus to allow direct visualisation of the fracture.

After the two windows were well-prepared, the fracture site was reduced and temporarily fixed. The metaphyseal plate was first applied on the radial side, followed by the application of the reconstruction plate on the ulnar side (Figure 2). Therefore, the ulnar nerve needed to be tension-free before wound closure.

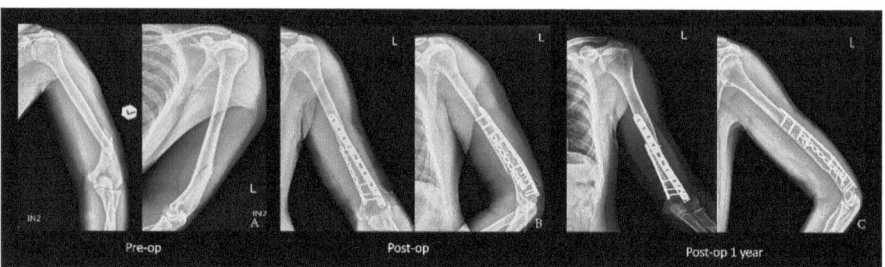

Figure 2. (**A**) Anteroposterior and lateral views showing a spiral fracture. (**B**) Postoperative radiographs showing the fixation with an AO LCP Metaphyseal Plate and AO Reconstruction LCP Plate using a triceps-sparing approach. (**C**) One-year postoperative radiographs revealing bone union. Abbreviations: LCP = locking compression plate. L = left.

2.4. Single Plating

In this group, only the radial window was exposed with the method described above. In brief, the fracture site was reduced and temporarily fixed. Subsequently, the metaphyseal plate was applied through the radial window (Figure 3).

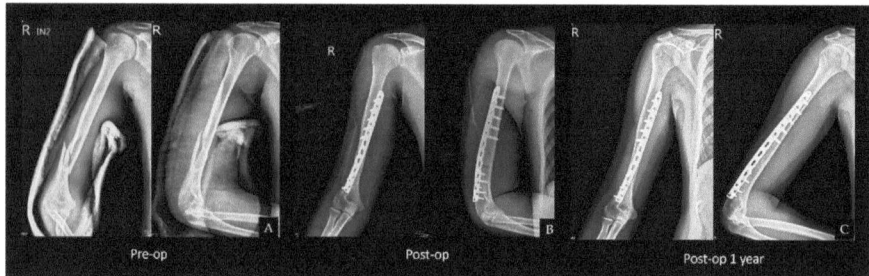

Figure 3. (**A**) Anteroposterior and lateral views showing a spiral fracture. (**B**) Postoperative radiographs showing the fixation with an AO LCP Metaphyseal Plate using a triceps-sparing approach. (**C**) One-year postoperative radiographs revealing bone union. Abbreviations: LCP = locking compression plate. R = right.

2.5. Postoperative Protocol

We carefully monitored the patients for postoperative distal circulation and neurological conditions. The wound dressings were regularly changed to avoid infections, and stitches were removed at 2 weeks postoperatively. The patients were followed up once a month to assess radiological union and complications (including wound infection, neuroplexia, and painful hardware, among others) until 1 year. Bone union was defined as the presence of three cortex unions on orthogonal radiographic images. At 3 weeks postoperatively, a sling was used for protection during the passive shoulder range of motion assessment, including flexion to 90° and external rotation to 30°, as tolerated. Active shoulder assistive range of motion and active elbow range of motion began at 3–6 weeks postoperatively. The active range of motion of the shoulder and elbow was continued at

6–12 weeks postoperatively when full weight bearing on the injured extremity was also allowed. Finally, we restricted patients from engaging in aggressive exercises until the radiographic union was achieved.

2.6. Variables, Data Sources, Measurement, Bias, and Study Size

The data obtained from medical records included basic demographics (age, sex, and underlying disease), fracture type (AO classification), blood loss, surgical duration, and complication rate. American Shoulder and Elbow Surgeons (ASES) score questionnaires were completed by every patient at 2 weeks, 1 month, 3 months, and 1 year postoperatively to assess the clinical and functional outcomes. Elbow flexion and extension range of motion were recorded at 3 and 6 months postoperatively.

2.7. Statistical Analysis

Baseline demographics were compared between the two groups using Fisher's exact test, and the treatment effects were analysed using the Mann–Whitney U test. The improvement rate was defined as the change over time, divided by the baseline values of each variable. All tests were two-tailed, and statistical significance was set at $p < 0.05$. Data were analysed using the Statistical Package for Social Sciences (SPSS) version 22 (SPSS Inc., Chicago, IL, USA).

3. Results

Thirty-four patients without underlying disease and preoperative radial nerve palsy who underwent surgery between January 2015 and December 2021 were enrolled. Among them, 18 and 16 patients were in group S and group D, respectively (Table 1). The mean follow-up period was 52 weeks (49–55 weeks). The fracture types included types 12-A, 12-B, and 12-C based on the AO/OTA classification. No significant differences were observed in the variables between the two groups.

Table 1. Patients' demographic data.

	Group S	Group D	*p*-Value
Numbers of patients	18	16	
Mean age (years)	27.56 ± 6.04	28.88 ± 6.12	0.532
Sex			0.732
Male	15 (83.33%)	14 (87.5%)	
Female	3 (16.67%)	2 (12.5%)	
BMI (kg/m^2)	24.78 ± 1.52	24.00 ± 1.27	0.117
Side			0.800
Right	12	10	
Left	6	6	
Fracture type (AO/OTA classification)			0.880
AO12A1	13	12	
AO12B1	3	3	
AO12C1	2	1	
Underlying disease	0	0	

Abbreviations: BMI = body mass index.

Group S had lesser estimated blood loss (205.56 ± 95.32 vs. 293.75 ± 125 mL, $p = 0.026$) and operative time (155.56 ± 36.40 vs. 196.13 ± 56.70 min, $p = 0.017$), which was found to be significant ($p < 0.05$) (Table 2). However, the hospital stay was not significantly different (4.78 ± 0.65 vs. 4.38 ± 0.89 days, $p = 0.137$).

Table 2. Perioperative characteristics.

	Group S	Group D	*p*-Value
Operative time (min)	155.56 ± 36.40	196.13 ± 56.70	0.017
Blood loss (mL)	205.56 ± 95.32	293.75 ± 125	0.026
Blood transfusion	0	0	
Complication	1 (5.56%)	3 (18.75%)	<0.05
Hospital stay (days)	4.78 ± 0.65	4.38 ± 0.89	0.137

Both group S (Figure 2) and group D (Figure 3) achieved 100% union without significant differences in the union time (90 ± 18.79 vs. 95 ± 16.33 days, $p = 0.416$) (Table 3).

Table 3. Clinical results.

	Group S	Group D	*p*-Value
Union rate	100%	100%	
Union time (days)	90 ± 18.79	95 ± 16.33	0.416
VAS			
2 weeks	4.44 ± 0.86	5.50 ± 0.73	0.001
1 month	2.11 ± 0.58	4.00 ± 0.52	<0.001
3 months	1.33 ± 0.49	2.13 ± 0.34	<0.001
1 year	0.33 ± 0.49	0.38 ± 0.50	0.807
ROM (3 months)			
Flexion (°)	118.33 ± 13.28	116.88 ± 17.31	0.783
Extension (°)	8.89 ± 12.31	6.25 ± 5.63	0.437
ROM (6 months)			
Flexion (°)	136.67 ± 10.85	133.75 ± 8.47	0.393
Extension (°)	3.89 ± 4.71	2.5 ± 2.58	0.303
ASES			
2 weeks	84.50 ± 5.01	61.70 ± 12.53	<0.001
1 month	96.20 ± 2.63	84.25 ± 14.56	0.002
3 months	100	94.76 ± 9.71	0.029
1 year	100	98.54 ± 3.99	0.13

Abbreviations: ROM = range of motion; VAS = visual analogue scale; ASES = American Shoulder and Elbow Surgeons.

The elbow range of motion was recorded at 3 and 6 months postoperatively. The mean elbow range of motion in flexion and extension was 118.33° ± 13.28° and 8.89° ± 12.31°, respectively, in group S at 3 months postoperatively. However, group D achieved 116.88° ± 17.31° and 6.25° ± 5.63° in flexion and extension, respectively. Furthermore, at 6 months postoperatively, the mean elbow range of motion was 136.67° ± 10.85° and 3.89° ± 4.71° in flexion and extension, respectively, in group S, whereas group D had 133.75° ± 8.47° and 2.5° ± 2.58° in flexion and extension, respectively. The elbow range of motion did not significantly differ in flexion or extension at 3 or 6 months postoperatively (Table 3).

The ASES score was higher (Figure 4), and the visual analogue scale score was lower (Figure 5) in group S, especially at 2 weeks, 1 month, and 3 months postoperatively. Group S had better pain scale and functional outcomes at 2 weeks, 1 month, and 3 months postoperatively than group D (84.50 ± 5.01 vs. 61.70 ± 12.53 at 2 weeks, 96.20 ± 2.63 vs. 84.25 ± 14.56 at 1 month, and 100.00 vs. 94.76 ± 9.71 at 3 months, $p < 0.05$). The two groups did not significantly differ at 1 year postoperatively (100.00 vs. 98.54 ± 3.99,

$p < 0.13$). Group S had better overall short-term outcomes than group D but showed no difference in long-term outcomes (Table 3).

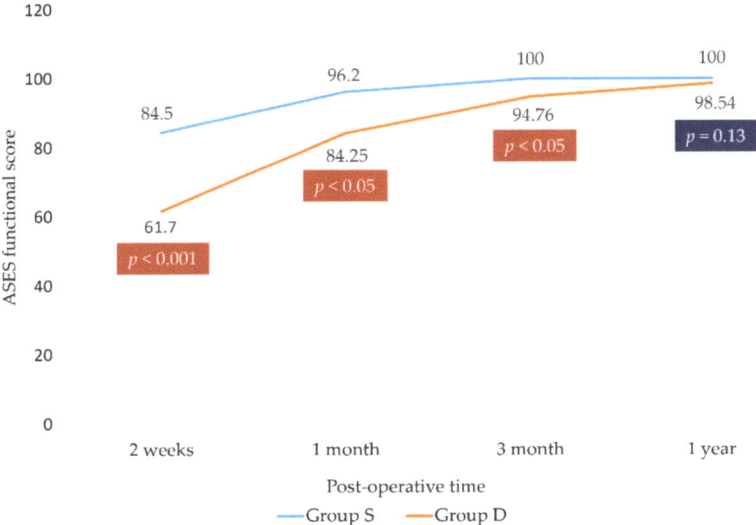

Figure 4. American Shoulder and Elbow Surgeons (ASES) score.

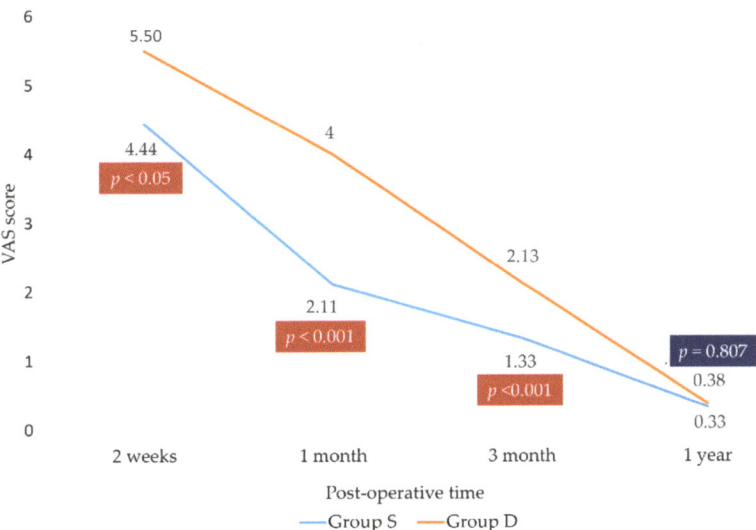

Figure 5. Visual analogue scale (VAS).

The overall complication rate was significantly higher in group D than in group S ($p < 0.05$). Three complications were noted in group D, of which two were due to painful hardware; the remaining patient had radial nerve palsy and recovered after 6 months. However, only one patient in group S developed radial nerve palsy and recovered after 8 months. Furthermore, no patients complained of implant irritation in group S.

4. Discussion

Here, in contrast with our hypothesis, single plating provided better short-term functional outcomes and similar union rates in distal-third humeral fractures caused by arm wrestling than double plating. The mechanism of humeral fracture caused by arm wrestling was first described by Brismar in 1975 [9]. Rotational failure due to the internal rotation countering the external rotation was the main cause of distal-third humeral fractures [5]. Ogawa et al. analysed 30 such cases, which were all spiral fractures. Of these, 83%, 16%, and 1% were located in the humeral lower third, middle third, and upper third, respectively [10]. Darren et al. similarly found that the most common injuries were spiral fractures of the distal third of the humerus, which is consistent with the results of our study [4]. Several studies compared the operative and non-operative treatments for humeral shaft fractures and found no differences in union time, ultimate range of motion, and complication rates [11,12]. Bumbaširević et al. presented six cases of humerus fractures caused by arm wrestling and demonstrated that both conservative and surgical approaches were successful treatment methods [3]. However, since most patients with this injury are young adults with high levels of daily activity, who want to return to work as soon as possible, most of them agreed to undergo surgery. To the best of our knowledge, only a few studies have compared surgical single and double plating for this type of injury. In other types of injury, which caused a distal humeral fracture, some studies have found that single plating is sufficient to effectively achieve bone union in extra-articular distal humeral fractures [13–21]. However, others showed that double plating provides rigid construction and optimal fracture union, allowing elderly patients to benefit from the early range of motion in intraarticular distal humeral fractures [22–25]. Prasarn et al. presented 15 cases of extra-articular distal humeral fractures treated with double plating, which achieved an optimal union rate and allowed early range of motion [26]. Consequently, it remains controversial whether single or double plating is the more appropriate method (Table 4).

Comparatively, the perioperative condition was better in patients with single plating than in those with double plating. Patients who were treated with double plating underwent a longer duration of surgery and had higher amounts of estimated blood loss than those treated with single plating. We assume this may be related to greater tissue exposure during the operation. Although the size of the surgical wound was similar in both groups, the ulnar window was exposed only in group D. In this window, it is important to carefully identify the ulnar nerve without causing damage. The fixation of the reconstruction plate also required additional time. After implant fixation, we ensured that the ulnar nerve was tension-free. However, despite the precaution we took with these two aspects, two patients still reported painful hardware. Only one patient developed complications in group S, and this complication was relatively severe. The patient developed radial nerve palsy and fortunately recovered 8 months later. We had assumed that better stability might be necessary when using only a single plate. Therefore, a longer metaphyseal plate was applied on the radial side. The radial nerve is located at the distal third of the humeral shaft, which may be damaged by the longer plate. Although the plate was carefully placed, palsy still occurred during traction. Meloy et al. conducted a retrospective study and showed a 31.25% complication rate in patients treated with double plating and 4.44% in those treated with single plating [13].

Both groups achieved comparable radiological outcomes with a 100% union rate within an average of 3 months. Patients in both groups had a comparable range of motion in the series follow-up. However, group S needed less time to recover and return to their daily activities. The functional score (ASES score) was strongly associated with the pain scale and daily activity. Therefore, we believe that the two groups were predominantly young men with good bone density. Furthermore, rigid fixation can be achieved with a single locking plate. The additional plate plays a minimal role in stability, and its application requires more dissection and exposure. Although we performed this procedure as minimally invasive as possible, dissection in group D resulted in soft tissue damage, which might have caused postoperative adhesions and pain. These may have affected the functional outcomes of these patients. Moreover, after starting a rehabilitation programme, patients showed steady improvement in functional outcomes.

Table 4. Summary of the literature review of distal-third humeral fractures.

Author	Year	Study Type	Management	Case Number	Conclusion
Gupta et al. [16]	2021	Retrospective study	EADHP	100	Complete union within 3 months: 95% Mean flexion: 123 ± 22° Mean extension: 4.031 ± 6.50°
Ali et al. [17]	2018	Prospective study	EADHP	20	Union time: 17.4 weeks Mean flexion: 127 ± 12.07°
Trikha et al. [18]	2017	Retrospective study	EADHP	36	Complete union within 3 months: 94.44% Mean flexion: 122.9 ± 23° Mean extension: 4.03 ± 6.5°
Kharbanda et al. [19]	2016	Retrospective study	EADHP	20	Mean time to union: 12 weeks Mean flexion: 125°
Scolaro et al. [20]	2014	Retrospective study	3.5-mm PL LCP	40	Achieved union: 95% Reoperation rate: 20%
Capo et al. [21]	2014	Retrospective study	EADHP	19	Union time: 7.3 months Mean flexion: 126° Mean extension: 7°
Meloy et al. [13]	2013	Retrospective comparative study	Double-column plating vs. single pre-contoured PL LCP	105	Single plating offers similar union rates and has significantly fewer complications with improved elbow range of motion
Mark L. Prasarn [26]	2011	Retrospective study	EADHP + 3.3/2.7-mm pelvic recon plate	15	Time to union: 11.5 weeks Mean elbow flexion: 4° Mean extension: 131° Reoperation rate: 13.3%
Watson et al. [25]	2014	Biomechanical study	Standard pre-contoured two-plate locked construct vs. single laterally-placed locked plate	NA	A single plate is biomechanically equivalent to two pre-contoured plates
Scolaro et al. [7]	2014	Biomechanical study	9-hole medial and lateral 3.5 mm DH LCP vs. 6-hole PL LCP	NA	Average bending stiffness and torsional stiffness were significantly greater in 6-hole posterolateral plate
Tejwani et al. [8]	2009	Biomechanical study	One LCP vs. Two reconstruction plates	NA	Double plating provides a more rigid fixation

EADPH = extra-articular distal humerus plating; LCP = locking compression plate; PL = posterolateral; DH = distal humerus; NA = not applicable.

The double-column plating technique is notorious for its high incidence of implant-related complications, such as painful hardware, ulnar neuritis, elbow stiffness, and iatrogenic radial nerve palsy [13]. Here, group D had more instances of painful hardware. We believe that less plating and limited surgical exposure would decrease postoperative implant irritation and soft tissue adhesion. Therefore, we selected a triceps-sparing approach based on the findings of Emmanuel et al., who reported a better elbow range of motion and triceps strength with this approach than those associated with a triceps-splitting approach [27]. Regarding plate configuration in treating distal humeral fractures, a systematic review and meta-analysis conducted by Yu et al. revealed that both the orthogonal and parallel plating methods could achieve successful outcomes with a similarly low number of complications [28]. Therefore, in our study, all patients underwent orthogonal plating.

Our study supports the use of single plating over double plating because the former sufficiently achieves rigid fixation, yields better early functional outcomes, and is associated with a shorter surgical duration, lower blood loss, and fewer complications.

Despite our study's comparative nature, some limitations need to be highlighted. First, the study was retrospective, and the surgeon selected the fixation strategies for each patient according to the different fracture patterns. Second, the study had a limited sample size.

5. Conclusions

In our study, single plating was found to provide similar union rates and elbow range of motion to double plating, with significantly lower surgical times and blood loss with improved early functional outcomes in patients with distal-third humeral fractures caused by arm wrestling.

Author Contributions: J.-T.M., H.-W.C., T.-L.L., C.-Y.L. and C.-J.H. contributed to the conception and design of the study. J.-T.M., H.-W.C. and T.-L.L. contributed to drafting the article. J.-T.M., H.-W.C., T.-L.L., C.-Y.L., I.-H.L. and C.-J.H. contributed to revising the article critically. All authors have read and agreed to the published version of the manuscript.

Funding: This research received no external funding.

Institutional Review Board Statement: The study was conducted in accordance with the guidelines of the Declaration of Helsinki and approved by the local Institutional Review Board of China Medical University & Hospital Research Ethics Committee (CMUH111-REC2-102).

Informed Consent Statement: Informed consent was obtained from all participants involved in the study.

Data Availability Statement: All the available data have been presented in this study. Details regarding the data supporting the reported results can be requested at the following e-mail address: jeffrey59835983@gmail.com.

Conflicts of Interest: The authors declare no conflict of interest.

References

1. Tytherleigh-Strong, G.; McQueen, M.M. The epidemiology of humeral shaft fractures. *J. Bone Jt. Surg. Br.* **1998**, *80*, 249–253. [CrossRef]
2. Kruczyński, J.; Jaszczur Nowicki, J.; Topoliński, T.; Srokowski, G.; Mańko, G.; Chantsoulis, M.; Frankowska, M.; Frankowski, P. Radiological and biomechanical analysis of humeral fractures occurring during arm wrestling. *Med. Sci. Monit.* **2012**, *18*, Cr303–Cr307. [CrossRef] [PubMed]
3. Bumbaširević, M.; Lešić, A.R.; Andjelković, S.Z.; Palibrk, T.D.; Milutinović, S.M. Fractures of the humerus during arm wrestling. *Vojnosanit. Pregl.* **2014**, *71*, 1144–1146. [CrossRef]
4. Moloney, D.P.; Feeley, I.; Hughes, A.J.; Merghani, K.; Sheehan, E.; Kennedy, M. Injuries associated with arm wrestling: A narrative review. *J. Clin. Orthop. Trauma* **2021**, *18*, 30–37. [CrossRef]
5. Mayfield, C.K.; Egol, K.A. Humeral fractures sustained during arm wrestling: A retrospective cohort analysis and review of the literature. *Orthopedics* **2018**, *41*, e207–e210. [CrossRef]
6. Sirbu, P.D.; Berea, G.; Asaftei, R.; Tudor, R.; Sova, R.; Bodescu, A. OS3-25 Minimally invasive plate osteosynthesis by anterior approach: An alternative in distal humeral shaft fractures produced by arm wrestling. *Injury* **2016**, *47* (Suppl. 10), S10. [CrossRef]
7. Scolaro, J.A.; Hsu, J.; Svach, D.; Mehta, S. Plate selection for fixation of extra-articular distal humerus fractures: A biomechanical comparison of three different implants. *Injury* **2014**, *45*, 2040–2044. [CrossRef] [PubMed]
8. Tejwani, N.C.; Murthy, A.; Park, J.; McLaurin, T.M.; Egol, K.A.; Kummer, F.J. Fixation of extra-articular distal humerus fractures using one locking plate versus two reconstruction plates: A laboratory study. *J. Trauma* **2009**, *66*, 795–799. [CrossRef]
9. Brismar, B.; Spangen, L. Fracture of the humerus from arm wrestling. *Acta Orthop. Scand.* **1975**, *46*, 707–708. [CrossRef]
10. Ogawa, K.; Ui, M. Humeral shaft fracture sustained during arm wrestling: Report on 30 cases and review of the literature. *J. Trauma* **1997**, *42*, 243–246. [CrossRef]
11. Mahabier, K.C.; Vogels, L.M.; Punt, B.J.; Roukema, G.R.; Patka, P.; Van Lieshout, E.M. Humeral shaft fractures: Retrospective results of non-operative and operative treatment of 186 patients. *Injury* **2013**, *44*, 427–430. [CrossRef] [PubMed]
12. Denard, A., Jr.; Richards, J.E.; Obremskey, W.T.; Tucker, M.C.; Floyd, M.; Herzog, G.A. Outcome of nonoperative vs operative treatment of humeral shaft fractures: A retrospective study of 213 patients. *Orthopedics* **2010**, *33*. [CrossRef]
13. Meloy, G.M.; Mormino, M.A.; Siska, P.A.; Tarkin, I.S. A paradigm shift in the surgical reconstruction of extra-articular distal humeral fractures: Single-column plating. *Injury* **2013**, *44*, 1620–1624. [CrossRef] [PubMed]
14. Moran, M.C. Modified lateral approach to the distal humerus for internal fixation. *Clin. Orthop. Relat. Res.* **1997**, *340*, 190–197. [CrossRef] [PubMed]
15. Levy, J.C.; Kalandiak, S.P.; Hutson, J.J.; Zych, G. An alternative method of osteosynthesis for distal humeral shaft fractures. *J. Orthop. Trauma* **2005**, *19*, 43–47. [CrossRef] [PubMed]
16. Gupta, A.K.; Samal, B.P.; Dalei, T.R. Functional and radiological outcome in distal third humerus fracture treated with extra-articular locking plate: A multicentric retrospective study. *J. Pharm. Bioallied. Sci.* **2021**, *13*, S1483–S1487. [CrossRef]

17. Ali, N.; Ahmad Mir, N.; Ahmad Dar, T.; Nawaz Rather, M.; Ahmad Mir, W.S.S.; Maajid, S. Outcome of extra-articular distal humerus fractures fixed by single column extra-articular distal humerus locking compression plate using triceps sparing postero-lateral approach. *Bull. Emerg. Trauma* **2018**, *6*, 306–312. [CrossRef]
18. Trikha, V.; Agrawal, P.; Das, S.; Gaba, S.; Kumar, A. Functional outcome of extra-articular distal humerus fracture fixation using a single locking plate: A retrospective study. *J. Orthop. Surg.* **2017**, *25*. [CrossRef]
19. Kharbanda, Y.; Tanwar, Y.S.; Srivastava, V.; Birla, V.; Rajput, A.; Pandit, R. Retrospective analysis of extra-articular distal humerus shaft fractures treated with the use of pre-contoured lateral column metaphyseal LCP by triceps-sparing posterolateral approach. *Strateg. Trauma Limb Reconstr.* **2017**, *12*, 1–9. [CrossRef]
20. Scolaro, J.A.; Voleti, P.; Makani, A.; Namdari, S.; Mirza, A.; Mehta, S. Surgical fixation of extra-articular distal humerus fractures with a posterolateral plate through a triceps-reflecting technique. *J. Shoulder Elb. Surg.* **2014**, *23*, 251–257. [CrossRef]
21. Capo, J.T.; Debkowska, M.P.; Liporace, F.; Beutel, B.G.; Melamed, E. Outcomes of distal humerus diaphyseal injuries fixed with a single-column anatomic plate. *Int. Orthop.* **2014**, *38*, 1037–1043. [CrossRef] [PubMed]
22. O'Driscoll, S.W. Optimizing stability in distal humeral fracture fixation. *J. Shoulder Elb. Surg.* **2005**, *14*, 186S–194S. [CrossRef] [PubMed]
23. Leigey, D.F.; Farrell, D.J.; Siska, P.A.; Tarkin, I.S. Bicolumnar 90-90 plating of low-energy distal humeral fractures in the elderly patient. *Geriatr. Orthop. Surg. Rehabil.* **2014**, *5*, 122–126. [CrossRef] [PubMed]
24. Korner, J.; Lill, H.; Müller, L.P.; Hessmann, M.; Kopf, K.; Goldhahn, J.; Gonschorek, O.; Josten, C.; Rommens, P.M. Distal humerus fractures in elderly patients: Results after open reduction and internal fixation. *Osteoporos. Int.* **2005**, *16*, S73–S79. [CrossRef] [PubMed]
25. Watson, J.D.; Kim, H.; Becker, E.H.; Shorofsky, M.; Lerman, D.; O'Toole, R.V.; Eglseder, W.A.; Murthi, A.M. Are two plates necessary for extraarticular fractures of the distal humerus? *Curr. Orthop. Pract.* **2014**, *25*, 462–466. [CrossRef]
26. Prasarn, M.L.; Ahn, J.; Paul, O.; Morris, E.M.; Kalandiak, S.P.; Helfet, D.L.; Lorich, D.G. Dual plating for fractures of the distal third of the humeral shaft. *J. Orthop. Trauma* **2011**, *25*, 57–63. [CrossRef] [PubMed]
27. Illical, E.M.; Farrell, D.J.; Siska, P.A.; Evans, A.R.; Gruen, G.S.; Tarkin, I.S. Comparison of outcomes after triceps split versus sparing surgery for extra-articular distal humerus fractures. *Injury* **2014**, *45*, 1545–1548. [CrossRef] [PubMed]
28. Yu, X.; Xie, L.; Wang, J.; Chen, C.; Zhang, C.; Zheng, W. Orthogonal plating method versus parallel plating method in the treatment of distal humerus fracture: A systematic review and meta-analysis. *Int. J. Surg.* **2019**, *69*, 49–60. [CrossRef]

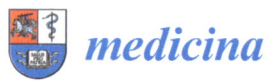

Article

Computed Tomography Does Not Improve Intra- and Interobserver Agreement of Hertel Radiographic Prognostic Criteria

Paulo Ottoni di Tullio [1], Vincenzo Giordano [1,*], William Dias Belangero [2], Robinson Esteves Pires [3], Felipe Serrão de Souza [1], Pedro José Labronici [4], Caio Zamboni [5], Felipe Malzac [1], Paulo Santoro Belangero [6], Roberto Yukio Ikemoto [7], Sergio Rowinski [8] and Hilton Augusto Koch [9]

[1] Serviço de Ortopedia e Traumatologia Prof. Nova Monteiro—Hospital Municipal Miguel Couto, Rio de Janeiro 22430-160, Brazil
[2] Departamento de Ortopedia, Reumatologia e Traumatologia—Universidade Estadual de Campinas (UNICAMP), Campinas 13083-970, Brazil
[3] Departamento do Aparelho Locomotor—Universidade Federal de Minas Gerais (UFMG), Belo Horizonte 31270-901, Brazil
[4] Departamento de Cirurgia Geral e Especializada—Universidade Federal Fluminense (UFF), Niteroi 24220-900, Brazil
[5] Departamento de Ortopedia—Santa Casa de São Paulo, São Paulo 01221-020, Brazil
[6] Departamento de Ortopedia e Traumatologia—Escola Paulista de Medicina, Universidade Federal de São Paulo (UNIFESP), São Paulo 04021-001, Brazil
[7] Grupo de Ombro e Cotovelo—Faculdade de Medicina do ABC, Santo André 09060-870, Brazil
[8] SUORT—Clínica Integrada, São Paulo 01258-010, Brazil
[9] Departamento de Radiologia—Universidade Federal do Rio de Janeiro (UFRJ), Rio de Janeiro 21941-901, Brazil
* Correspondence: v_giordano@me.com; Tel.: +55-(21)-99751-6859

Abstract: *Background and Objectives*: Proximal humerus fractures are the second most frequent site of avascular necrosis (AVN), occurring in up to 16% of cases. The Hertel criteria have been used as a reference for the prediction of humerus head ischemia. However, these are based solely on the use of radiographs, which can make interpretation extremely difficult due to several reasons, such as the overlapping fragments, severity of the injury, and noncompliant acute pain patients. The objectives of the study were to evaluate the role of computed tomography (CT) in the interpretation of the Hertel criteria and to evaluate the intra- and interobserver agreement of orthopedic surgeons, comparing their area of expertise. *Materials and Methods*: The radiographs and CT scans of 20 skeletally mature patients who had fractures of the proximal humerus were converted to jpeg and mov, respectively. All images were evaluated by eight orthopedic surgeons (four trauma surgeons and four shoulder surgeons) in two different occasions. The intra- and interobserver agreement was assessed by using the Kappa coefficient. The level of significance was 5%. *Results*: There was a weak-to-moderate intraobserver agreement ($\kappa < 0.59$) for all examiners. Only the medial metaphyseal hinge greater than 2 mm was identified by 87.5% of evaluators both in the radiographic and CT examinations in the two rounds of the study ($p < 0.05$). There was no significant interobserver agreement ($\kappa < 0.19$), as it occurred only in some moments of the second round of evaluation. *Conclusions*: The prognostic criteria for humeral head ischemia evaluated in this study showed weak intra- and interobserver agreement in both the radiographic and tomographic evaluation. CT did not help surgeons in the primary interpretation of Hertel prognostic criteria used in this study when compared to the radiographic examination.

Keywords: proximal humerus fracture; humerus head necrosis; avascular necrosis risk factors; posttraumatic avascular necrosis; Hertel criteria

1. Introduction

Fractures of the proximal humerus represent 4 to 5% of all fractures, being the third most common in the human body [1]. Approximately 85% of patients can be treated non-surgically, particularly older patients with fractures involving the surgical neck of the humerus [2]. However, fractures considered more complicated require surgical treatment, especially in younger patients. Indeed, about 13 to 16% of all fractures of the proximal humerus are in three, four, or more parts, including the humerus head, greater tuberosity, lesser tuberosity, and shaft, and present unacceptable displacements [3]. Although a good functional outcome has been reported both after non-surgical treatment and after internal fixation [4], several postoperative complications have been described as a result of proximal humerus fractures, including avascular necrosis (AVN) of the humeral head [5].

Regardless of the type of treatment, proximal humerus fractures are the second most frequent site of AVN, occurring in up to 16% of cases [6]. The main risk factors for AVN are a greater number of fragments, head-split fracture, short segment of the humeral calcar, rupture of the medial hinge, displaced tuberosities, glenohumeral fracture/dislocation, and significant angular displacement of the head [7,8]. Other factors, such as the surgical approach and poor anatomical reduction, have also been implicated as risk factors [8]. Hertel et al. [7] radiographically evaluated 100 fractures of the proximal humerus in 98 patients who underwent internal fixation over a period of four years. These authors observed that good predictors of ischemia were posteromedial metaphyseal extension of the head less than 8.0 mm, medial hinge rupture (>2.0 mm), and fracture patterns involving the anatomical neck. The combination of these three factors led to a positive predictive value of 97% for the development of AVN of the humeral head.

Shortly after its publication, other studies from the same group observed high intra- and interobserver reliability of the Hertel classification, providing a more adequate description of proximal humerus fractures compared to the systems described by the Neer system and the AO group (Arbeitsgmenischaft für Osteosynthesefragen) [9,10]. However, there are some potential confounding factors in the study by Hertel et al. [7], such as the use of radiographs alone and the adoption of deltopectoral approach in all surgical procedures. In particular, the use of radiographs can make interpretation extremely difficult due to the overlapping fragments, severity of the injury, and noncompliant acute pain patients, making it impossible to perform all the shoulder standard views and not allowing substantial agreement [11].

We hypothesized that the adoption of computed tomography (CT) images, including three-dimensional reconstruction (3D CT), to radiographs of the proximal humerus in patients with fractures increases the reproducibility of the Hertel criteria, thus improving intra- and interobserver agreement among orthopedic surgeons. The objective of the study was to evaluate the role of CT in the interpretation of the Hertel criteria, using the radiographic evaluation of the same cases as a standard to identify the criteria described by these authors as prognostics for AVN of the humeral head.

2. Materials and Methods

Radiographs and CT scans of 20 skeletally mature patients who had fractures of the proximal humerus treated at the Institution between January and December 2020 were selected. Patients were chosen at random. We included patients older than 18 years, with a confirmed diagnosis of proximal humerus fractures, and who signed the Informed Consent form. We excluded patients with missing demographic data; inaccurate imaging exams; and presenting a pathological fracture or previous fracture history, surgical history, congenital deformities, or degenerative changes at the same region.

Patients' privacy and security during the acquisition, storage, and transmission of their medical information were protected. The identity of the patients was not revealed. All patients were surgically treated and had standard preoperative radiographic and CT studies. The age ranged from 52 to 70 years, with a mean of 59.4 (SD ± 6.21882) years. Fifteen (75%) patients were female, and the right side was affected in 12 (60%) cases. The main injury mechanism was a fall to the ground in 17 (85.0%) cases (Table 1). The imaging evaluation comprised a true AP (Grashey), scapular Y, and axillary view [12]. In patients with limited abduction of the glenohumeral joint due to pain or joint incongruity, the modified axillary view was performed [13]. The CT evaluation comprised 5 mm axial, coronal, and sagittal slices and a 3D reconstruction. Both radiographic and tomographic images were kept anonymous for the purpose of this study.

Table 1. Patient demographics and STANDARD assessment ($n = 20$).

Case	Age (Years)	Gender	Side	Mechanism of Trauma	Neer (Parts)	Hertel					
						X-ray C1	X-ray C2	X-ray C3	CT C1	CT C2	CT C3
1	58	M	R	MCA	III (H, GT, S)	P	A	A	P	A	A
2	53	F	R	Fall to the ground	II (GT)	A	A	A	A	A	A
3	52	F	R	Fall to the ground	III (H GT, S)	P	P	A	P	P	A
4	68	M	R	Fall to the ground	II (LT)	P	P	A	P	P	A
5	57	F	L	Fall to the ground	IV	A	A	I	A	A	A
6	65	F	L	Fall to the ground	IV	I	A	A	A	A	A
7	55	F	L	Fall to the ground	IV	A	A	I	A	A	P
8	64	F	R	Fall to the ground	IV	P	P	A	P	P	A
9	67	F	R	Fall to the ground	IV	A	A	I	A	A	P
10	59	M	L	MCA	III (H, GT, S)	P	A	A	P	A	A
11	53	M	R	MVA	III (H, GT, S)	P	A	A	P	A	A
12	56	F	L	Fall to the ground	II (H)	P	A	A	P	P	A
13	52	F	R	Running over	III (H, GT, S)	P	P	A	P	P	A
14	70	F	R	Fall to the ground	IV	P	A	A	P	A	A
15	66	F	L	Fall to the ground	II (LT)	P	P	A	P	P	A
16	58	F	R	Fall to the ground	III (H, GT, S)	I	A	A	A	A	A
17	54	F	L	Fall to the ground	II (LT)	P	P	A	A	A	A
18	69	M	R	Fall to the ground	II (H)	P	A	A	P	A	A
19	53	F	L	Fall to the ground	II (H)	A	A	A	A	A	A
20	59	F	R	Fall to the ground	III (H, GT, S)	A	A	A	A	A	A

Source: SOT-Nova, HMMC, 2022. Legends: M—male; F—female; L—left; R—right; II—two parts; III—three parts; IV—four or more parts; H—head; GT—greater tuberosity; LT—lesser tuberosity; S—shaft; X-ray—radiography; CT—computed tomography; C1—Criterion A; C2—Criterion B; C3—Criterion C; P—present; A—absent; I—inconclusive; MCA: motorcycle accident.

Fractures were classified radiographically, according to the Neer system [12,14]. In addition, three of the Hertel criteria were evaluated on radiographs and on CT (Figure 1). All images were initially evaluated independently by two consultants who were fellowship-trained in orthopedic trauma and with more than 10 years of experience. In cases of disagreement, a senior consultant (with more than 20 years of experience in orthopedic trauma) evaluated the images. There were only 2 cases of disagreement, Cases 10 and 11. Both were further classified after the third evaluator as Neer 3-parts (head, greater tuberosity, and shaft), with medial metaphyseal extension < 8 mm observed on both the X-ray and CT. The standard (namely STANDARD) was considered when an absolute agreement was encountered between at least two evaluators.

The Standards for Reporting of Diagnostic Accuracy (STARD) questionnaire was used to determine surgeons' perception of their accuracy in identifying each of the three criteria [15,16]. The selection was evidence-based whenever possible; therefore, the "inconclusive" category was added. Thus, both the evaluators defined as STANDARD and the respondents invited to participate in the study were asked to answer whether each of these three criteria was "present", "absent" or "inconclusive" (cannot be evaluated) in the radiographic and tomographic examinations.

The radiographic images of the 20 cases were extracted from the DICOM (Digital Imaging and Communications in Medicine) disk, which was developed by the American College of Radiology (ACR) and the National Electrical Manufacturers Association (NEMA—Arlington, VA, USA); converted to jpeg (Joint Photographic Experts Group) with 1000 × 1000 pixels and 300 DPI resolution; and stored case by case in individual folders, from 01 to 20 [17]. In the same way, the tomographic images of the 20 cases were extracted from the DICOM disk, recorded as individual frames, and saved in the mov (Multimedia

Container File) format, a file name extension for the QuickTime multimedia file format (Apple Inc., Cupertino, CA, USA), with a resolution of 1228 × 657 ppi [18]. Figures 2–4 illustrate some of the cases used in the study.

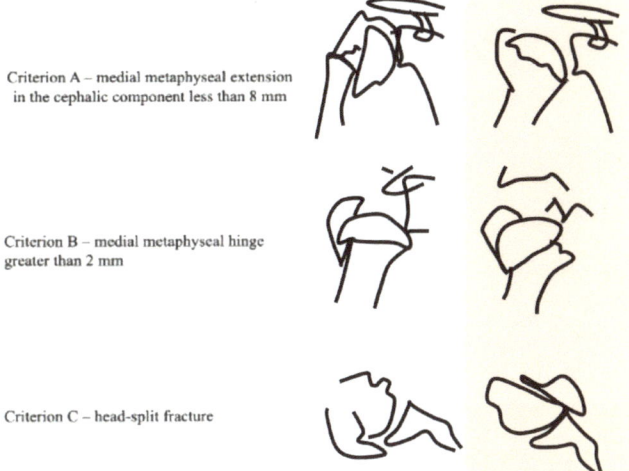

Figure 1. The three Hertel criteria adopted in the study. Criterion A represents the medial metaphyseal extension < 8 mm; Criterion B represents the medial metaphyseal hinge < 2 mm; and Criterion C represents the humerus head-split fracture. (Image produced on computer and from the author's personal archive VG).

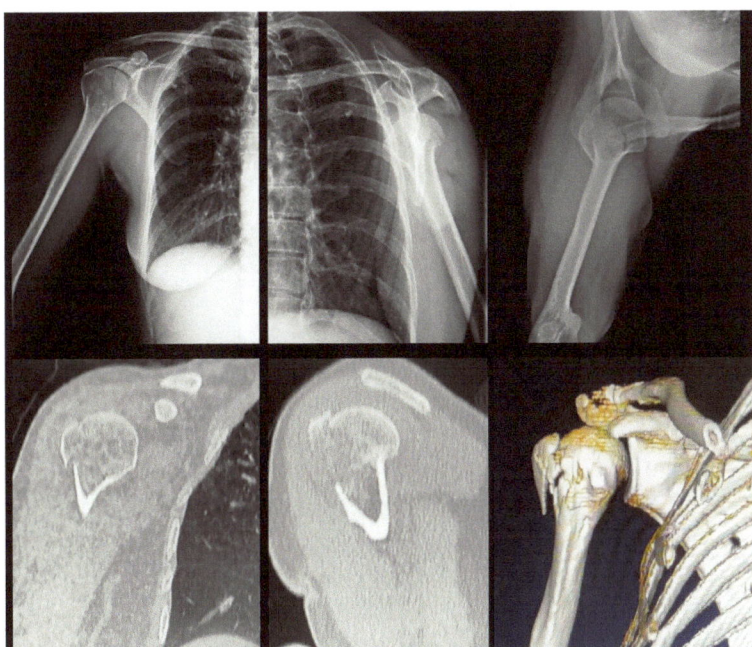

Figure 2. Radiographic and CT images of a 53-year-old female patient with a right proximal humerus fracture (Case 2). Note that none of Hertel's prognostic criteria is present in either of the two imaging exams. The fracture was classified as Neer 2-parts (greater tuberosity).

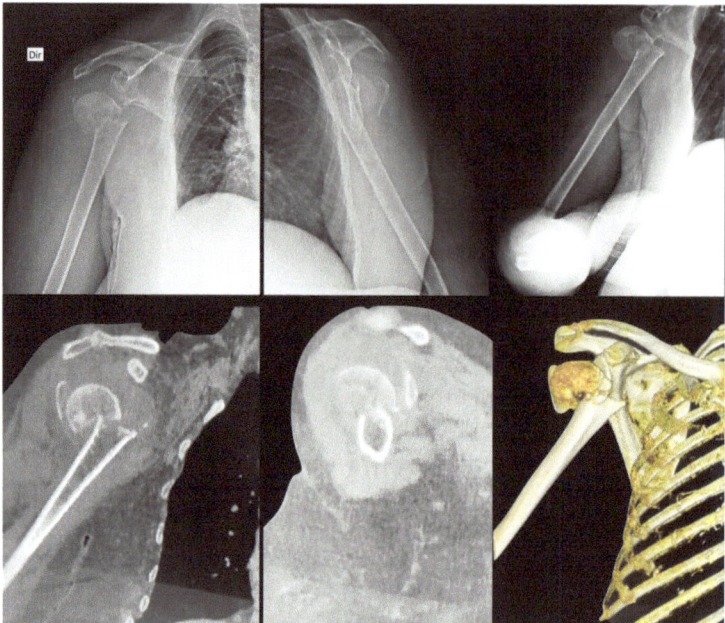

Figure 3. Radiographic and CT images of a 52-year-old female patient with a right proximal humerus fracture (Case 3). Note that the medial metaphyseal extension in the cephalic component less than 8 mm (Criterion A) and the medial metaphyseal hinge greater than 2 mm (Criterion B) are present and easily identified in both imaging exams. The fracture was classified as Neer 3-parts (head, greater tuberosity, and shaft).

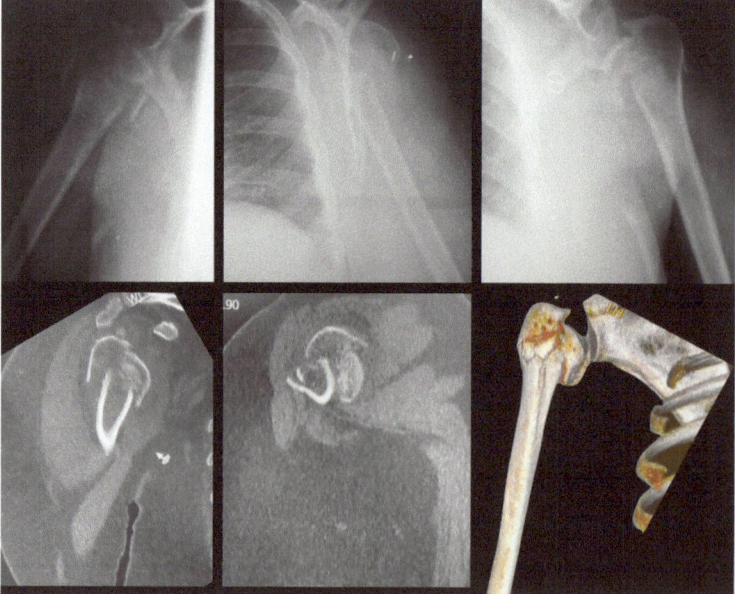

Figure 4. Radiographic and CT images of a 67-year-old female patient with a right proximal humerus fracture (Case 9). Note that it is possible to observe the split-head fracture of the head (Criterion C) only on CT, especially in 3D reconstruction. The fracture was classified as Neer 4-parts.

The images were sent by email to eight board-certified orthopedic surgeons with more than 10 years of experience in the treatment of proximal humerus fractures (Observers 1–8), in 20 individual folders, along with instructions on how to respond (Appendix A). All possible data that could identify the patients, such as name, initials, and date of birth, were removed from the exams so that their confidentiality was fully preserved. Four surgeons with fellowship in orthopedic trauma (namely TRAUMA 1 to TRAUMA 4) and four surgeons with fellowship in shoulder and elbow (namely, SHOULDER 1 to SHOULDER 4) were invited. Surgeons were asked to determine whether each of the Hertel prognostic criteria used in the study was "present", "absent", or "inconclusive" on radiographic and CT imaging. Respondents received the illustration of the prognostic criteria used in the study. They were asked to start with the radiographic images and not store images on their computers. Images were evaluated on two occasions, separated by 15 days—Round 1 (R1) and Round 2 (R2). For R2, the 20 folders were randomized and sent back to respondents by email, with the same guidelines as in R1.

The inferential analysis consisted of the Kappa coefficient (κ) to assess intraobserver agreement in the criteria (positive, negative, and inconclusive) according to radiographic and tomographic images [19]. Landis and Koch [19] suggest the following interpretation: $\kappa < 0.19$—no/very poor agreement; $0.20 < \kappa < 0.39$—weak agreement; $0.40 < \kappa < 0.59$—moderate agreement; $0.60 < \kappa < 0.79$—good agreement; and $\kappa \geq 0.80$—very good (excellent) agreement. The interobserver agreement was defined by the level of concordance (positive/negative/inconclusive) in the cases divided by the total number of cases ($n = 20$) and multiplied by 100 (% of concordant cases). The interobserver agreement of the eight surgeons and the STANDARD was provided by four percentages of concordant cases (positive/negative/inconclusive/general). The significance level adopted was 5%. Statistical analysis was performed by using SPSS version 26 software (IBM, New York, NY, USA).

3. Results

3.1. Intraobserver Agreement

There was a weak-to-moderate intraobserver agreement for all examiners. For analytical consistency, the percentage of agreement was judged useful only when the Kappa coefficient was significant (Supplementary Materials Table S1). Only the medial metaphyseal hinge greater than 2 mm (Criterion B) was identified by all evaluators both in the radiographic and CT examinations in the two rounds of the study ($p < 0.05$), except by the evaluator SHOULDER 4. Both Criteria A and C were identified significantly less frequently in the two rounds of the study, with no difference between radiographic and tomographic evaluations ($p > 0.05$). The SHOULDER 4 evaluator showed no intraobserver agreement for any of the criteria evaluated in R1 and R2.

3.2. Interobserver Agreement

The percentage of "inconclusive" concordant cases by CT in R1 and R2 was not processed due to improper operation (division by zero), as there were no "inconclusive" cases by CT observed according to the STANDARD. There was practically no significant agreement with the STANDARD, as it occurred only in some moments of R2. Interobserver agreement was seen as weak in both R1 and R2. Despite this, it was observed that there is strong agreement between the imaging methods used in the study. There was significant agreement at a level of 5% for the criteria between the radiographic and tomographic exams of moderate-to-strong degree for almost all evaluators, regardless of the moment (R1 and R2). However, it was observed that the radiographic evaluation presented a higher number of the "inconclusive" category than the CT, regardless of the criterion (Criteria A, B, and C) and the moment (R1 and R2), although there was no statistical significance. Supplementary Materials Tables S2 and S3 provide the percentage of concordant cases in R1 and R2, respectively.

4. Discussion

Overall, it was observed that intra- and interobserver agreement was weak in both R1 and R2. Analyzing individually each of the prognostic criteria used in this study, it was observed that only the presence of a medial metaphyseal hinge greater than 2 mm (Criterion B) was identified by all evaluators both in the radiographic examination and in the CT in the two rounds of the study as statistically significant, meaning that there is no evidence supporting our hypothesis. There was practically no significant agreement with the STANDARD, occurring only in some moments of R2. Nevertheless, there was a strong agreement between the imaging methods used in the study for almost all the evaluators, regardless of the moment (R1 and R2), with the CT evaluation showing a lower number of the "inconclusive" responses than the radiography evaluation, regardless of the criterion (A, B, and C) and moment (R1 and R2).

It is known that posttraumatic osteonecrosis of the proximal humerus is the most common complication after fractures in this anatomic region, occurring in up to 16% of patients, and represents a problem for both the patient and the surgeon [6,8,20]. In this context, surgeons must be able to assess the risk factors for AVN of the humeral head to influence not only decision-making, but also to guide them regarding the prognosis in relation to this complication [13,14,21]. Hertel et al. [7] described some predictors of humeral head ischemia after fracture; however, little is discussed about the difficulty of interpreting these criteria in the presence of numerous factors that potentially make it difficult to evaluate the radiographic examination.

The guidelines recommend that radiographic screening should be the first imaging investigation in the emergency department [22]. However, a high rate of suboptimal shoulder radiographs has been identified, particularly in AP and axillary views, resulting in increased workload, increased radiation to patients, inconvenience and decreased patient satisfaction, and increased risk of incorrect or missed diagnoses [23]. The variability in interpretation and the questioned reliability of this test have led some authors to independently assess its effectiveness. Martínez-Sola et al. [24] found a low-to-moderate degree of interobserver agreement, using a single AP radiograph of the shoulder, denoting the difficulty of interpretation by orthopedic surgeons of various levels of experience of some of the currently most used classifications for fractures of the proximal humerus. Likewise, Iordens et al. [25] found weak intra- and interobserver agreement by using radiographs of the proximal end of the humerus for the Hertel criteria. Most likely because of this difficulty in radiographic evaluation, which can be understood as a confusing diagnostic and prognostic factor, some authors observed that the Hertel criteria were not sufficient to determine a greater chance of progression to osteonecrosis of the humeral head [11]. Analyzing specifically the three prognostic criteria evaluated in this study, we can see that the presence of a medial metaphyseal hinge greater than 2 mm (Criterion B) was identified in a statistically significant way by all evaluators, except the evaluator SHOULDER 4. Interestingly, from this evaluator, we observed that there was an almost symmetrical pattern of inversion of his responses between R1 and R2, thus leading us to believe that an attention bias may have occurred during the responses. Thereby, what was considered to be a bad prognostic factor in R1 was considered to be a good prognostic factor in R2, and vice versa.

It is known that there is a strong correlation between AVN of the humeral head and medial metaphyseal hinge [7,20,26]. Hertel et al. [7] found an accuracy of 0.79 for ischemia when the medial hinge was interrupted by more than 2 mm. Solberg et al. [20] noted the occurrence of osteonecrosis in all patients in whom the medial hinge was initially less than 2 mm in length. However, these authors [20] were unable to identify whether medial hinge extension or a history of dislocation was the specific cause of osteonecrosis. Humeral head AVN has been reported in up to 33% of patients, and late surgery (>48 h) appears to be an important prognostic factor for ischemia [27]. However, while a history of dislocation associated with a proximal humerus fracture could be expected to lead to osteonecrosis from capsular injury and direct vascular damage, this is not fully supported in the literature [8,26,28–31]. Interestingly and antagonistically, Neviaser et al. [29], in a series of 34 patients treated with open reduction and internal fixation of fractures of the proximal humerus, showed that the posteromedial hinge length was not an accurate parameter to predict the risk of osteonecrosis of the humeral head, although it has been shown to be useful for surgical planning, especially as it involves an important support region (calcar) for internal fixation, greatly reducing the incidence of cut-out and/or cut-through [31].

The prognostic ability of the other two criteria evaluated in this study (medial metaphyseal extension in the cephalic component less than 8 mm—Criterion A; and fracture by partition of the head—Criterion C) is even more controversial and, probably, is mainly due to the inability to fully assess the proximal humerus morphology in a fractured segment with radiographs alone, as pointed out before. In this sense, the use of CT gains importance, as it allows the surgeon and the radiologist to perform the reconstruction of the proximal humerus in different planes, with slices of small sizes and in a three-dimensional perspective; however, in the light of current knowledge, there is no evidence of that 3D CT is superior to 2D CT [32]. Campochiaro et al. [11] suggested that all fractures involving the calcar should be studied with CT, as an accurate assessment of the fracture in three planes is necessary. In this study, only the presence of a medial metaphyseal hinge greater than 2 mm (Criterion B) was identified in a statistically significant way by all evaluators in the CT, except for the SHOULDER 4 evaluator; meanwhile, the other two criteria showed little uniformity between evaluators. There was a trend toward greater identification of Criteria A and C by TRAUMA surgeons on CT; however, this was not statistically significant.

This study has some limitations. Although not evaluated in the study, there are other factors that may represent risk factors for AVN of the humeral head—such as the surgical approach and the quality of reduction—and generate confusion in its epidemiological estimate, which is illustrated by the widely varying rates of posttraumatic osteonecrosis between studies [8]. In addition, the reported rate of humeral head AVN depends, among other risk factors already mentioned, on the duration of patient follow-up, the intensity of the resulting symptoms, and the imaging methods used to diagnose its presence [4–6,33,34]. In addition, the study design did not include the follow-up of patients, thus making it impossible to observe which patients developed AVN of the humeral head and to correlate this complication with the findings of both the evaluators and the STANDARD. This information would be important to assess the accuracy of the prognostic criteria investigated in the study and to understand the lack of interobserver agreement with the STANDARD. Moreover, the use of images in JPEG format is biased due to zoom or brightness adjustments compared to dedicated software for viewing radiographs. Furthermore, more dedicated software for the MOV file would allow all CT planes to be viewed simultaneously, and this would theoretically increase accuracy and orientation when viewing a CT scan. The adoption of these measures could theoretically increase intraobserver agreement, which can be tested in future studies. Finally, the objective was to evaluate the role of both two- and three-dimensional CT in the interpretation of the three criteria described by Hertel, using the radiographic evaluation of the same cases as a standard. Unlike other studies [25,35–38], our study did not seek to assess whether there was a difference between 2D and 3D tomography. In the current study, we showed some usefulness for both the 2D and 3D tomography to help surgeons in the primary interpretation of Hertel prognostic criteria, with moderate intraobserver agreement, without, however, statistical difference when compared to the radiographic examination. Recent studies have shown that the use of other imaging modalities, such as segmented 3D CT [39] and 3D printed models [40,41], adds value to the understanding of the morphology of the proximal humerus fracture, which was not evaluated in the current study.

Some strengths of the study deserve to be highlighted. The main one was to show that none of Hertel prognostic criteria evaluated in this study present interobserver agreement, regardless of whether the assessment is performed by using radiographs, CT, or both. Other authors have already observed the same, including employing more modern imaging methods than those used in this study [11,25,39,41]. The main limitation of the study by Hertel et al. [7] was the assessment of the fracture pattern by a single observer, which obviously lacks objectivity and reproducibility. The prognostic value of the Hertel criteria for decision-making has been questioned in particular because it has been reported that the humeral head can survive even in the initial absence of proximal flow from the anterior and posterior branches of the humeral circumflex artery [42]. Thus, our findings (and those of others) indicate that Hertel prognostic predictors should be used cautiously and sparingly when defining the eventual risk of AVN of the humeral head due to their low interobserver agreement.

5. Conclusions

The prognostic criteria for humeral head ischemia evaluated in this study showed weak intra- and interobserver agreement in both radiographic and tomographic evaluation. CT did not help surgeons in the primary interpretation of Hertel prognostic criteria used in this study when compared to radiographic examination.

Supplementary Materials: The following supporting information can be downloaded at https://www.mdpi.com/article/10.3390/medicina58101489/s1. Table S1. Distribution of criterion A, B, and C by radiographic and CT images between rounds R1 and R2. Table S2. Interobserver analysis in relation to STANDARD: percentage of cases in agreement with prognostic criteria A, B, and C by radiography and CT of the evaluators in round R1. Table S3. Interobserver analysis in relation to STANDARD: percentage of cases in agreement with prognostic criteria A, B, and C by radiography and CT of the evaluators in round R2.

Author Contributions: Conceptualization, V.G. and P.O.d.T.; methodology, V.G. and P.O.d.T.; software, P.O.d.T.; validation, V.G., P.O.d.T., H.A.K. and W.D.B.; formal analysis, V.G., P.O.d.T. and H.A.K.; investigation, P.O.d.T. and V.G.; resources, P.O.d.T.; data curation, V.G., P.O.d.T. and H.A.K.; writing—original draft preparation, V.G.; writing—review and editing, P.O.d.T., V.G. and H.A.K.; visualization, P.O.d.T., V.G., H.A.K., W.D.B., R.E.P., F.S.d.S., P.J.L., C.Z., F.M., P.S.B., R.Y.I. and S.R.; supervision, V.G.; project administration, P.O.d.T.; funding acquisition, P.O.d.T. All authors have read and agreed to the published version of the manuscript.

Funding: This research received no external funding.

Institutional Review Board Statement: The study was conducted in accordance with the Declaration of Helsinki and approved by the Institutional Review Board of Hospital Municipal Miguel Couto (protocol code 002/2021, 1 Feburary 2021).

Informed Consent Statement: Patient consent was waived due to the lockdown imposed by the COVID-19 pandemic, which prevented patients from going to the hospital to sign the document.

Data Availability Statement: Not applicable.

Acknowledgments: The authors would like to acknowledge Edson Marchiori, José Sérgio Franco, Antonio Carlos Pires Carvalho, and César Fontenelle from the Universidade Federal do Rio de Janeiro (UFRJ) for their invaluable comments and suggestions.

Conflicts of Interest: The authors declare no conflict of interest.

Appendix A. Individual Folders with Instructions on How to Respond the Survey

- This study seeks to evaluate Hertel's radiographic criteria using computed tomography (CT);
- We separated 20 cases of fractures of the proximal humerus, with X-rays and CT images, individualized in a separate folder;
- Randomization was performed, and the cases were numbered from 1 to 20;
- We ask that each examiner define which Hertel criteria are present by evaluating the radiographs and then their respective CT scans;
- At the end of the evaluation, each examiner will have made 40 evaluations. 2 for each case;
- In the folder with the files there is a photo explaining each of the 3 Hertel criteria, (reproduced from these author original article);

- We kindly ask you to return these results for each patient. Example:

  Case 1:
  X-ray 1
- criterion A present/absent/cannot evaluate;
- criterion B present/absent/cannot evaluate;
- criterion C present/absent/cannot evaluate;

  CT 1
- criterion A present/absent/cannot evaluate;
- criterion B present/absent/cannot evaluate;
- criterion C present/absent/cannot evaluate;
- The annotation of these results can be done in the way that suits the examiner. Annotated on a sheet of paper, or in an Excell table, or in a .doc text;
- After ending with the document, please send it to the emails: p_tullio@hotmail.com and v_giordano@me.com;
- Very soon we will send the same cases again but with a new randomization for a second evaluation, allowing us to make an intra and interobserver agreement comparison.

  Thanks a lot in advance.
  Best regards.
  Paulo and Vincenzo

References

1. Jabran, A.; Peach, C.; Ren, L. Biomechanical analysis of plate systems for proximal humerus fractures: A systematic literature review. *Biomed. Eng. Online* **2018**, *17*, 47. [CrossRef] [PubMed]
2. Hageman, M.G.; Jayakumar, P.; King, J.D.; Guitton, T.G.; Doornberg, J.N.; Ring, D.; Science of Variation Group. The factors influencing the decision making of operative treatment for proximal humeral fractures. *J. Shoulder Elb. Surg.* **2015**, *24*, e21–e26. [CrossRef] [PubMed]
3. Keding, A.; Handoll, H.; Brealey, S.; Jefferson, L.; Hewitt, C.; Corbacho, B.; Torgerson, D.; Rangan, A. The impact of surgeon and patient treatment preferences in an orthopaedic trauma surgery trial. *Trials* **2019**, *20*, 570. [CrossRef] [PubMed]
4. Maccagnano, G.; Solarino, G.; Pesce, V.; Vicenti, G.; Coviello, M.; Nappi, V.S.; Giannico, O.V.; Notarnicola, A.; Moretti, B. Plate vs reverse shoulder arthroplasty for proximal humeral fractures: The psychological health influence the choice of device? *World J. Orthop.* **2022**, *13*, 297–306. [CrossRef] [PubMed]
5. Belayneh, R.; Lott, A.; Haglin, J.; Konda, S.; Zuckerman, J.D.; Egol, K.A. Osteonecrosis after surgically repaired proximal humerus fractures is a predictor of poor outcomes. *J. Orthop. Trauma* **2018**, *32*, e387–e393. [CrossRef] [PubMed]
6. Rutherford, C.S.; Cofield, R.H. Osteonecrosis of the shoulder. *Orthop Trans.* **1987**, *11*, 239.
7. Hertel, R.; Hempfing, A.; Stiehler, M.; Leunig, M. Predictors of humeral head ischemia after intracapsular fracture of the proximal humerus. *J. Shoulder Elb. Surg.* **2004**, *13*, 427–433. [CrossRef]
8. Patel, S.; Colaco, H.B.; Elvey, M.E.; Lee, M.H. Post-traumatic osteonecrosis of the proximal humerus. *Injury* **2015**, *46*, 1878–1884. [CrossRef]
9. Majed, A.; Macleod, I.; Bull, A.M.; Zyto, K.; Resch, H.; Hertel, R.; Reilly, P.; Emery, R.J. Proximal humeral fracture classification systems revisited. *J. Shoulder Elb. Surg.* **2011**, *20*, 1125–1132. [CrossRef]
10. Sukthankar, A.V.; Leonello, D.T.; Hertel, R.W.; Ding, G.S.; Sandow, M.J. A comprehensive classification of proximal humeral fractures: HGLS system. *J. Shoulder Elb. Surg.* **2013**, *22*, e1–e6. [CrossRef]
11. Campochiaro, G.; Rebuzzi, M.; Baudi, P.; Catani, F. Complex proximal humerus fractures: Hertel's criteria reliability to predict head necrosis. *Musculoskelet. Surg.* **2015**, *99*, S9–S15. [CrossRef]
12. Neer, C.S., 2nd. Displaced proximal humeral fractures. I. Classification and evaluation. *J. Bone Joint Surg. Am.* **1970**, *52*, 1077–1089. [CrossRef]
13. Senna, L.F.; Pires, E.; Albuquerque, R. Modified axillary radiograph of the shoulder: A new position. *Rev. Bras. Ortop.* **2016**, *52*, 115–118. [CrossRef]
14. Neer, C.S., 2nd. Displaced proximal humeral fractures. II. Treatment of three-part and four-part displacement. *J. Bone Joint Surg. Am.* **1970**, *52*, 1090–1103. [CrossRef]
15. Bossuyt, P.M.; Reitsma, J.B.; Bruns, D.E.; Gatsonis, C.A.; Glasziou, P.P.; Irwig, L.M.; Lijmer, J.G.; Moher, D.; Rennie, D.; de Vet, H.C.; et al. Towards complete and accurate reporting of studies of diagnostic accuracy: The STARD initiative. *Clin. Radiol.* **2003**, *58*, 575–580. [CrossRef]

16. Giordano, V.; Gomes, A.F.; Amaral, N.P.; Albuquerque, R.P.; Pires, R.E. Preventing surgical complications: A survey on surgeons' perception of intra-articular malleolar screw misplacement in a cadaveric study. *Patient Saf. Surg.* **2011**, *5*, 24. [CrossRef]
17. Oladiran, O.; Gichoya, J.; Purkayastha, S. Conversion of JPG image into DICOM image format with one click tagging. In *Digital Human Modeling. Applications in Health, Safety, Ergonomics, and Risk Management: Health and Safety*; Duffy, V., Ed.; Springer: Cham, Switzerland, 2017; pp. 61–70. [CrossRef]
18. El-Boghdadly, K.; Onwochei, D.N.; Millhoff, B.; Ahmad, I. The effect of virtual endoscopy on diagnostic accuracy and airway management strategies in patients with head and neck pathology: A prospective cohort study. *Can. J. Anaesth.* **2017**, *64*, 1101–1110. [CrossRef]
19. Landis, J.R.; Koch, G.G. The measurement of observer agreement for categorical data. *Biometrics* **1977**, *33*, 159–174. [CrossRef]
20. Solberg, B.D.; Moon, C.N.; Franco, D.P.; Paiement, G.D. Surgical treatment of three and four-part proximal humeral fractures. *J. Bone Joint Surg. Am.* **2009**, *91*, 1689–1697. [CrossRef]
21. Leyshon, R.L. Closed treatment of fractures of the proximal humerus. *Acta Orthop. Scand.* **1984**, *55*, 48–51. [CrossRef]
22. Sandstrom, C.K.; Kennedy, S.A.; Gross, J.A. Acute shoulder trauma: What the surgeon wants to know. *Radiographics* **2015**, *35*, 475–492. [CrossRef]
23. Richards, B.; Riley, J.; Saithna, A. Improving the diagnostic quality and adequacy of shoulder radiographs in a District General Hospital. *BMJ Qual. Improv. Rep.* **2016**, *5*, u209855.w3501. [CrossRef]
24. Martínez-Sola, R.; León-Muñoz, V.J.; Najem-Rizk, A.N.; Soler-Vasco, B.; Arrieta-Martínez, C.J.; López-Sorroche, E.; Cárdenas-Grande, E.; Salmerón-Vélez, G.; Ruiz-Molina, J.Á.; Martínez-Martínez, F.; et al. 'Absolute' inter-observer classifications agreement for proximal humeral fractures with a single shoulder anteroposterior X-ray. *J. Orthop. Surg.* **2021**, *29*, 23094990211010520. [CrossRef] [PubMed]
25. Iordens, G.I.; Mahabier, K.C.; Buisman, F.E.; Schep, N.W.; Muradin, G.S.; Beenen, L.F.; Patka, P.; van Lieshout, E.M.; sen Hartog, D. The reliability and reproducibility of the Hertel classification for comminuted proximal humeral fractures compared with the Neer classification. *J. Orthop. Sci.* **2016**, *21*, 596–602. [CrossRef]
26. Robinson, C.M.; Khan, L.A.; Akhtar, M.A. Treatment of anterior fracture-dislocations of the proximal humerus by open reduction and internal fixation. *J. Bone Joint Surg. Br.* **2006**, *88*, 502–508. [CrossRef]
27. Schnetzke, M.; Bockmeyer, J.; Loew, M.; Studier-Fischer, S.; Grützner, P.A.; Guehring, T. Rate of avascular necrosis after fracture dislocations of the proximal humerus: Timing of surgery. *Obere Extrem.* **2018**, *13*, 273–278. [CrossRef]
28. Lee, C.K.; Hansen, H.R. Post-traumatic avascular necrosis of the humeral head in displaced proximal humeral fractures. *J. Trauma* **1981**, *21*, 788–791. [CrossRef]
29. Neviaser, A.S.; Hettrich, C.M.; Dines, J.S.; Lorich, D.G. Rate of avascular necrosis following proximal humerus fractures treated with a lateral locking plate and endosteal implant. *Arch. Orthop. Trauma Surg.* **2011**, *131*, 1617–1622. [CrossRef]
30. Trupka, A.; Wiedemann, E.; Ruchholtz, S.; Brunner, U.; Habermeyer, P.; Schweiberer, L. Dislozierte Mehrfragmentfrakturen des Humeruskopfes. Bedeutet die Luxation des Kopffragments eine Prognoseverschlechterung? *Unfallchirurg* **1997**, *100*, 105–110. [CrossRef]
31. Thompson, J.H.; Attum, B.; Rodriguez-Buitrago, A.; Yusi, K.; Cereijo, C.; Obremskey, W.T. Open reduction and internal fixation with a locking plate via deltopectoral approach for the treatment of three and four-part and proximal humeral fractures. *JBJS Essent. Surg. Tech.* **2018**, *8*, e26. [CrossRef]
32. Berkes, M.B.; Dines, J.S.; Little, M.T.; Garner, M.R.; Shifflett, G.D.; Lazaro, L.E.; Wellman, D.S.; Dines, D.M.; Lorich, D.G. The impact of three-dimensional CT imaging on intraobserver and interobserver reliability of proximal humeral fracture classifications and treatment recommendations. *J. Bone Joint Surg. Am.* **2014**, *96*, 1281–1286. [CrossRef]
33. Greiner, S.; Kääb, M.J.; Haas, N.P.; Bail, H.J. Humeral head necrosis rate at mid-term follow-up after open reduction and angular stable plate fixation for proximal humeral fractures. *Injury* **2009**, *40*, 186–191. [CrossRef] [PubMed]
34. Sakai, T.; Sugano, N.; Nishii, T.; Hananouchi, T.; Yoshikawa, H. Extent of osteonecrosis on MRI predicts humeral head collapse. *Clin. Orthop. Relat. Res.* **2008**, *466*, 1074–1080. [CrossRef] [PubMed]
35. Bahrs, C.; Rolauffs, B.; Südkamp, N.P.; Schmal, H.; Eingartner, C.; Dietz, K.; Pereira, P.L.; Weise, K.; Lingenfelter, E.; Helwig, P. Indications for computed tomography (CT-) diagnostics in proximal humeral fractures: A comparative study of plain radiography and computed tomography. *BMC Musculoskelet. Disord.* **2009**, *10*, 33. [CrossRef]
36. Chelli, M.; Gasbarro, G.; Lavoué, V.; Gauci, M.O.; Raynier, J.L.; Trojani, C.; Boileau, P. The reliability of the Neer classification for proximal humerus fractures: A survey of orthopedic shoulder surgeons. *JSES Int.* **2022**, *6*, 331–337. [CrossRef]
37. Jia, X.; Chen, Y.; Qiang, M.; Zhang, K.; Li, H.; Jiang, Y.; Zhang, Y. Compared to X-ray, three-dimensional computed tomography measurement is a reproducible radiographic method for normal proximal humerus. *J. Orthop. Surg. Res.* **2016**, *11*, 82. [CrossRef]
38. Stirma, G.A.; Secundino, A.R.; Gonzalez, F.G.; Sola, W.C.; de Souza, G.A.L.; Dau, L. Inter/intra-observer evaluation between radiographs and tomographies for proximal humerus fracture. *Acta Ortop. Bras.* **2020**, *28*, 36–39. [CrossRef]
39. Dauwe, J.; Mys, K.; Putzeys, G.; Schader, J.F.; Richards, R.G.; Gueorguiev, B.; Varga, P.; Nijs, S. Advanced CT visualization improves the accuracy of orthopaedic trauma surgeons and residents in classifying proximal humeral fractures: A feasibility study. *Eur. J. Trauma Emerg. Surg.* **2020**, 1–7. [CrossRef]
40. Cocco, L.F.; Aihara, A.Y.; Lopes, F.P.P.L.; Werner, H.; Franciozi, C.E.; Dos Reis, F.B.; Luzo, M.V.M. Three-dimensional printing models increase inter-rater agreement for classification and treatment of proximal humerus fractures. *Patient Saf. Surg.* **2022**, *16*, 5. [CrossRef]

41. Puglisi, G.; Montemagno, M.; Denaro, R.; Condorelli, G.; Caruso, V.F.; Vescio, A.; Testa, G.; Pavone, V. 3D-printed models versus CT scan and X-rays imaging in the diagnostic evaluation of proximal humerus fractures: A triple-blind interobserver reliability comparison study. *Adv. Orthop.* **2022**, *2022*, 5863813. [CrossRef]
42. Lambert, S.M. Ischaemia, healing and outcomes in proximal humeral fractures. *EFORT Open Rev.* **2018**, *3*, 304–315. [CrossRef] [PubMed]

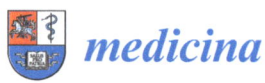

Review

Overtraining Syndrome as a Risk Factor for Bone Stress Injuries among Paralympic Athletes

Tomislav Madzar [1], Tonci Masina [2], Roko Zaja [2], Snjezana Kastelan [2], Jasna Pucarin Cvetkovic [2], Hana Brborovic [2], Matija Dvorski [2], Boris Kirin [3,4], Andreja Vukasovic Barisic [3,4], Ivan Cehok [5] and Milan Milosevic [2,*]

[1] Polyclinic Life, Trpinjska 5, 10000 Zagreb, Croatia; tomislav_madzar@yahoo.com
[2] School of Medicine, University of Zagreb, Salata 3, 10000 Zagreb, Croatia; tonci.masina@mef.hr (T.M.); roko.zaja@snz.hr (R.Z.); snjezana.kastelan@mef.hr (S.K.); jpucarin@snz.hr (J.P.C.); hana.brborovic@snz.hr (H.B.); matija.dvorski@snz.hr (M.D.)
[3] Croatian Paralympic Committee, Savska Cesta 137, 10000 Zagreb, Croatia; boris.kirin@bj.ht.hr (B.K.); andreja.vukasovic@yahoo.com (A.V.B.)
[4] General County Hospital Bjelovar, Antuna Mihanovica 8, 43000 Bjelovar, Croatia
[5] Department of Nursing, University North, 104 Brigade 3, 42000 Varazdin, Croatia; icehok@unin.hr
* Correspondence: milan.milosevic@snz.hr; Tel.: +385-1-4590-167

Abstract: *Background and Objectives:* In this review, we have explored the relationship between overtraining syndrome (OTS) and bone stress injuries among paralympic athletes. OTS is a complex condition that arises from an imbalance between training volume, nutrition, and recovery time, leading to significant negative effects on paralympic athlete's performance and overall well-being. On the other hand, bone stress injuries occur when abnormal and repetitive loading is applied to normal bone, resulting in microdamage accumulation and potential. The prevalence of overtraining syndrome and bone stress injuries among athletes highlights the need for a better understanding of their relationship and implications for prevention and management strategies. *Methods:* A literature review from the PubMed, Web of Science, and Google Scholar databases including the MeSH keywords "overtraining syndrome", "bone", and "paralympic athletes". *Results:* Studies have consistently shown that athletes engaged in endurance sports are particularly susceptible to overtraining syndrome. The multifactorial nature of this condition involves not only physical factors, but also psychological and environmental determinants. In addition, the diagnosis and management of OTS and bone stress injuries present challenges in clinical practice. *Conclusions:* Currently, there are no definitive biochemical markers for overtraining syndrome. The diagnosis is based on a combination of subjective measures such as questionnaires, symptoms checklists, and objective biomarkers, including hormone levels, inflammatory markers, and imaging studies. However, these diagnostic approaches have limitations regarding their specificity and sensitivity.

Keywords: overtraining syndrome; risk factor; bone stress injuries; paralympic athletes

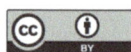

1. Introduction

Overtraining syndrome (OTS) and associated bone stress injuries are significant concerns among athletes, with a subsequent profound impact on their performance and overall health. OTS refers to a state of chronic fatigue and decreased performance resulting from an imbalance between training load, nutrition, and recovery time [1]. On the other hand, bone stress injuries are a common type of overuse injury characterized by the accumulation of microdamage in bone tissue due to repetitive loading [2].

The prevalence of OTS and bone stress injuries among athletes is a growing concern in the field of sports medicine. Currently, varying rates of overtraining syndrome have been reported, even up to 30% among young athletes. Additionally, around 10–20% of all sports medicine injuries were stress fractures. These conditions can have significant consequences for athletes, leading to decreased performance, prolonged recovery periods, and even long-term health implications [1,2].

OTS can also affect paralympic athletes just as it can impact athletes in other sports. Paralympic athletes face unique challenges due to their disabilities, but the principles of overtraining and risk factors remain largely the same. Paralympic athletes often participate in intensive training programs to enhance their physical performance and excel in their respective sports. However, when the training load exceeds the body's ability to recover, OTS can occur. Diagnosing OTS can be challenging as it involves a combination of subjective and objective measures. There is no specific medical test that can definitively diagnose OTS. Instead, healthcare professionals rely on a comprehensive evaluation of an athlete's symptoms, training history, and performance changes.

Detailed understanding of the relationship between OTS and bone stress injuries is crucial for the development of effective prevention and management strategies. The interplay between training load, energy availability, hormonal imbalances, genetic factors, neuromuscular control, biomechanics, inflammatory markers, and psychosocial factors has been explored as they are potential contributors to the development of both conditions [3–6]. In this review article, our aim was to contribute to the body of knowledge surrounding OTS as a risk factor for bone stress injuries among paralympic athletes by encompassing risk factors, mechanism of action explanations, diagnostic possibilities, and prevention strategies. Due to the nature and classification of paralympic athletes there are high possibilities of overtraining in disability compensation compared to non-paralympic athletes.

2. Methods

A literature review from the PubMed, Web of Science, and Google Scholar databases including the MeSH (Medical Subject Headings) keywords "overtraining syndrome", "bone", and "paralympic athletes" has been made. Out of 37 found papers, we included 28 papers in the English language with full-text availability covering the last 20 years (from 2003 to 2023).

3. Risk Factors and their Mechanism of Action

Age has been identified as an intrinsic factor that may influence an athlete's risk of developing OTS. Younger athletes are often more susceptible due to their higher training intensities and inadequate recovery periods [1]. However, the role of age as a risk factor for OTS remains controversial. While some studies suggested that younger athletes are at higher risk [7], others did not report a significant association between age and the incidence of OTS [8].

Gender is another important intrinsic factor that appears to influence the prevalence of OTS among athletes. Females have been found to be at a higher risk compared to males [1]. Hormonal fluctuations throughout the menstrual cycle may contribute to this increased vulnerability among women. For example, estrogen levels during certain phases of the menstrual cycle have been associated with decreased exercise performance and increased fatigue [9]. Armento et al. investigated gender differences in physiological responses to training load among endurance runners and found that female athletes exhibited different patterns of hormonal responses compared to males during periods of high training load. This highlights the importance of considering gender-specific factors when studying overtraining syndrome and bone stress injuries [4].

A medical history of previous injury has also been suggested as a potential risk factor for developing OTS. Athletes with previous injuries may have altered movement patterns or imbalances that can contribute to overuse and overtraining [1]. However, there is limited research that specifically examines the relationship between previous injury history and OTS incidence.

Extrinsic factors related to training volume/intensity, recovery periods, and nutrition are crucial contributors to the risk of developing OTS in an athlete. A high training volume/intensity without adequate recovery periods is a common cause of OTS [1]. Numerous studies have emphasized the importance of periodization in training programs by incorporating appropriate rest periods [10,11].

OTS is a complex condition influenced by various intrinsic and extrinsic factors that can increase an athlete's susceptibility to its development.

3.1. Inflammatory Cytokines

In recent years, there has been an emerging interest in investigating the role of inflammatory markers in the pathogenesis of OTS and bone stress injuries among athletes [3,5]. Inflammation plays a crucial role in tissue repair processes, but excessive or prolonged inflammation may contribute to tissue damage, highlighting the potential role of inflammatory cytokines, such as interleukin-6 (IL-6), tumor necrosis factor-alpha (TNF-α), and C-reactive protein (CRP), in OTS. Studies have proposed that elevated levels of these markers may contribute to the development of fatigue, muscle damage, and impaired immune function commonly observed in athletes with OTS. Schwellnus et al. discussed the possible involvement of inflammation in bone stress injuries among athletes. They suggested that pro-inflammatory cytokines and chemokines released during repetitive loading can lead to an imbalance between bone resorption and formation processes, ultimately increasing the risk of stress fractures [3]. Furthermore, it was thoroughly described how IL-6 and other pro-inflammatory cytokines stimulate osteoblasts to express receptor activator of nuclear factor kappa-B ligand (RANKL), which then binds to receptor activator of nuclear factor kappa-B (RANK) in osteoclasts, leading to the stimulation of bone resorption [12]. Although these studies provided information on the potential role of inflammation in both OTS and bone stress injuries, further research is needed to elucidate the underlying mechanisms and establish causality.

3.2. Genetic Factors

Genetic factors have also been implicated as potential contributors to individual susceptibility to OTS and bone stress injuries. Tenforde et al. discussed the importance of neuromuscular control in preventing excessive loading on bones and highlighted the potential benefits of targeted strength training programs to improve neuromuscular function [5]. Furthermore, investigating potential genetic factors that influence susceptibility to OTS could provide valuable information on individual variations in response to training loads. Understanding genetic predispositions may help identify athletes at higher risk for developing OTS or bone stress injuries.

Several genetic variations have been investigated for their potential association with overtraining-related outcomes such as fatigue resistance, muscle damage markers, and inflammatory responses. For example, polymorphisms in genes related to collagen synthesis, such as COL5A1 and COL1A1, have been studied in the context of OTS and bone stress injuries. However, the specific genetic factors that contribute to the risk of OTS are still not well understood, and more research is required to elucidate their role [13,14].

3.3. Nutritional Deficiencies and Energy Availability

Nutritional deficiencies or imbalances can significantly impact an athlete's susceptibility to both OTS and bone stress injuries. Inadequate energy intake, particularly low energy availability (LEA), has emerged as a significant risk factor for the development of both conditions [15]. LEA occurs when an athlete's energy intake does not meet the energy demands of training and normal physiological functions, leading to negative consequences on various body systems including hormonal regulation, immune function, metabolic processes, and bone health [15,16]. Studies have shown that athletes with LEA are at increased risk for developing both OTS and bone stress injuries [4,5]. Cupka and Sedliak reviewed the impact of low energy availability on the performance and testosterone levels of male endurance athletes. This metabolic disturbance can contribute to the onset of OTS symptoms [17]. Energy availability refers to the amount of dietary energy intake available for physiological functions after accounting for energy expended during exercise. It is influenced by factors such as caloric intake, exercise expenditure, thermoregulation, growth, repair processes, and reproductive function [15]. The balance between energy intake and expenditure is crucial to maintaining optimal health and performance among athletes. This imbalance can have significant consequences for various physiological systems in the body. In the context of athletics, low energy availability often arises from intentional or unintentional restrictions in food intake due to concerns about body weight or composition [16].

The influence of energy availability, a key component in the development of OTS, has also been explored in relation to bone stress injuries. Low energy availability can lead to a condition known as relative energy deficiency in sport (RED-S), characterized by hormonal imbalances, impaired bone health, and increased risk of injury [5]. Mountjoy et al. proposed that RED-S encompasses a range of adverse health outcomes resulting from inadequate energy availability, including suppression of metabolic rates, menstrual disturbances in women, decreased testosterone levels in men, impaired bone health, cardiovascular dysfunction, immunological impairments, psychological disturbances, gastrointestinal problems, hematological abnormalities, and impaired growth and development in adolescents [15]. Several studies have examined the association between RED-S/LEA and an increased risk of bone stress injuries among athletes. A narrative review by Hamstra-Wright et al. highlighted the importance of a holistic approach to monitoring training load in relation to bone stress injuries. The authors emphasized the need for a personalized assessment that considers individual risk factors and cumulative risks associated with the training load capacity [18].

The relationship between low energy availability and bone health has been extensively studied. LEA can disrupt hormonal balance, leading to menstrual irregularities in female athletes and decreased testosterone levels in male athletes [16]. These hormonal changes can have detrimental effects on bone health, resulting in decreased bone mineral density and increased susceptibility to fractures [15]. In a study by Tenforde et al., female college distance runners with LEA were found to have significantly lower bone mineral density in the lumbar spine compared to their counterparts with normal EA. Furthermore, LEA can affect bone remodeling processes by affecting both osteoblasts and osteoclast activity [5]. Armento et al. discussed how LEA may lead to decreased osteoblast function through alterations in insulin-like growth factor-1 (IGF-1), estrogen levels, leptin signaling pathways, and mechanical loading responses. Furthermore, reduced estrogen concentrations resulting from LEA can enhance osteoclast activity, leading to excessive bone resorption [4].

Carbohydrate intake predicts quick hormonal responses to stress and improves explosion responses during exercise when above 5.0 g/kg/day, higher carbohydrate intake stimulates chronic growth hormone release (despite its acute suppressive effects); together, carbohydrate and protein intake predicted the late prolactin response (30 min after hypoglycemia), muscle recovery speed was directly predicted by overall calorie intake, regardless of the proportion of macronutrients, protein intake prevents body and visceral fat accumulation and increases basal metabolism rate when above 1.6 g/kg/day, sleep patterns are the major determinants of mood states, and excessive concurrent physical and cognitive effort decreases fat oxidation, increases muscle catabolism, and impairs libido [19].

3.4. Psychological and Psychosocial Factors

Although the role of physical factors in OTS has been extensively studied, there is growing recognition of the importance of psychological factors in its development among athletes. Psychosocial factors have also gained attention as potential contributors to both OTS and bone stress injuries among athletes. Psychological stressors associated with high-performance sports may impact an athlete's risk of these conditions through various mechanisms, including altered immune function, disrupted sleep patterns, or maladaptive coping strategies [6]. OTS is a complex condition that arises from an imbalance between training load, nutrition, and recovery time. It is characterized by a decrease in training performance and persistent fatigue, which can have detrimental effects on an athlete's physical and mental well-being. This section aims to dive into the physiological changes associated with OTS by incorporating additional research studies [1].

Psychological stressors have been identified as crucial contributors to the onset and progression of OTS. These stressors can arise from multiple sources such as training demands, competition pressure, personal life stressors, and perfectionistic tendencies. The review highlights how these stressors can lead to increased levels of anxiety and depression symptoms among athletes with OTS. However, it is important to note that not all athletes who experience high levels of psychological distress develop OTS. This suggests that individual differences play a role in determining susceptibility to OTS [1].

To gain a deeper understanding of the relationship between psychological factors and OTS, recent research has proposed approaching OTS as a complex system phenomenon. This perspective acknowledges the intricate interactions between various biological systems involved in OTS development. Authors have suggested employing techniques like transomics analyses and machine learning for comprehensive evaluation of individuals with suspected or diagnosed OTS. They have also highlighted that future research should focus on the analysis of brain neural networks in relation to the prevention and management of OTS. Neuroimaging studies could provide information on how prolonged exposure to psychological stress affects brain structure and function among athletes with, or at risk of developing, OTS. Furthermore, investigating hypothalamic–pituitary–adrenal responses to stress may elucidate hormonal imbalances associated with excessive training loads and inadequate recovery periods in athletes prone to developing OTS. Although psychological interventions have shown promise in managing various mental health conditions among athletes, their effectiveness specifically in preventing or managing OTS remains an area that needs further exploration. Valovich McLeod et al. suggest that cognitive behavior therapy (CBT) and stress management techniques could be valuable approaches to address psychological distress associated with OTS [20].

As pointed out by Maccagnano at al., for shoulder arthroplasty it is very important to perform a psychological analysis of each patient in order to choose the appropriate treatment [21]. This rule can also be applied to injured paralympic athletes.

Psychological factors play a significant role in the development of overtraining syndrome among athletes. Psychological stressors arising from training demands, competition pressure, and stressors of personal life can contribute to increased levels of anxiety and depression symptoms among individuals with OTS. Recent research suggests approaching OTS as a complex system phenomenon that involves interactions between multiple biological systems.

3.5. Hormonal Status, Oxidative Stress, and Immune System

Hormonal imbalances play an important role in the pathophysiology of OTS. Cadegiani and Kater conducted a study investigating the predictive value of basal hormones in male athletes with OTS. Their findings revealed lower levels of testosterone and higher levels of estradiol in athletes with OTS compared to healthy individuals. These hormonal alterations may contribute to the fatigue and decreased performance observed in OTS [22].

Immune system dysfunction has been identified as a contributing factor to both OTS and bone stress injuries. Schwellnus et al. discussed the relationship between the training load in sports and the risk of illness and overtraining. They highlighted that excessive training load can lead to immunosuppression, making athletes more susceptible to infections and other immune-related disorders. This compromised immune function may further exacerbate fatigue symptoms and impair the ability of an athlete to recover [3].

Collectively, exploring the physiology and mechanisms underlying overtraining syndrome is crucial to unraveling its complexities. Hormonal imbalances such as altered testosterone–estradiol ratios have been observed in individuals with OTS. Oxidative stress resulting from the production of reactive oxygen species in exercise can contribute to fatigue symptoms seen in athletes with OTS. Inflammation and immune system dysfunction also play a significant role in both overtraining syndrome and bone stress injuries among athletes.

4. Diagnostic Approaches to Overtraining Syndrome and Bone Stress Injuries

The accurate and timely diagnosis of OTS and bone stress injuries is crucial for effective management and prevention of long-term complications among athletes. This section aims to critically review current diagnostic methods for OTS and bone stress injuries, considering additional research from various articles.

Differences between OTS, functional and non-functional overreaching, that are crucial in an appropriate approach to diagnosing OTS are shown in Figure 1.

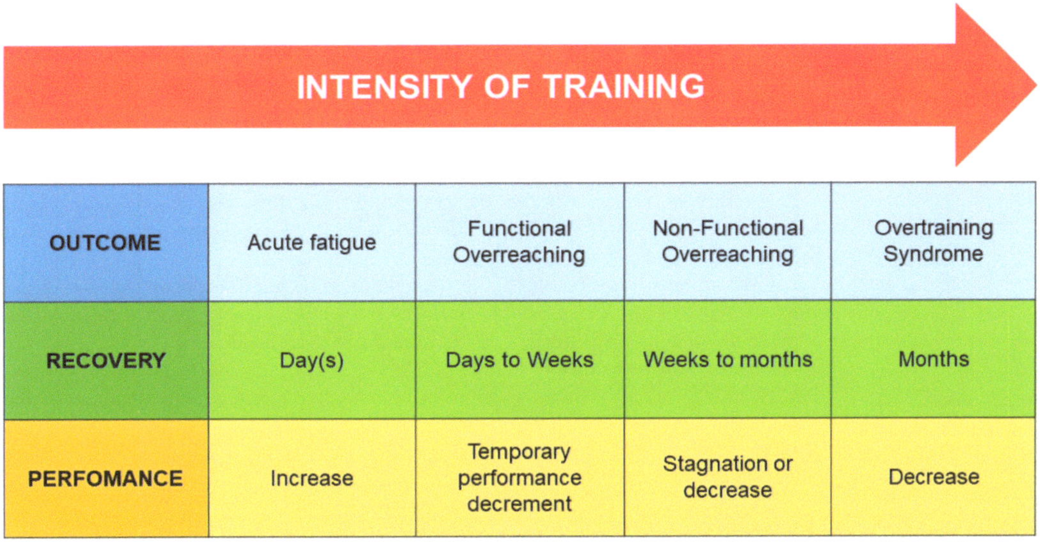

INTENSITY OF TRAINING →

OUTCOME	Acute fatigue	Functional Overreaching	Non-Functional Overreaching	Overtraining Syndrome
RECOVERY	Day(s)	Days to Weeks	Weeks to months	Months
PERFOMANCE	Increase	Temporary performance decrement	Stagnation or decrease	Decrease

Figure 1. Differences between overreaching and overtraining [23].

The diagnosis of OTS involves a combination of subjective measures, such as questionnaires and symptoms checklists, along with objective biomarkers, including hormone levels and inflammatory markers [24,25]. Subjective measures provide information on an athlete's perception of their training load, fatigue, mood states, recovery status, and overall well-being. Various validated questionnaires have been developed to assess different aspects related to OTS. For example, the Recovery-Stress Questionnaire for Athletes (RESTQ-Sport) evaluates an athlete's balance between recovery demands and stressors [24]. On the other hand, the Profile of Mood States (POMSs) assesses various mood dimensions that may be affected by overreaching or excessive training loads [26].

Objective biomarkers offer physiological insights into an athlete's response to training load and recovery status. Hormonal imbalances have been observed in athletes with overtraining syndrome; decreased testosterone levels and increased estradiol levels are commonly reported findings. Furthermore, alterations in cortisol secretion patterns have been associated with the development of OTS. However, it is important to note that hormonal changes can be influenced by factors such as age, sex, phase of the menstrual cycle in women, time of day when samples were collected, individual variations in hormonal responses to exercise stressors, or other factors unrelated to the OTS itself [25].

Inflammatory markers also play a role in the diagnosis of OTS. Studies have reported elevated levels of C-reactive protein (CRP) and interleukin-6 (IL-6) in athletes experiencing OTS [25]. These markers reflect the systemic inflammatory response to excessive training loads, indicating a potential link between chronic inflammation and the development of OTS. However, it is important to interpret these findings with caution as exercise-induced inflammation can also occur in response to acute bouts of intense exercise, without necessarily indicating the presence of OTS.

Despite the progress made in diagnostic approaches for OTS, there are still limitations that need to be addressed. Subjective measures are prone to individual interpretation and reporting bias. Athletes may underreport symptoms due to fear of negative consequences, desire to continue training, or lack of awareness of the severity of their condition [24]. Additionally, subjective measures are heavily based on self-reporting, which can introduce variability into the assessment process.

Objective biomarkers show promise but require further validation and standardization for clinical use. Hormonal changes observed in athletes with OTS may not be specific enough for accurate diagnosis as hormonal fluctuations can occur due to various factors other than overtraining alone [25]. Similarly, inflammatory markers are influenced by multiple factors, including acute bouts of exercise or infection/inflammation unrelated to OTS itself.

Additionally, advances in technology offer opportunities for real-time monitoring of training load and recovery status using wearable devices or mobile applications [3]. These technologies can provide objective data on training volume, intensity, heart rate variability, sleep quality, and other relevant factors to aid in the diagnosis of OTS. Integrating these technological advances with subjective and objective measures can improve diagnostic accuracy and facilitate early intervention.

Collectively, diagnosing OTS requires a multifaceted approach that combines subjective measures and objective biomarkers. Subjective measures, such as questionnaires, provide insights into an athlete's perception of their training load and well-being. Objective biomarkers offer physiological information but require further validation for clinical use. Future research should focus on integrating multiple biomarkers with advanced technology to enhance diagnostic accuracy and facilitate timely intervention for athletes at risk of developing OTS.

5. Prevention and Management Strategies for OTS and Bone Stress Injuries

Understanding and implementing effective prevention and management strategies for OTS and bone stress injuries is crucial to optimizing athletes' health and performance. This section will review current strategies for preventing overtraining syndrome among athletes, the role of strength training and conditioning programs in reducing the risk of bone stress injuries and explore treatment options for both overtraining syndrome and bone stress injuries.

To prevent overtraining syndrome among athletes, various strategies have been proposed. One approach is periodization of training, which involves planned variations in training volume and intensity to optimize performance while minimizing the risk of overtraining [1]. By carefully manipulating training variables such as load, frequency, duration, and recovery periods throughout different phases of a training program, coaches can ensure that athletes achieve optimal adaptations without exceeding their recovery capacity. Periodization has been shown to improve athletic performance in various sports by balancing workload with adequate rest [27].

In addition to periodization, monitoring biomarkers during preseason training may help identify early signs of overreaching or overtraining. A study by Clemente et al. investigated hematological and biochemical markers in professional soccer players during the preseason period. The results showed an increase in platelet levels, but decreased absolute neutrophil counts, absolute monocyte counts, and calcium levels after preseason training. Furthermore, there were significant increases in creatinine, alkaline phosphatase, C-reactive protein, cortisol, and testosterone levels. Monitoring these blood measurements could provide valuable insight into an athlete's physiological response to changes in training load [28].

In terms of bone stress injury prevention, strength training and conditioning programs play a crucial role. Resistance training has been shown to improve sport performance, improve body composition, and reduce the rate of sport-related injuries. By incorporating exercises that target specific muscle groups and movements relevant to the sport of the athlete, strength training helps improve biomechanics and reduce the risk of overuse injuries [1].

Furthermore, nutritional support plays a vital role in both preventing OTS and promoting recovery from bone stress injuries. Adequate energy intake is crucial to meet energy demands during intense training periods [3]. Low energy availability can lead to relative energy deficiency in sport (RED-S), which has severe health consequences if not addressed properly [4]. Adequate intake of macronutrients (carbohydrates, proteins, fats) and micronutrients (vitamins, minerals) is crucial to meet the metabolic demands of exercise and promote recovery processes. Athletes should work with sports nutrition professionals to ensure that they meet their nutritional needs based on their activity levels.

When OTS occurs despite preventive measures, appropriate treatment strategies are essential for recovery. Rest is crucial to allow the body to recover from the accumulated fatigue and stress associated with OTS [28]. Rehabilitation protocols should focus on gradually reintroducing training while considering individual responses to treatment. Physical therapy interventions such as manual therapy techniques, therapeutic exercises tailored to specific needs, and modalities can help promote healing, restore function, and prevent future injuries [20]. Medications such as non-steroidal anti-inflammatory drugs can help manage pain and inflammation associated with bone stress injuries [2]. However, it is essential to consider possible side effects and consult with healthcare professionals before using pharmacological interventions.

Participation in physical training can be highly skeletally demanding, particularly during periods of rapid growth in adolescence, and when competition and training demands are heaviest. Sports involving running and jumping are associated with a higher incidence of bone stress injuries and some athletes appear to be more susceptible than others. Maintaining a very lean physique in aesthetic sports (gymnastics, figure skating and ballet) or a prolonged negative energy balance in extreme endurance events (long distance running and triathlon) may compound the risk of bone stress injuries with repetitive mechanical loading of bone, due to the additional negative effects of hormonal disturbances [29].

Finally, effective prevention and management strategies for OTS and bone stress injuries require a comprehensive approach that includes periodic training, monitoring biomarkers during training periods, incorporating strength training programs, ensuring adequate nutritional support, promoting rest, and rehabilitation protocols when needed. By implementing these strategies in a customized manner while considering personalized athlete characteristics, coaches, sports medicine professionals, and athletes themselves can optimize performance outcomes while minimizing the risk of OTS and subsequent bone stress injuries in athletic populations. More research is needed to explore additional preventive measures, as well as to refine existing strategies to improve athlete health and performance.

6. Limitation, Strength, and Future Aspects

The relationship between OTS and bone stress injuries among athletes has been extensively studied, but there are still several areas that require further research to enhance our understanding of this complex relationship. This section will critically review the literature and identify key research gaps, highlighting the need for additional investigations in specific populations and aspects of OTS and bone stress injuries.

An area that requires further research is the identification of specific risk factors and mechanisms underlying the development of OTS and its association with bone stress injuries. Although some intrinsic and extrinsic risk factors have been identified, such as age, sex, training volume/intensity, inadequate recovery periods, there is a need for more comprehensive studies that consider multiple factors simultaneously. For example, a study by Matos et al. investigated various potential risk factors for overuse injuries in young athletes aged 12–17 years. They found that LEA, menstrual dysfunction in female athletes, a previous history of injuries, low body mass index, and high intensity of training load were significant predictors of developing overuse injuries [1].

Furthermore, it is essential to explore the impact of psychological stressors on the development of OTS and subsequent bone stress injuries among athletes. Psychological factors play a crucial role in an athlete's overall well-being and performance. A study by Costa et al. examined the relationship between psychosocial variables (e.g., perceived stress levels) and bone health outcomes in elite female artistic gymnasts. The findings highlighted how psychosocial factors can influence hormonal balance, nutritional status, and energy availability, ultimately affecting bone health outcomes [2].

More research is needed to understand the long-term consequences of OTS on bone health outcomes among athletes. Longitudinal studies that evaluate changes in bone mineral density, bone turnover markers, and fracture risk over extended periods can provide valuable information on the recovery process and long-term effects of OTS on bone health. A study by Barrack et al. followed a group of male endurance athletes for two years to assess changes in BMD and incidence of stress fractures. The findings revealed that LEA was associated with decreased bone mineral density and increased risk of stress fractures [30].

Also, research should focus on specific populations that may be more susceptible to OTS and bone stress injuries. For example, youth athletes have unique physiological characteristics that may influence their response to training and injury [1]. Understanding the specific needs and vulnerabilities of these populations will help tailor prevention and management strategies accordingly. Studies are necessary to examine the impact of gender-specific factors on the development of overtraining syndrome among female athletes [31]. Female athletes face distinct challenges related to menstrual status, energy availability, and hormonal fluctuations, which may contribute to their increased susceptibility to both OTS and bone stress injuries.

In addition, there is a need for standardized diagnostic criteria and objective measures that can accurately identify overtraining syndrome from other conditions with similar symptoms. Currently, diagnosis is based on subjective measures such as questionnaires or checklists of symptoms combined with objective biomarkers such as hormone levels or inflammatory markers [20,22]. However, more research is needed to validate these diagnostic approaches against gold standard methods while considering individual variations in response to training load.

In terms of prevention strategies for OTS and bone stress injuries, future research should investigate the effectiveness of targeted interventions beyond traditional approaches, such as training periodization or adequate recovery periods. For example, studies exploring the potential benefits of psychological interventions, including mindfulness-based training or cognitive behavioral therapy, could provide valuable information on the management of psychological stressors and the reduction in the risk of developing OTS.

Lastly, research should explore novel methodologies to assess bone health and injury risk in athletes with overtraining syndrome. Advanced imaging techniques, such as magnetic resonance imaging, can offer more accurate evaluations of bone microarchitecture and early detection of stress fractures [22]. Incorporating biomechanical analyses, such as gait analysis or motion capture systems, could provide further insight into the movement patterns and loading mechanics that contribute to bone stress injuries.

While significant progress has been made in understanding the relationship between OTS and bone stress injuries among athletes, there are still several areas that require further investigation. Future research should focus on identifying specific risk factors and mechanisms underlying these conditions, exploring the impact of psychological stressors, understanding long-term consequences on bone health outcomes, investigating the vulnerabilities of specific populations, establishing standardized diagnostic criteria, evaluating targeted prevention strategies beyond traditional approaches, and exploring novel methodologies for assessing bone health and injury risk. Addressing these research gaps will improve our understanding of this complex relationship and improve the prevention and management of overtraining syndrome and bone stress injuries among athletes. This paper could be useful as a step for a consensus on pathology in other clinical areas [32].

7. Conclusions

In conclusion, various intrinsic and extrinsic factors contribute to an athlete's susceptibility to developing OTS. Age, sex, genetics, previous injury history, training volume/intensity, inadequate recovery periods, and nutritional deficiencies or imbalances all play a role in increasing the risk of OTS among athletes. Understanding these risk factors is crucial for implementing appropriate preventive strategies tailored to individual athletes' needs. Further research should focus on elucidating the underlying mechanisms through which these risk factors influence the development of OTS while considering their potential interaction with other variables, such as psychological factors. In general, a comprehensive approach that combines physical and psychological evaluations, together with individualized training programs and support systems, is necessary to effectively prevent and manage OTS among athletes.

Author Contributions: Conceptualization, T.M. (Tomislav Madzar), M.M., R.Z., T.M. (Tonci Masina), M.D., J.P.C., H.B., S.K., I.C., B.K. and A.V.B.; methodology, T.M. (Tomislav Madzar) and M.M.; writing—original draft preparation, T.M. (Tomislav Madzar) and M.M.; writing—review and editing, T.M. (Tomislav Madzar), M.M., R.Z., T.M. (Tonci Masina), M.D., J.P.C., H.B., S.K., I.C., B.K. and A.V.B.; supervision, M.M. All authors have read and agreed to the published version of the manuscript.

Funding: This research received no external funding.

Data Availability Statement: Data used for analysis are contained within the article.

Acknowledgments: The authors thank Ivo Dumic-Cule for help in the initial conceptualization of the paper and review.

Conflicts of Interest: The authors declare no conflicts of interest.

References

1. Matos, N.; Winsley, R.J. Trainability of young athletes and overtraining. *J. Sports Sci. Med.* **2007**, *6*, 353–367. [PubMed]
2. Costa, J.A.; Rago, V.; Brito, P.; Figueiredo, P.; Sousa, H.; Abade, E.; Brito, J. Training in women soccer players: A systematic review on training load monitoring. *Front. Psychol.* **2022**, *13*, 943857. [CrossRef] [PubMed]
3. Schwellnus, M.; Soligard, T.; Alonso, J.M.; Bahr, R.; Clarsen, B.; Dijkstra, H.P.; Gabbett, T.J.; Gleeson, M.; Hagglund, M.; Hutchinson, M.R.; et al. How much is too much? (Part 2) International Olympic Committee consensus statement on load in sport and risk of illness. *Br. J. Sports Med.* **2016**, *50*, 1043–1052. [CrossRef] [PubMed]
4. Armento, A.; Heronemus, M.; Truong, D.; Swanson, C. Bone Health in Young Athletes: A Narrative Review of the Recent Literature. *Curr. Osteoporos. Rep.* **2023**, *21*, 447–458. [CrossRef] [PubMed]
5. Tenforde, A.S.; Carlson, J.L.; Sainani, K.L.; Chang, A.O.; Kim, J.H.; Golden, N.H.; Fredericson, M. Sport and Triad Risk Factors Influence Bone Mineral Density in Collegiate Athletes. *Med. Sci. Sports Exerc.* **2018**, *50*, 2536–2543. [CrossRef] [PubMed]
6. Gabbett, T.J.; Hulin, B.; Blanch, P.; Chapman, P.; Bailey, D. To Couple or not to Couple? For Acute: Chronic Workload Ratios and Injury Risk, Does it Really Matter? *Int. J. Sports Med.* **2019**, *40*, 597–600. [CrossRef] [PubMed]
7. De Oliveira, D.F.; Lopes, L.S.; Gomes-Filho, E. Metabolic changes associated with differential salt tolerance in sorghum genotypes. *Planta* **2020**, *252*, 34. [CrossRef]
8. Rietjens, I.; Vervoort, J.; Maslowska-Gornicz, A.; Van den Brink, N.; Beekmann, K. Use of proteomics to detect sex-related differences in effects of toxicants: Implications for using proteomics in toxicology. *Crit. Rev. Toxicol.* **2018**, *48*, 666–681. [CrossRef]
9. Jurimae, J.; Maestu, J.; Jurimae, T.; Mangus, B.; von Duvillard, S.P. Peripheral signals of energy homeostasis as possible markers of training stress in athletes: A review. *Metabolism* **2011**, *60*, 335–350. [CrossRef]
10. Meeusen, R.; Duclos, M.; Foster, C.; Fry, A.; Gleeson, M.; Nieman, D.; Raglin, J.; Rietjens, G.; Steinacker, J.; Urhausen, A.; et al. Prevention, diagnosis, and treatment of the overtraining syndrome: Joint consensus statement of the European College of Sport Science and the American College of Sports Medicine. *Med. Sci. Sports Exerc.* **2013**, *45*, 186–205. [CrossRef]
11. Soligard, T.; Schwellnus, M.; Alonso, J.M.; Bahr, R.; Clarsen, B.; Dijkstra, H.P.; Gabbett, T.; Gleeson, M.; Hagglund, M.; Hutchinson, M.R.; et al. How much is too much? (Part 1) International Olympic Committee consensus statement on load in sport and risk of injury. *Br. J. Sports Med.* **2016**, *50*, 1030–1041. [CrossRef] [PubMed]
12. Dumic-Cule, I.; Brkljacic, J.; Rogic, D.; Bordukalo Niksic, T.; Tikvica Luetic, A.; Draca, N.; Kufner, V.; Trkulja, V.; Grgurevic, L.; Vukicevic, S. Systemically available bone morphogenetic protein two and seven affect bone metabolism. *Int. Orthop.* **2014**, *38*, 1979–1985. [CrossRef] [PubMed]

13. Buxens, A.; Ruiz, J.R.; Arteta, D.; Artieda, M.; Santiago, C.; Gonzalez-Freire, M.; Martinez, A.; Tejedor, D.; Lao, J.I.; Gomez-Gallego, F.; et al. Can we predict top-level sports performance in power vs endurance events? A genetic approach. *Scand. J. Med. Sci. Sports* **2011**, *21*, 570–579. [CrossRef] [PubMed]
14. Ahmetov, I.I.; Egorova, E.S.; Gabdrakhmanova, L.J.; Fedotovskaya, O.N. Genes and Athletic Performance: An Update. *Med. Sport. Sci.* **2016**, *61*, 41–54. [CrossRef]
15. Mountjoy, M.; Sundgot-Borgen, J.K.; Burke, L.M.; Ackerman, K.E.; Blauwet, C.; Constantini, N.; Lebrun, C.; Lundy, B.; Melin, A.K.; Meyer, N.L.; et al. IOC consensus statement on relative energy deficiency in sport (RED-S): 2018 update. *Br. J. Sports Med.* **2018**, *52*, 687–697. [CrossRef]
16. Loucks, A.B.; Kiens, B.; Wright, H.H. Energy availability in athletes. *J. Sports Sci.* **2011**, *29* (Suppl. S1), S7–S15. [CrossRef]
17. Cupka, M.; Sedliak, M. Hungry runners—Low energy availability in male endurance athletes and its impact on performance and testosterone: Mini-review. *Eur. J. Transl. Myol.* **2023**, *33*, 11104. [CrossRef]
18. Hamstra-Wright, K.L.; Huxel Bliven, K.C.; Napier, C. Training Load Capacity, Cumulative Risk, and Bone Stress Injuries: A Narrative Review of a Holistic Approach. *Front. Sports Act. Living* **2021**, *3*, 665683. [CrossRef]
19. Cadegiani, F. Clinical, Metabolic, and Biochemical Behaviors in Overtraining Syndrome and Overall Athletes. In *Overtraining Syndrome in Athletes*; Springer: Cham, Switzerland, 2020. [CrossRef]
20. Valovich McLeod, T.C.; Decoster, L.C.; Loud, K.J.; Micheli, L.J.; Parker, J.T.; Sandrey, M.A.; White, C. National Athletic Trainers' Association position statement: Prevention of pediatric overuse injuries. *J. Athl. Train.* **2011**, *46*, 206–220. [CrossRef]
21. Maccagnano, G.; Solarino, G.; Pesce, V.; Vicenti, G.; Coviello, M.; Nappi, V.S.; Giannico, O.V.; Notarnicola, A.; Moretti, B. Plate vs reverse shoulder arthroplasty for proximal humeral fractures: The psychological health influence the choice of device? *World J. Orthop.* **2022**, *13*, 297–306. [CrossRef]
22. Cadegiani, F.A.; Kater, C.E. Novel causes and consequences of overtraining syndrome: The EROS-DISRUPTORS study. *BMC Sports Sci. Med. Rehabil.* **2019**, *11*, 21. [CrossRef] [PubMed]
23. Schorb, A.; Niebauer, J.; Aichhorn, W.; Schiepek, G.; Scherr, J.; Claussen, M.C. Overtraining from a sports psychiatry perspective. *Dtsch. Z. Sportmed.* **2021**, *72*, 271–279. [CrossRef]
24. Kellmann, M.; Bertollo, M.; Bosquet, L.; Brink, M.; Coutts, A.J.; Duffield, R.; Erlacher, D.; Halson, S.L.; Hecksteden, A.; Heidari, J.; et al. Recovery and Performance in Sport: Consensus Statement. *Int. J. Sports Physiol. Perform.* **2018**, *13*, 240–245. [CrossRef] [PubMed]
25. Cadegiani, F.A.; da Silva, P.H.L.; Abrao, T.C.P.; Kater, C.E. Diagnosis of Overtraining Syndrome: Results of the Endocrine and Metabolic Responses on Overtraining Syndrome Study: EROS-DIAGNOSIS. *J. Sports Med.* **2020**, *2020*, 3937819. [CrossRef]
26. Morgan, W.P. Selected psychological factors limiting performance: A mental health model. In *Limits of Human Performance*; Clarke, D., Eckert, H.M., Eds.; Human Kinetics: Champaign, IL, USA, 1985; pp. 70–80.
27. Issurin, V.B. Biological Background of Block Periodized Endurance Training: A Review. *Sports Med.* **2019**, *49*, 31–39. [CrossRef] [PubMed]
28. Cabre, H.E.; Moore, S.R.; Smith-Ryan, A.E.; Hackney, A.C. Relative Energy Deficiency in Sport (RED-S): Scientific, Clinical, and Practical Implications for the Female Athlete. *Dtsch. Z. Sportmed.* **2022**, *73*, 225–234. [CrossRef]
29. Beck, B.; Drysdale, L. Risk Factors, Diagnosis and Management of Bone Stress Injuries in Adolescent Athletes: A Narrative Review. *Sports* **2021**, *9*, 52. [CrossRef]
30. Barrack, M.T.; Fredericson, M.; Tenforde, A.S.; Nattiv, A. Evidence of a cumulative effect for risk factors predicting low bone mass among male adolescent athletes. *Br. J. Sports Med.* **2017**, *51*, 200–205. [CrossRef]
31. Ackerman, K.E.; Collomp, K.; Kater, C.E.; Cadegiani, F.A. Editorial: New Perspectives on the Endocrinology of Physical Activity and Sport. *Front. Endocrinol.* **2021**, *12*, 728756. [CrossRef]
32. Moretti, L.; Coviello, M.; Rosso, F.; Calafiore, G.; Monaco, E.; Berruto, M.; Solarino, G. Current Trends in Knee Arthroplasty: Are Italian Surgeons Doing What Is Expected? *Medicina* **2022**, *58*, 1164. [CrossRef]

Disclaimer/Publisher's Note: The statements, opinions and data contained in all publications are solely those of the individual author(s) and contributor(s) and not of MDPI and/or the editor(s). MDPI and/or the editor(s) disclaim responsibility for any injury to people or property resulting from any ideas, methods, instructions or products referred to in the content.

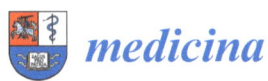

Review

Bone Remodeling in Osteoarthritis—Biological and Radiological Aspects

Luka Dudaric [1], Ivo Dumic-Cule [2,3], Eugen Divjak [4], Tomislav Cengic [5,*], Boris Brkljacic [4,6] and Gordana Ivanac [4,6]

1. Croatia Poliklinika, Rijeka Radiology Unit, Vukovarska 7A, 51000 Rijeka, Croatia; lukadudaric@yahoo.com
2. Clinical Department of Diagnostic and Interventional Radiology, University Hospital Centre Zagreb, Kispaticeva 12, 10000 Zagreb, Croatia; ivodc1@gmail.com
3. Department of Nursing, University North, 104 Brigade 3, 42000 Varazdin, Croatia
4. Department of Diagnostic and Interventional Radiology, University Hospital Dubrava, Avenija Gojka Suska 6, 10000 Zagreb, Croatia; edivjak@gmail.com (E.D.); boris@brkljacic.com (B.B.); gordana.augustan@gmail.com (G.I.)
5. Department of Orthopedics and Traumatology, University Hospital Centre Sestre Milosrdnice, Draskoviceva 19, 10000 Zagreb, Croatia
6. School of Medicine, University of Zagreb, Salata 3, 10000 Zagreb, Croatia
* Correspondence: cengict@me.com; Tel.: +385-98-1655-686

Abstract: Among available papers published on the given subject over the last century, various terms have been used as synonyms for one, now generally accepted—osteoarthritis, in some countries called "wear and tear" or "overload arthritis". The opsolent terms—hypertrophic arthritis, degenerative arthritis, arthritis deformans and osteoarthrosis—sought to highlight the dominant clinical signs of this ubiquitous, polymorph disease of the whole osteochondral unit, which by incidence and prevalence represents one of the leading chronic conditions that cause long-term pain and incapacity for work. Numerous in vitro and in vivo research resulted in broadened acknowledgments about osteoarthritis pathophysiology and pathology on both histological and cellular levels. However, the cause of osteoarthritis is still unknown and is currently the subject of a hypothesis. In this paper, we provide a review of recent findings on biological phenomena taking place in bone tissue during osteoarthritis to the extent useful for clinical practice. Choosing a proper radiological approach is a conditio sine qua non to the early diagnosis of this entity.

Keywords: osteoarthritis; osteophyte; bone remodeling

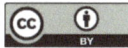

1. Introduction

Bone morphogenesis (osteogenesis) is the process of formation and maintenance of bone tissue and is the result of bone formation and bone resorption. Both processes, bone formation (osteoproduction) and bone resorption (osteoresorption), are functionally balanced in the creation and maintenance of optimal functional structure, or homeostasis, of the skeletal system according to functional demands. Deviation from the physiological balance of these processes is manifested in pathological osteogenesis. One morphological substrate of pathological osteogenesis is osteophyte formation in osteoarthritis (OA).

In other words, physiological and pathological osteogenesis are essentially similar processes as they are based on the same basic principles of bone tissue biology—osteoinduction and osteoconduction. The principle of osteoinduction is based on molecular factors that act on the proliferation and differentiation of bone phenotype cells [1–4]. The purpose of lifelong continuous internal reconstruction of bone tissue and the skeletal system is to achieve and maintain optimal skeletal architecture according to mechanical, static, and humoral circumstances. During prenatal, neonatal, and infantile stages, bones undergo development and growth. Intensive development of all systems of the musculoskeletal system occurs in early childhood and school age, which ends around 14 years of age. The maturation period, from 15 to 20 years of age, is characterized by the overall growth of the body, with bones rapidly growing in length and reaching their anatomical norm, definitive shape, and size through bone modeling. At the end of this period and entering adulthood, the processes of organ development conclude, and bone growth ceases. The intensity of bone production decreases and balances with bone resorption, and the total mass of bone tissue stabilizes and undergoes permanent lifelong remodeling. During aging, bone resorption intensifies, bones atrophy, lose strength and elasticity, and degenerative changes and senile osteoporosis occur.

Histomorphological osteogenic changes occur through processes that are always identical, regardless of the circumstances or phases of growth and development and the modeling or remodeling of bones. During the embryonic period, bones develop from embryonic connective tissue. The organization and morphology of the skeleton in development are determined by a series of programmed and induced processes. The process of osteogenesis or ossification occurs in two ways: intramembranous and endochondral ossification. Ossification also occurs postnatally [1–4].

In mature human individuals, approximately 25% of cancellous bone tissue and about 3% of compact bone tissue are replaced by remodeling each year [5]. The purpose of bone remodeling is to optimize the architecture of the skeletal system and adapt it to biomechanical demands. It is a dynamic lifelong process that achieves and maintains homeostasis of the skeletal system according to changing biomechanical and metabolic circumstances. Haapasalo et al. demonstrated the great capacity for modifying bone architecture in their study of changes in size, shape, and distribution of bone mass in the humerus of professional tennis players [6]. Significant differences were found between the right and left arms of the subjects. The dominant arm of tennis players had increased bone strength due to increased bone size, while bone volume density did not contribute to this difference compared to the non-dominant arm. In other words, the biomechanical optimization of the dominant arm's humerus was not the result of increased bone mass but rather specific architecture achieved through bone mass remodeling in accordance with the biomechanical demands of playing tennis. Similar conclusions were drawn by Bass et al. in their study of biomechanical loading of the humerus in pre- and post-pubertal girls playing tennis [7]. Biomechanical loading before puberty led to increased bone mass and resistance to bending. The increased resistance to bending and torsion was primarily achieved by changing the shape and mass of individual bone parts, rather than changing the volumetric bone density or its total mass. The dominant humerus adapted to the increased load through increased bone resorption in the endocortical area.

Bone remodeling achieves optimal biomechanical adaptation of bone with a minimal amount of bone material. If bone strength was achieved solely by increasing bone mass, an excessively massive skeletal system would burden the organism in all aspects of its biological functionality (energy and substance expenditure, mobility, etc.). In their study on the shape of the femoral neck in women, Zebaze et al. showed that its fragility in older age is not solely due to bone loss but also inadequate remodeling of existing bone mass [8].

2. Bone Modeling and Remodeling in Osteoarthritis

Two layers can be distinguished in the subchondral bone tissue histomorphologically. The layer of bone tissue (thickness 1–3 mm) that continues from the calcified layer of articular cartilage is composed of homogeneous compact bone material. Mechanically and physiologically, this layer corresponds to compact bone tissue in other parts of the bone [8–12]. This layer is followed by a more porous and metabolically active layer of trabecular bone tissue, which has lower density and volume. When studying osteoarthritic changes in the subchondral bone tissue, both layers should be distinguished due to their different biological responses in later stages of osteoarthritis [13–15]. Morphological changes during the progression of osteoarthritis also affect the articular cartilage. Changes in the zone of calcified cartilage differ from those affecting its more superficial zones separated by the tidemark.

In the early stages of osteoarthritis, there is a significant increase in remodeling of the subchondral bone tissue. The mineral apposition rate exceeds 3.5 μm/day, which is about five times higher compared to physiological remodeling. The consequences of increased remodeling during osteoarthritis include a temporary reduction in bone mass, increased porosity, and decreased bone density. Additionally, the number of areas in the subchondral bone that undergo remodeling increases [16]. In an experiment on mice, Zhu et al. demonstrated that osteoclasts in the affected subchondral bone tissue produce netrin-1, which contributes to pain induction by stimulating sensory nerve fibers in the subchondral bone tissue [17].

Significant thinning of the subchondral bone tissue layer has been observed in an experimental model of osteoarthritis in dogs. This finding was accompanied by significant destruction of the articular cartilage and reduced production of glycosaminoglycans within it [18]. Similar changes were reported by Bellido et al. in an experimental model of osteoarthritis in rabbits [19]. Comparable changes can also be found in humans in the early stages of progressive cartilage degeneration. In a cohort study of women aged 45–64 years, a significant increase in bone resorption markers was observed in individuals with progressive osteoarthritis [20]. High levels of bone resorption markers have also been found in middle-aged individuals (aged 27–56 years) in the early stages of osteoarthritis without clinically manifested disease symptoms [21]. The causes of increased remodeling in the early stages of osteoarthritis are not fully understood but are believed to involve humoral interaction between damaged articular cartilage and subchondral bone tissue mediated by vascular invasion and communication channels between cartilage and bone.

Increased levels of transforming growth factor β (TGF-β), insulin-like growth factor (IGF), interleukins 1 and 6 (IL-1 and IL-6), and prostaglandin E2 (PGE2) have been found in altered articular cartilage. These factors are involved in the humoral regulation of bone remodeling. An experiment on osteoblast cell cultures showed that osteoblasts in osteoarthritic knee joints produce six times more IL-6 and PGE2 than osteoblasts in healthy joints [22,23]. It has been confirmed that changes in mineralization and volume of subchondral bone tissue occur below areas of articular cartilage that exhibit significant damage [24]. Microscopic lesions in subchondral bone tissue, even in healthy joints, can stimulate osteocytes to increase the production of receptor activator of nuclear factor-κB ligand (RANKL) and decrease osteoprotegerin (OPG), leading to increased bone resorption [25,26]. Decreased RANKL/OPG ratio and increased bone remodeling have been found in animals with induced OA development [19].

Remodeling of the subchondral bone tissue is accompanied by vascular invasion into the area of calcified cartilage. Increased vascularity is the result of the stimulation of blood vessels in the subchondral bone tissue by angiogenic factors, such as endothelial growth factor. Its concentration is significantly increased in the synovial fluid of OA patients [27]. Angiogenic factors stimulate chondrocytes in articular cartilage to synthesize and secrete matrix metalloproteinases and catabolic enzymes that prevent the interaction of metalloproteinases with their inhibitors. The combination of vascular invasion into the articular cartilage and increased influx of catabolic factors without inhibition of metalloproteinases ensures the progression of cartilage destruction. Consequently, these events diminish the mechanical integrity of the articular cartilage and promote remodeling as an attempt at joint adaptation to increased load. The existence of physiological communication between subchondral bone tissue and articular cartilage has been demonstrated in rats [28]. An experimental model of osteoarthritis in mice confirmed an increase in the caliber and number of these communications [29,30].

In the later stages of osteoarthritis, the intensity of remodeling decreases. Morphological features of such remodeling include increased bone volume and increased bone density, known as bone sclerosis. Both changes are clearly visible on X-ray images. By comparing the bone volume and density of OA patients with those of healthy individuals, it has been determined that OA patients have a 15% increase in bone density and a 30% increase in bone volume [31–33]. Analysis of subchondral bone tissue in OA patients has shown increased volume and reduced mineralization [34]. The inverse relationships of these bone tissue parameters can be interpreted as an adaptive attempt to compensate for decreased mineralization by increasing the volume of bone tissue [24]. Reduced mineralization of bone tissue during OA is associated with the structure of collagen produced by osteoblasts in osteoarthritic joints. It involves collagen type I composed of $\alpha 1$ chains, which distinguishes it from normal collagen type I composed of two $\alpha 1$ chains and one $\alpha 2$ chain [35,36]. Such collagen structure contributes to reduced mineralization during OA. Reduced bone resorption in the later stages of osteoarthritis is not accompanied by a decrease in osteoproduction, resulting in an overall increase in the volume and density of the subchondral bone tissue.

The described changes have secondary effects on surrounding joint tissues, particularly on the synovial membrane. In the later stages of OA, synovial membrane hyperplasia can occur without an inflammatory process.

3. Osteophytes Morphology and Development

Roland and Moskowitz consider osteoarthritis (OA) as the final stage of heterogeneous etiopathogenetic events affecting the joints [37]. In joints affected by OA changes, in addition to disturbances in the structure of the articular cartilage and subchondral bone tissue, osteophytes develop [38]. Osteophytes are bony outgrowths covered with a fibrocartilaginous cap (from Greek "osteo" = bone + "phyton" = plant, vegetation). Genuine osteophytes (osteochondrophytes) grow under the periosteum, along the edge of the articular cartilage or the insertion of the synovial membrane. In this regard, osteochondrophytes are called marginal osteophytes. The position of marginal osteophytes corresponds to the area where three different joint structures come into contact (articular cartilage, synovial membrane, and periosteum). The synovial fluid enables an additional indirect relationship between these tissues. Marginal osteophytes are a common finding in degenerative OA.

In addition to genuine osteophytes, traction and inflammatory osteophytes have been described. Traction osteophytes develop in the areas of tendon insertions (enthesophytes), while inflammatory osteophytes (syndesmophytes) are characteristic of ankylosing spondylitis. Osteophytes that appear further from the edge of the articular cartilage are called central osteophytes. Their position corresponds to the areas of damaged articular cartilage.

Osteophytes are clearly visible on X-ray images of joints affected by OA. Their distribution and dimensions can be precisely analyzed on appropriate joint radiographs.

The cause that triggers the development of osteophytes has not been established. The development of osteophytes involves morphogenetic processes from the early stages of skeletal development (endochondral and intramembranous ossification). Cytomorphologically and according to gene expression patterns, chondrogenesis and the formation of new bone tissue during osteophyte development particularly resemble identical processes in fracture healing with callus formation [39]. Possible causes of osteophyte development include mechanical overload of the joint and humoral factors. Experimental models of OA are based on these factors, such as cruciate ligament transection in the knee joint (biomechanical) and the administration of TGF-β1 and bone morphogenetic protein 2 (BMP-2) (humoral) into the joint cavity [40,41]. Destruction of the articular cartilage and the development of osteophytes have also been found in biomechanically unloaded joints during immobilization [42]. Therefore, previous notions that osteoarthritis is a causal consequence of aging have been rejected because cartilage atrophy alone does not always result in osteoarthritis. BMPs are a subset of the TGF-β superfamily of signaling molecules, and play a crucial role in regulating various cellular processes, particularly in the development and maintenance of bones, cartilage, and other tissues. BMP-2 promotes bone formation by stimulating the differentiation of mesenchymal stem cells into osteoblasts, facilitating the creation of new bone tissue [43,44].

Since the cause of osteophyte development has not been determined, despite the existence of experimental models, the question arises whether it is a functional adaptation of the joint or a pathological change. The answer still relies on assumptions. One theory suggests that osteophytes are the organism's attempt to stabilize a biomechanically insufficient joint by increasing the surface area of the articular cartilage [45]. As OA progresses and articular cartilage degenerates, it is believed that osteophytes represent an adaptive attempt by the organism to repair the degenerated cartilage rather than a degenerative change [46]. It is probable that the local humoral milieu, established through certain biomechanical stimuli, stimulates chondrogenesis and endochondral ossification, leading to osteophyte formation [45].

In animal experimental models of OA, stages of osteophyte development have been described. The dominant mechanism of osteophyte formation is endochondral ossification, in which osteogenic cells mainly originate from the periosteum. Areas of intramembranous ossification appear during the definitive shaping of osteophytes, where osteogenic cells mainly originate from the synovial membrane. The expression of numerous growth factors has been investigated in osteophytes [45]. Research results regarding the expression of bone morphogenetic proteins in osteophytes are ambiguous. In rat periosteal stem cells, TGF-β did not induce chondrogenesis, while treatment of these cells with BMP-2 resulted in the production of collagen type II and aggrecan. Chondrocytes treated with BMP-2 showed markers of chondrocyte hypertrophy (collagen type X, osteocalcin), while in the culture treated with a combination of BMP-2 and TGF-β, chondrocyte hypertrophy was absent [47]. However, Uuistalo et al. showed that BMP-2 stimulates chondrogenesis from mouse periosteal stem cells and supports further endochondral ossification [48]. In a study on avian species, BMP-2 did not exhibit a chondrogenic effect on periosteal cells [49]. Chondrogenic differentiation of human mesenchymal stem cells from the synovial membrane was observed after the addition of TGF-β to the culture. Joyce et al., studying periosteal ossification in rats, found that depending on the dosage, TGF-β directs ossification in an endochondral or intramembranous direction. High doses of exogenous TGF-β introduced into the periosteum support endochondral ossification, while at lower doses, ossification mainly occurs intramembranously [50,51].

4. Radiological Characteristics of Osteoarthritis

It is believed that changes in subchondral bone tissue play a crucial role in the pathogenesis of osteoarthritis and can be detected early, long before clinical signs appear [52,53]. In the early stages of osteoarthritis, radiological signs are sparse, so depending on the stage of osteoarthritis, it is necessary to choose the appropriate radiological examination method. The expression of the radiological signs depends on the biomechanical characteristics of the affected joint.

As degenerative changes progress, the articular cartilage deteriorates, and the joint space decreases, which is evident on X-rays as a narrowing of the joint space. The joint surfaces become deformed, flattened, uneven, or irregularly shaped. The latter is the result of focal cartilage proliferation that calcifies, leading to double or triple contour deformities on X-rays (Figure 1). Subchondral sclerosis of the joint surfaces can progress to eburnation (ivory-like appearance). Convex joint bodies lose their convexity, while concave joint bodies become shallower and flattened. Hypertrophic changes in the form of osteophytes develop chronically along the edges of the joint surfaces. Increasing osteophytes can result in a bony bridging between the articulating joint surfaces. Bone pseudocysts appear as cyst-like, marginally sclerotic transparencies in the subchondral area, varying in size and shape. Enlarged pseudocysts can cause subluxation of the joint bodies and the presence of loose bone fragments, called joint mice, in the joint space. Fracture of the bony wall of a pseudocyst can create communication between the joint cavity and the denuded joint body. Since 1957, the Kellgren and Lawrence classification has been used for the assessment of osteoarthritis changes in radiological practice. The radiological analysis includes osteophytes, periarticular ossifications, changes in articular cartilage associated with subchondral sclerosis of bone tissue, and pseudocysts in the subchondral bone tissue. According to the radiological findings, osteoarthritis changes are graded into five stages (0–4) [54].

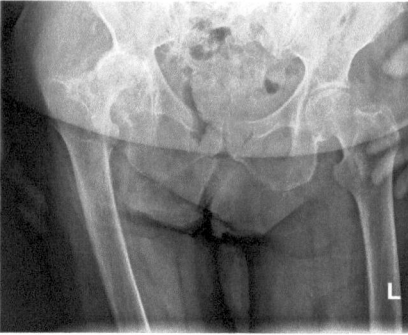 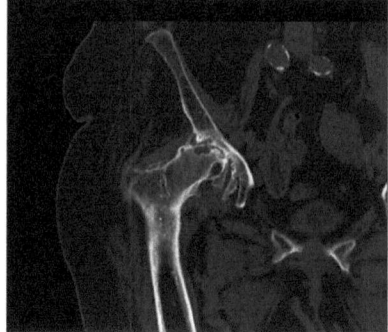

Figure 1. Sagittal X-ray of the pelvis and computerized tomography of the right hip (same patient). Severe right-sided coxarthrosis deformans. Grossly reduced joint space. Dense, sclerotic subchondral bone tissue of the deformed articular bodies interspersed with cyst-like transparencies of bone. Abundant marginal osteophytes of the articular surfaces and femoral head subluxation with consequent higher position of the right half of the pelvis. L—left side.

Complete joint ankylosis as a result of osteoarthritis is rarely seen today. Cartilaginous elements in some joints often become calcified (chondrocalcinosis which should be differentiated from calcium pyrophosphate dihydrate deposition disease), such as the menisci in the knee joint or the glenoid labrum in the shoulder joint. The radiographic findings often do not correspond to the subjective complaints of the patients, so in the presence of a rich physical examination and clinical picture, the radiographic findings may be only minimally altered. Computed tomography, compared to conventional radiographic imaging of joints affected by osteoarthritis, provides richer data on the extent of the pathoanatomical substrate.

In early osteoarthritis changes, visible on magnetic resonance imaging (MRI), there are subchondral sclerosis and cysts in the bone tissue, lesions in the surrounding bone marrow, fissures in the articular cartilage (Figure 2), and changes in the synovial membrane [55].

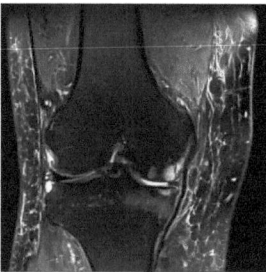 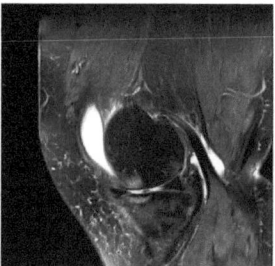 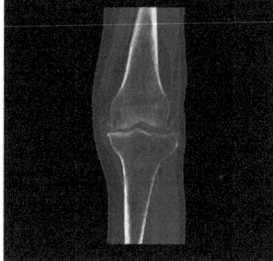

Figure 2. Mild deforming gonarthrosis visualized by MRI (proton-density fat saturated sequences in sagittal and coronal plane) and by CT (multiplanar reconstruction, coronal plane). Patchy areas of subchondral bone edema of femoral and tibial articulations with numerous marginal osteophytes. Articular cartilage is denuded in medial compartment, while in lateral compartment I-II degree hondromalacic changes are seen. Narrowed articular spaces with reactive effusion propagating to suprapatellar bursa are seen. High signal intensity of menisci and cruciate ligaments suggestive of degenerative changes. Ruptured medial meniscus. Reactive edema of periarticular and subcutaneous soft tissues.

The role of ultrasound examination of the joints primarily relates to non-skeletal tissues (periosteum, synovial membrane, tendons, ligaments, etc.). Ultrasound can differentiate marginal bone appositions on joint bodies (osteophytes) and the width of the joint space, as well as its expansion due to effusion (Figure 3). Some components of the accessory structure of the joint, such as the meniscus in the knee joint, can be partially visualized with ultrasound (Figure 4). Synovial bursae adjacent to joints affected by osteoarthritis serve as an anatomical substrate for the development of cysts that can be well examined by ultrasound. Examples include the bursae in the popliteal fossa (bursae mucosae regionis genus posterioris), among which the bursa musculi semimembranosi and the bursa subtendinea musculi gastrocnemii medialis, often combined into one, from which a Baker's cyst develops in 10–20% of cases of knee osteoarthritis. When a Baker's cyst communicates with the joint space of the knee joint, inflammatory processes from the cyst can directly transfer to the knee joint (Figure 5).

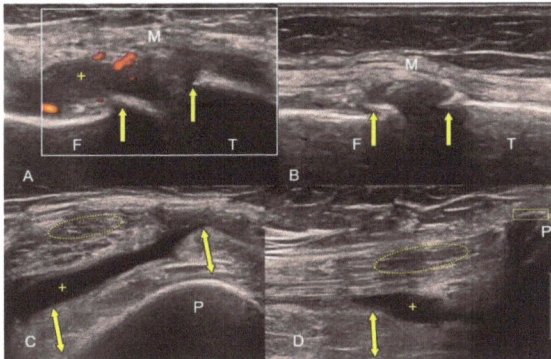

Figure 3. (**A–D**) Ultrasound of the knee joint in exacerbation of osteoarthritis (high-frequency linear probe: B-mode and Power Doppler). Irregular echoes from the femoral (F) and tibial (T) articular surfaces corresponding to marginal osteophytes (**A,B**). Hyperemia (red color in white rectangle) and edema of the thickened, hypertrophic synovial membrane (yellow bidirectional arrows) with effusion (+) in the suprapatellar bursa are signs of reactive inflammation. Loss of tension and fine linear echostructure of the medial collateral ligament (M). Absence of linear echostructure and decreased echogenicity (yellow ellipse) in the distal part of the quadriceps muscle tendon. Enthesophyte (yellow rectangle) at the base of the patella (P) (**C,D**).

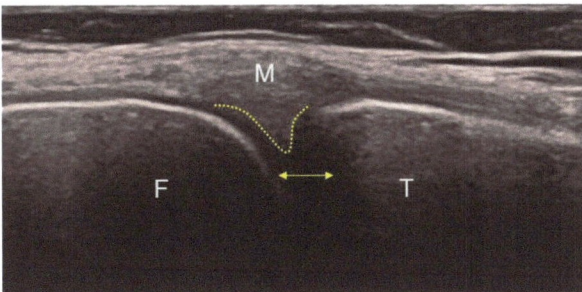

Figure 4. Ultrasound of the medial part of a healthy knee. Regular echoes from the femoral (F) and tibial (T) articular surfaces. The peripheral part of the medial meniscus (yellow dotted line) without a visible boundary continues into the posterior (oblique) fibers of the medial collateral ligament (M) that insert into it. The other (anterior) fibers of the medial collateral ligament continue vertically toward their insertion on the proximal tibia. Normal distance between the articular bodies indicates preserved thickness of the articular cartilages (yellow bidirectional line).

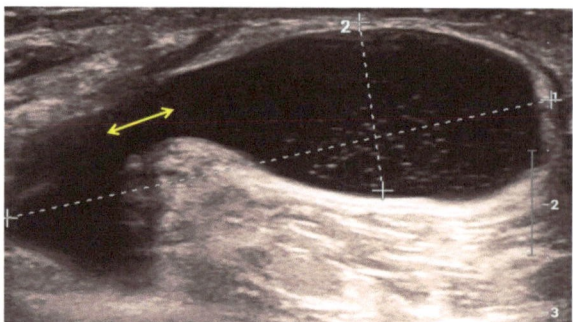

Figure 5. Sonographic image of a Baker's cyst in the medial part of the popliteal fossa. Punctiform internal echoes from the cyst lumen which communicate with the joint space of the knee joint (yellow bidirectional arrow). Fluid within the cyst enhances the ultrasound beam posteriorly.

Numerous national and international guidelines have been developed for the diagnosis of osteoarthritis, which has been well-received by primary healthcare physicians. According to the British national guidelines from 2022, the diagnosis of osteoarthritis is made in individuals over 45 years of age with joint pain associated with physical activity, if they do not have morning stiffness of the joints or if it does not last longer than 30 min. The routine use of imaging diagnostic methods is not recommended, except in atypical cases that suggest a different diagnosis. This recommendation is supported by the lack of evidence for the contribution of imaging methods in diagnosing osteoarthritis, considering that anamnesis and physical examination of the patient are sufficient for diagnosis, while reducing unnecessary use of healthcare and financial resources [56]. A somewhat different point of view is held by a group of international experts, who believe that a positive clinical and typical radiographic finding is sufficient for diagnosing knee osteoarthritis, and further diagnostic imaging with magnetic resonance imaging is not recommended [57].

5. Conclusions

Contemporary experimental and clinical studies on osteoarthritis (OA) provide findings that are practically applicable to the pharmacological curative and rehabilitative approach to patients. Experts in this field unanimously emphasize the importance of a multidisciplinary and multimodal approach to OA casuistry, as well as an individualized approach to the patient. Interdisciplinary collaboration places significant demands on clinical radiology. It is expected to provide radiological diagnosis and data on the characteristics of the pathoanatomical substrate not only of the skeletal system but also of other affected locomotor apparatus systems. Radiology also includes the classification of OA changes, which, in addition to its diagnostic significance, serves as a starting point for deciding on a curative approach. The quantification of the effects of treatment and rehabilitation is also within the domain of radiological examination.

In recent times, human life expectancy has been increasing, as well as the duration of degenerative changes, which amplifies and complicates their consequences, affecting not only the health but also the economic status of patients and the entire community. For this reason, research in the field under discussion gains a broader foundation and deeper significance.

Author Contributions: Conceptualization, L.D. and B.B.; methodology, L.D., G.I., T.C. and E.D.; writing—original draft preparation, I.D.-C. and G.I.; writing—review and editing, E.D., T.C., I.D.-C. and B.B.; supervision, G.I. and B.B. All authors have read and agreed to the published version of the manuscript.

Funding: This research received no external funding.

Institutional Review Board Statement: Not applicable.

Informed Consent Statement: Not applicable.

Data Availability Statement: Data used for analysis are contained within the article.

Acknowledgments: The authors thank the Department of Diagnostic and Interventional Radiology, University Hospital Dubrava, for the radiological images that improved the manuscript.

Conflicts of Interest: The authors declare no conflict of interest.

References

1. Đudarić, L. Izražaj Osteoniduktivnih Proteina I Njihovih Inhibitora Tijekom Osteogeneze. Ph.D. Thesis, Medicinski Fakultet Sveučilišta u Rijeci, Rijeka, Croatia, 2014.
2. Lian, J.B.; Stein, G.S. Osteoblast Biology. In *Osteoporosis*; Marcus, R., Feldman, D., Kelsey, J., Eds.; Academic Press Inc.: San Diego, CA, USA, 1996; pp. 23–35.
3. Đudarić, L.; Zoričić Cvek, S.; Cvijanović, O.; Fužinac-Smojver, A.; Ćelić, T.; Martinović, D. Osnove biologije koštanog tkiva. *Med. Flum.* **2014**, *50*, 21–38.
4. Zoričić Cvek, S.; Bobinac, D.; Đudarić, L.; Cvijanović, O. Pregradnja koštanog sustava. *Med. Flum.* **2015**, *51*, 482–493.
5. Becker, K.L. *Principles and Practice of Endocrinology and Metabolism*; Lippincott Williams & Wilkins: Philadelphia, PA, USA, 2001.
6. Haapasalo, H.; Kontulainen, S.; Sievänen, H.; Kannus, P.; Järvinen, M.; Vuori, I. Exercise-induced bone gain is due to enlargement in bone size without a change in volumetric bone density: A peripheral quantitative computed tomography study of the upper arms of male tennis players. *Bone* **2000**, *27*, 351–357. [CrossRef]
7. Bass, S.L.; Saxon, L.; Daly, R.M.; Turner, C.H.; Robling, A.G.; Seeman, E.; Stuckey, S. The effect of mechanical loading on the size and shape of bone in pre-, peri-, and postpubertal girls: A study in tennis players. *J. Bone Miner. Res.* **2002**, *17*, 2274–2280. [CrossRef]
8. Zebaze, R.M.; Jones, A.; Knackstedt, M.; Maalouf, G.; Seeman, E. Construction of the femoral neck during growth determines its strength in old age. *J. Bone Miner. Res.* **2007**, *22*, 1055–1061. [CrossRef] [PubMed]
9. Milz, S.; Putz, R. Quantitative morphology of the subchondral plate of the tibial plateau. *J. Anat.* **1994**, *185*, 103–110.
10. Eckstein, F.; Milz, S.; Hermann, A.; Putz, R. Thickness of the subchondral mineralised tissue zone (SMZ) in normal male and female and pathological human patellae. *J. Anat.* **1998**, *192*, 81–90. [CrossRef]
11. Clark, J.M.; Huber, J.D. The structure of the human subchondral plate. *J. Bone Jt. Surg.* **1990**, *72*, 866–873. [CrossRef]
12. Brown, T.D.; Vrahas, M.S. The apparent elastic modulus of the juxtarticular subchondral bone of the femoral head. *J. Orthop. Res.* **1984**, *2*, 32–38. [CrossRef]
13. Brandt, K.D.; Myers, S.L.; Burr, D.; Albrecht, M. Osteoarthritic changes in canine articular cartilage, subchondral bone, and synovium fifty-four months after transaction of the anterior cruciate ligament. *Arthritis Rheum.* **1991**, *34*, 1560–1570. [CrossRef]
14. Dedrick, D.K.; Goldstein, S.A.; Brandt, K.D.; O'Connor, B.L.; Goulet, R.W.; Albrecht, M. A longitudinal study of subchondral plate and trabecular bone in cruciate-deficient dogs with osteoarthritis followed up for 54 months. *Arthritis Rheum.* **1993**, *36*, 1460–1467. [CrossRef] [PubMed]
15. Burr, D.B.; Gallant, M.A. Bone remodelling in osteoarthritis. *Nat. Rev. Rheumatol.* **2012**, *8*, 665–673. [CrossRef] [PubMed]
16. Intema, F.; Sniekers, Y.H.; Weinans, H.; Vianen, M.E.; Yocum, S.A.; Zuurmond, A.M.M.; DeGroot, J.; Lafeber, F.P.; Mastbergen, S.C. Similarities and discrepancies in subchondral bone structure in two differently induced canine models of osteoarthritis. *J. Bone Miner. Res.* **2010**, *25*, 1650–1657. [CrossRef]
17. Zhu, S.; Zhu, J.; Zhen, G.; Hu, Y.; An, S.; Li, Y.; Zheng, Q.; Chen, Z.; Yang, Y.; Wan, M.; et al. Subchondral bone osteoclasts induce sensory innervation and osteoarthritis pain. *J. Clin. Investig.* **2019**, *129*, 1076–1093. [CrossRef] [PubMed]
18. Sniekers, Y.H.; Intema, F.; Lafeber, F.P.; van Osch, G.J.; van Leeuwen, J.P.; Weinans, H.; Mastbergen, S.C. A role for subchondral bone changes in the process of osteoarthritis; a micro-CT study of two canine models. *BME Musculoskelet. Disord.* **2008**, *9*, 20. [CrossRef] [PubMed]
19. Bellido, M.; Lugo, L.; Roman-Blas, J.A.; Castañeda, S.; Caeiro, J.R.; Dapia, S.; Calvo, E.; Largo, R.; Herrero-Beaumont, G. Subchondral bone microstructural damage by increased remodeling aggravates experimental osteoarthritis preceded by osteoporosis. *Arthritis Res. Ther.* **2010**, *12*, R152. [CrossRef]
20. Bettica, P.; Cline, G.; Hart, D.J.; Meyer, J.; Spector, T.D. Evidence for increased bone resorption in patients with progressive knee osteoarthritis: Longitudinal results from the Chingford study. *Arthritis Rheum.* **2002**, *46*, 3178–3184. [CrossRef]
21. Bolbos, R.I.; Zuo, J.; Banerjee, S.; Link, T.M.; Ma, C.B.; Li, X.; Majumdar, S. Relationship between trabecular bone structure and articular cartilage morphology and relaxation times in early OA of the knee joint using parallel MRI at 3T. *Osteoarthr. Cartil.* **2008**, *16*, 1150–1159. [CrossRef]
22. Mansell, J.P.; Collins, C.; Bailey, A.J. Bone, not cartilage, should be the major focus in osteoarthritis. *Nat. Clin. Pract. Rheum.* **2007**, *3*, 306–307. [CrossRef]
23. Massicotte, F.; Lajeunesse, D.; Benderdour, M.; Pelletier, J.P.; Hilal, G.; Duval, N.; Martel-Pelletier, J. Can altered production of interleukin-1β, interleukin-6, transforming growth factor-β, and prostaglandin E2 by isolated human subchondral osteoblasts identify two subgroups of osteoarthritic patients. *Osteoarthr. Cartil.* **2002**, *10*, 491–500. [CrossRef]

24. Cox, L.G.E.; van Donkelaar, C.C.; van Rietbergen, B.; Emans, P.J.; Ito, K. Decreased bone tissue mineralization can partly explain subchondral sclerosis observed in osteoarthritis. *Bone* **2012**, *50*, 1152–1161. [CrossRef] [PubMed]
25. Nakashima, T.; Hayashi, M.; Fukunaga, T.; Kurata, K.; Oh-Hora, M.; Feng, J.Q.; Bonewald, L.F.; Kodama, T.; Wutz, A.; Wagner, E.F.; et al. Evidence for osteocyte regulation of bone homeostasis through RANKL expression. *Nat. Med.* **2011**, *17*, 1231–1234. [CrossRef] [PubMed]
26. Kennedy, O.D.; Herman, B.C.; Laudier, M.D. Activation of resorption in fatigue-loaded bone involves both apoptosis and active pro-osteoclastogenic signaling by distinct osteocyte cell populations. *Bone* **2012**, *50*, 1115–1122. [CrossRef] [PubMed]
27. Brown, R.A.; Tomlinson, I.W.; Hill, C.R.; Weiss, J.B.; Phillips, P.; Kumar, S. Relationship of angiogenesis factor in synovial fluid to various joint diseases. *Ann. Rheum. Dis.* **1983**, *42*, 301–307. [CrossRef]
28. Pan, J.; Zhou, X.; Li, W. In situ measurement of transport between subchondral bone and articular cartilage. *J. Orthop. Res.* **2009**, *27*, 1347–1352. [CrossRef]
29. Hwang, J.; Bae, W.C.; Shieu, W.; Lewis, C.W.; Bugbee, W.D.; Sah, R.L. Increased hydraulic conductance of human articular cartilage and subchondral bone plate with progression of osteoarthritis. *Arthritis Rheum.* **2008**, *58*, 3831–3842. [CrossRef]
30. Pan, J.; Wang, B.; Li, W.; Zhou, X.; Scherr, T.; Yang, Y.; Price, C.; Wang, L. Elevated cross-talk between subchondral bone and cartilage in osteoarthritic joints. *Bone* **2012**, *51*, 212–217. [CrossRef]
31. Fazzalari, N.; Parkinson, I.H. Fractal properties of subchondral cancellous bone in severe osteoarthritis of the hip. *J. Bone Miner. Res.* **1997**, *12*, 632–640. [CrossRef]
32. Arden, N.K.; Griffiths, G.O.; Hart, D.J.; Doyle, D.V.; Spector, T.D. The association between osteoarthritis and osteoporotic fracture: The Chingford study. *Br. J. Rheumatol.* **1996**, *35*, 1299–1304. [CrossRef]
33. Hannan, M.T.; Anderson, J.J.; Zhang, Y.; Levy, D.; Felson, D.T. Bone mineral density and knee osteoarthritis in elderly men and women. The Framingham Study. *Arthritis Rheum.* **1993**, *36*, 1671–1680. [CrossRef]
34. Grynpas, M.; Alpert, B.; Katz, I.; Lieberman, I.; Pritzker, K.P.H. Subchondral bone in osteoarthritis. *Calcif. Tissue Int.* **1991**, *49*, 20–26. [CrossRef]
35. Chan, T.F.; Couchourel, D.; Abed, E.; Delalandre, A.; Duval, N.; Lajeunesse, D. Elevated Dickkopf-2 levels contribute to the abnormal phenotype of human osteoarthritic osteoblasts. *J. Bone Miner. Res.* **2011**, *26*, 1399–1410. [CrossRef] [PubMed]
36. Li, X.; Liu, P.; Liu, W.; Maye, P.; Zhang, J.; Zhang, Y.; Hurley, M.; Guo, C.; Boskey, A.; Sun, L.; et al. Dkk2 has a role in terminal osteoblast differentiation and mineralized matrix formation. *Nat. Genet.* **2005**, *37*, 945–952. [CrossRef]
37. Moskowitz, R.W. Bone remodeling in osteoarthritis: Subchondral and osteophytic responses. *Osteoarthr. Cartil.* **1999**, *7*, 323–324. [CrossRef]
38. Bullough, P. The pathology of osteoarthritis. In *Osteoarthritis*; Moskowitz, R., Howell, D., Goldberg, V., Mankin, H., Eds.; W.B. Saunders: Philadelphia, PA, USA, 1992; pp. 39–69.
39. Matyas, J.R.; Sandell, L.J.; Adams, M.E. Gene expression of type II collagens in chondro-osteophytes in experimental osteoarthritis. *Osteoarthr. Cartil.* **1997**, *5*, 99–105. [CrossRef] [PubMed]
40. Tardif, G.; Pelletier, J.P.; Boileau, C.; Martel-Pelletier, J. The BMP antagonists follistatin and gremlin in normal and early osteoarthritic cartilage: An immunohistochemical study. *Osteoarthr. Cartil.* **2009**, *17*, 263–270. [CrossRef] [PubMed]
41. van Beuningen, H.M.; Glansbeek, H.L.; van der Kraan, P.M.; van den Berg, W.B. Differential effects of local application of BMP-2 or TGF-beta 1 on both articular cartilage composition and osteophyte formation. *Osteoarthr. Cartil.* **1998**, *6*, 306–317. [CrossRef]
42. Langenskiöld, A.; Michelsson, J.E.; Videman, T. Osteoarthritis of the knee in the rabbit produced by immobilization. Attempts to achieve a reproducible model for studies on pathogenesis and therapy. *Acta Orthop. Scand.* **1979**, *50*, 1–14. [CrossRef]
43. Dumic-Cule, I.; Brkljacic, J.; Rogic, D.; Bordukalo Niksic, T.; Tikvica Luetic, A.; Draca, N.; Kufner, V.; Trkulja, V.; Grgurevic, L.; Vukicevic, S. Systemically available bone morphogenetic protein two and seven affect bone metabolism. *Int. Orthop.* **2014**, *38*, 1979–1985. [CrossRef] [PubMed]
44. Dumic-Cule, I.; Peric, M.; Kucko, L.; Grgurevic, L.; Pecina, M.; Vukicevic, S. Bone morphogenetic proteins in fracture repair. *Int. Orthop.* **2018**, *42*, 2619–2626. [CrossRef]
45. van der Kraan, P.M.; van den Berg, W.B. Osteophytes: Relevance and biology. *Osteoarthr. Cartil.* **2007**, *15*, 237–244. [CrossRef] [PubMed]
46. Neuman, P.; Hulth, A.; Lindén, B.; Johnell, O.; Dahlberg, L. The role of osteophytic growth in hip osteoarthritis. *Int. Orthop.* **2003**, *27*, 262–266. [CrossRef] [PubMed]
47. Hanada, K.; Solchaga, L.A.; Caplan, A.I.; Hering, T.M.; Goldberg, V.M.; Yoo, J.U.; Johnstone, B. BMP-2 induction and TGF-beta 1 modulation of rat periosteal cell chondrogenesis. *J. Cell Biochem.* **2001**, *81*, 284–294. [CrossRef]
48. Uusitalo, H.; Hiltunen, A.; Ahonen, M.; Kahari, V.M.; Aro, H.; Vuorio, E. Induction of periosteal callus formation by bone morphogenetic protein-2 employing adenovirusmediated gene delivery. *Matrix Biol.* **2001**, *20*, 123–127. [CrossRef]
49. Iwasaki, M.; Nakahara, H.; Nakase, T.; Kimura, T.; Takaoka, K.; Caplan, A.I.; Ono, K. Bone morphogenetic protein 2 stimulates osteogenesis but does not affect chondrogenesis in osteochondrogenic differentiation of periosteum-derived cells. *J. Bone Miner. Res.* **1994**, *9*, 1195–1204. [CrossRef] [PubMed]
50. Shirasawa, S.; Sekiya, I.; Sakaguchi, Y.; Yagishita, K.; Ichinose, S.; Muneta, T. In vitro chondrogenesis of human synovium-derived mesenchymal stem cells: Optimal condition and comparison with bone marrowderived cells. *J. Cell Biochem.* **2006**, *97*, 84–97. [CrossRef] [PubMed]

51. Joyce, M.E.; Roberts, A.B.; Sporn, M.B.; Bolander, M.E. Transforming growth factor-beta and the initiation of chondrogenesis and osteogenesis in the rat femur. *J. Cell Biol.* **1990**, *110*, 2195–2207. [CrossRef]
52. Anderson-MacKenzie, J.M.; Quasnichka, H.L.; Starr, R.L.; Lewis, E.J.; Billingham, M.E.; Bailey, A.J. Fundamental subchondral bone changes in spontaneous knee osteoarthritis. *Int. J. Biochem. Cell Biol.* **2005**, *37*, 224–236. [CrossRef]
53. Hayami, T.; Pickarski, M.; Zhuo, Y.; Wesolowski, G.A.; Rodan, G.A.; Duong, L.T. Characterization of articular cartilage and subchondral bone changes in the rat anterior cruciate ligament transection and meniscectomized models of osteoarthritis. *Bone* **2006**, *38*, 234–243. [CrossRef]
54. Xu, L.; Hayashi, D.; Roemer, F.W.; Felson, D.T.; Guermazi, A. Magnetic resonance imaging of subchondral bone marrow lesions in association with osteoarthritis. *Semin. Arthritis Rheum.* **2012**, *42*, 105–118. [CrossRef]
55. Kellgren, J.H.; Lawrence, J.S. Radiological assessment of osteo-arthrosis. *Ann. Rheum. Dis.* **1957**, *16*, 494–502. [CrossRef] [PubMed]
56. NICE. *Osteoarthritis in over 16s: Diagnosis and Management*; National Institute for Health and Care Excellence (NICE): London, UK, 2022.
57. Martel-Pelletier, J.; Maheu, E.; Pelletier, J.P.; Alekseeva, L.; Mkinsi, O.; Branco, J.; Monod, P.; Planta, F.; Reginster, J.Y.; Rannou, F. A new decision tree for diagnosis of osteoarthritis in primary care: International consensus of experts. *Aging Clin. Exp. Res.* **2019**, *31*, 19–30. [CrossRef] [PubMed]

Disclaimer/Publisher's Note: The statements, opinions and data contained in all publications are solely those of the individual author(s) and contributor(s) and not of MDPI and/or the editor(s). MDPI and/or the editor(s) disclaim responsibility for any injury to people or property resulting from any ideas, methods, instructions or products referred to in the content.

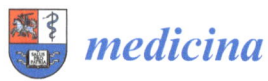

Review

Complications of Percutaneous Vertebroplasty: A Pictorial Review

Mislav Cavka [1,†], Domagoj Delimar [2,3,†], Robert Rezan [1], Tomislav Zigman [3,4], Kresimir Sasa Duric [3,5], Mislav Cimic [3], Ivo Dumic-Cule [1,6,*] and Maja Prutki [1,3]

[1] Clinical Department of Diagnostic and Interventional Radiology, University Hospital Centre Zagreb, Kispaticeva 12, 10000 Zagreb, Croatia; mislav.cavka@yahoo.com (M.C.); rrezan@gmail.com (R.R.); maja.prutki@gmail.com (M.P.)
[2] Department of Orthopaedic Surgery, University Hospital Centre Zagreb, Kispaticeva 12, 10000 Zagreb, Croatia; domagoj.delimar@kbc-zagreb.hr
[3] School of Medicine, University of Zagreb, Salata 3, 10000 Zagreb, Croatia; zigman.tomislav@gmail.com (T.Z.); kresimir.sasa.djuric@kbc-zagreb.hr (K.S.D.); cimicmislav@gmail.com (M.C.)
[4] Department of Surgery, University Hospital Centre Zagreb, Kispaticeva 12, 10000 Zagreb, Croatia
[5] Department of Neurosurgery, University Hospital Centre Zagreb, Kispaticeva 12, 10000 Zagreb, Croatia
[6] Department of Nursing, University North, 104 Brigade 3, 42000 Varazdin, Croatia
* Correspondence: ivodc1@gmail.com; Tel.: +385-98-1655-686
† These authors contributed equally to this work.

Abstract: Percutaneous vertebroplasty is a minimally invasive treatment technique for vertebral body compression fractures. The complications associated with this technique can be categorized into mild, moderate, and severe. Among these, the most prevalent complication is cement leakage, which may insert into the epidural, intradiscal, foraminal, and paravertebral regions, and even the venous system. The occurrence of a postprocedural infection carries a notable risk which is inherent to any percutaneous procedure. While the majority of these complications manifest without symptoms, they can potentially lead to severe outcomes. This review aims to consolidate the various complications linked to vertebroplasty, drawing from the experiences of a single medical center.

Keywords: vertebroplasty; complication; cement leakage; spondylodiscitis

Citation: Cavka, M.; Delimar, D.; Rezan, R.; Zigman, T.; Duric, K.S.; Cimic, M.; Dumic-Cule, I.; Prutki, M. Complications of Percutaneous Vertebroplasty: A Pictorial Review. *Medicina* **2023**, *59*, 1536. https://doi.org/10.3390/medicina59091536

Academic Editor: Cory Xian

Received: 13 June 2023
Revised: 7 August 2023
Accepted: 24 August 2023
Published: 25 August 2023

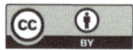

Copyright: © 2023 by the authors. Licensee MDPI, Basel, Switzerland. This article is an open access article distributed under the terms and conditions of the Creative Commons Attribution (CC BY) license (https://creativecommons.org/licenses/by/4.0/).

1. Introduction

Percutaneous vertebroplasty is a minimally invasive procedure wherein bone cement is percutaneously injected directly into a fractured vertebral body. While various types of bone cement are accessible, polymethyl methacrylate (PMMA) is the most commonly utilized and is considered a reliable stabilizing agent for vertebroplasty [1]. Some growth factors, such as bone morphogenetic proteins, have undergone preclinical testing for similar applications, suggesting a potential alternative to PMMA in the future [2–4]. Typically, this procedure is guided by fluoroscopy, although occasionally CT scans are employed for precise needle placement and post-injection monitoring.

Vertebral compression fractures arise from trauma or the weakening of the bone structure due to conditions like osteoporosis or neoplasia, which are furthermore associated with an increased morbidity and mortality [5,6]. The practice of vertebroplasty is widespread for treatments on the lumbar and thoracic spine. In contrast, cervical vertebroplasty is executed by more skilled practitioners due to the smaller size of vertebral bodies and pedicles. Percutaneous vertebroplasty is recommended for cases of osteoporotic vertebral body compression fractures that persistently exhibit symptoms despite nonsurgical interventions, as well as for pathological fractures attributed to osteolytic metastases, spinal myeloma lesions, or vascular neoplasms. Absolute contraindications include local infection and untreated hematogenous infection [1].

Complications arising from vertebroplasty are stratified according to three levels of severity. Within the realm of mild complications, there are instances of temporary exacerbation of pain and transient episodes of hypotension. Moving on to moderate complications, these encompass occurrences such as infections and the seepage of cement into foraminal, epidural, or dural space. Severe complications emerge when the extravasation of cement takes place within paravertebral veins, potentially leading to pulmonary embolism, cardiac perforation, cerebral embolism, or even fatality [7]. Factors such as cortical destruction, the presence of soft-tissue masses in the epidural region, lesions exhibiting heightened vascularity, and significant vertebral collapse collectively contribute to an elevated likelihood of encountering complications. As a result, the frequency of complications is notably higher in cases of neoplastic vertebral collapse as opposed to osteoporotic collapse [8].

In this review, based on experiences from our center, we aimed to provide useful information which included practical advice that would help primarily in preventing potential complications when performing percutaneous vertebroplasty.

2. Mild Complications

Uncommon complications of vertebroplasty include a temporary rise in pain and fever. These occurrences are attributed to an inflammatory response triggered by the heat generated during the polymerization of polymethyl methacrylate [9]. Typically, postprocedure pain is mainly linked to the fracture itself, procedural complications, or the development of a vertebral body fracture at an adjacent level. Pain existing prior to the procedure is more likely associated with alternate conditions, such as undiagnosed degenerative disk disease preceding the vertebroplasty [1]. The management of pain and fever can be effectively achieved through the use of analgesics and antipyretics [2,8].

Transient arterial hypotension is an infrequent complication with unclear pathogenic mechanisms, although some hypotheses involve potential toxicity, vasodilatation, or allergic effects of the cement or bone marrow micro-emboli. It showed a satisfactory response to supportive measures and is considered self-limiting [2,10].

Fractures of the ribs, along with potential linked radiculopathy and pneumothorax, may arise. The most significant vulnerability to intraprocedural rib fractures is observed in patients with advanced osteoporosis, where fractures develop due to downward pressure applied to the chest wall of the patient during needle insertion. Radiculopathy is generally treatable using conservative approaches involving analgesics and is typically anticipated to subside within a few months [11].

3. Extravasation of Cement

Leakage of cement is a relatively common outcome of vertebroplasty and is identified as a main contributor to complications [5,12]. This occurrence can transpire through a cortical opening into the intervertebral disc space or adjacent paravertebral soft tissues, through the paravertebral veins, via the basivertebral foramen, or along the needle channel. Factors that influence the flow of cement into or out of a vertebral body can be grouped into three categories: parameters associated with the bone and fracture, attributes of the cement itself, and aspects of the injection technique (including parameters like volume, velocity, pressure, and needle placement). The density and properties of the vertebral bone play a significant role in determining cement flow. Higher bone density and increased bone quality provide a more stable environment for cement placement and reduce the risk of leakage. Osteoporotic or severely weakened bone may have compromised structural integrity, and thereby an increased risk of cement extravasation. The type and configuration of the vertebral fracture can impact cement flow. For example, in cases of a simple compression fracture, cement tends to flow more readily into the fractured region. In complex fractures with multiple fracture lines or clefts, it may be challenging to achieve uniform cement distribution, leading to potential leakage [13]. The viscosity of the cement affects its flow characteristics. Therefore, higher viscosity may resist easy flow, requiring higher injection pressures and potentially increasing the risk of leakage. In contrast, lower viscosity cements may flow more easily but can also be associated with increased leakage risk if not controlled properly. The setting time of the cement determines the duration during which it remains injectable, while the mechanical properties of the cement, such as its elasticity and compressive strength, can impact its ability to stabilize the fractured vertebral body and resist dislodgment or fracture [14]. The volume of injected cement affects the distribution and potential leakage. Injecting an excessive volume of cement can increase the pressure within the vertebral body and lead to unwanted extravasation. The rate of cement injection and the applied pressure influence how well the cement fills the voids within the vertebral body. Thus, excessive pressure can force cement into unintended spaces, while slower injection may allow for more controlled distribution [15]. Some of these parameters have already been studied, although the interaction of cement with the structure of the vertebral body and details regarding how the cement extravasates from the vertebral body are still poorly understood [5].

The leakage of cement material into the spinal canal or neural foramen has been described as epidural leakage, a phenomenon that can manifest not only via defects in the posterior wall of the vertebrae or through the basivertebral foramina, but also through the anterior internal venous plexus. Certain observations suggest that the incidence of epidural leakage is most pronounced in the upper thoracic vertebral bodies, irrespective of the quantity of PMMA injected. When it comes to vertebroplasty procedures above the T-7 level, it is crucial that these are undertaken by a skilled and experienced specialist, given the smaller size of the vertebral bodies and pedicles [16]. The higher rate of cement extravasation is expected following administration of the larger amount of PMMA. Identifying leakage by fluoroscopy or X-ray is difficult and inter-observer agreement dependent. Therefore, a CT scan is the method of choice for precise assessment of the rate of cement extravasation and could help with detecting whether postoperative clinical symptoms are associated with leakage [12]. Most cement leakages are asymptomatic but can also cause compression and subsequently lead to a severe clinical consequence such as paraplegia, spinal cord compression, cement pulmonary embolism, and even death. Neurologic symptoms may be temporary, probably due to local inflammation, or may be caused by the direct compression by the cement [5,17]. Delayed onset of neurological symptoms, manifested as L4 radiculopathy following cement leakage, was recently reported [18].

3.1. Epidural and Foraminal Cement Leakage

Cement leakage into the foraminal or epidural spaces may lead to compromised neurological status due to spinal cord or nerve root damage, which is dependent on the volume of the leakage (Figure 1). Most cases remain clinically asymptomatic or with negligible symptoms [2].

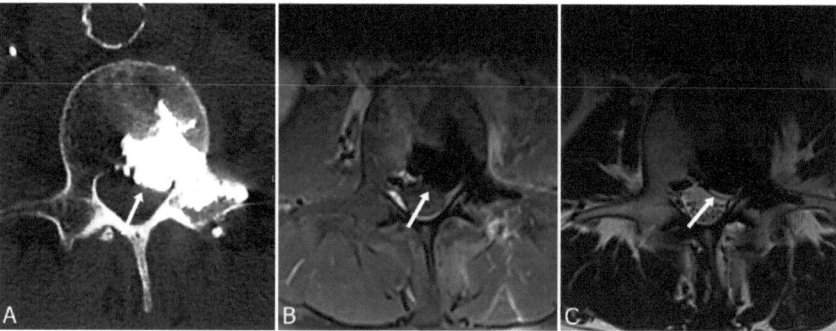

Figure 1. Cement leakage into epidural space with compression of the dural sac (arrows) seen on axial CT image (**A**), T1-weighted (**B**), and T2-weighted (**C**) MRI images, following vertebroplasty of L2 vertebrae in a 67-year-old man.

Cement leakage into the epidural space can be classified into three distinct categories: type B entails leakage via the basivertebral vein, type S involves the segmental vein route, and type C arises through a cortical breach. Leaks of type B originate from the vascular foramen and advance into the spinal canal, disseminating along the epidural venous plexus.

Type S leaks usually follow a horizontal trajectory, tracing alongside the segmental veins. On the other hand, type C leakage emerges from a cortical disruption encircling a vertebral body, potentially extending into the spinal canal (refer to Figure 2) [19].

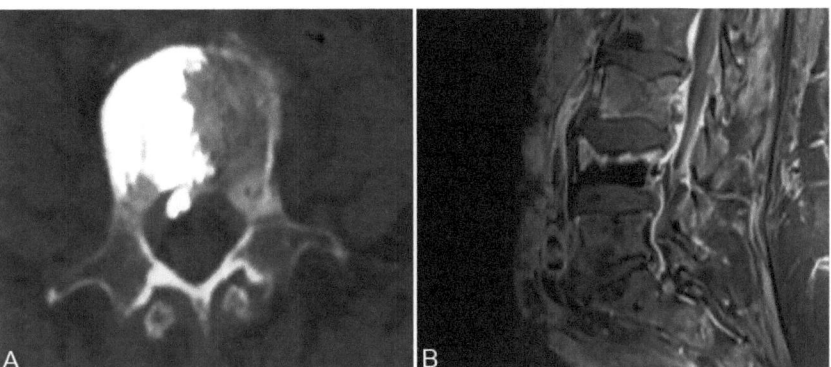

Figure 2. Axial CT image (**A**) and T2 weighted sagittal MRI image (**B**) show discrete intraspinal bone cement leakage.

3.2. New Vertebral Fractures

Leakage of cement into the intervertebral disc space during vertebroplasty increases the risk of subsequent fractures in neighboring vertebral bodies. Hence, it is recommended to position the needle laterally and away from the vertebra's central axis, especially in cases of fractures located at the vertebra's center. Moreover, adjustments to the cement's viscosity and volume are advisable to enhance its consistency and reduce the likelihood of leakage [2]. It is vital to highlight that the literature lacks a prospective randomized study on the occurrence of new vertebral fractures in osteoporotic patients with vertebral collapses, comparing those treated with vertebroplasty with those treated with conservative management [7]. Some researchers have concluded that adjacent-level fractures subsequent to vertebroplasty are more likely attributable to underlying osteoporosis rather than the procedure itself [1].

3.3. Paravertebral Soft Tissue Leakage

Cement leakage into the paravertebral soft tissues typically lacks clinical significance. Such leakage might stem from preexisting cortical damage or from the cortical breach occurring during the biopsy preceding the vertebroplasty (see Figure 3) [7]. While instances are infrequent, there have been reports of temporary femoral neuropathy and instances requiring surgical removal of cement deposited within the paravertebral soft tissues [11].

3.4. Venous System Cement Leakage and Pulmonary Embolism

Leakage was more frequently observed within the perivertebral venous plexus in comparison to the nearby intervertebral discs or the surrounding soft tissues (see Figure 3). The venous network traversing the vertebral column consists of three primary interconnected systems: the internal venous plexus, the external venous plexus, and the basivertebral system. Originating within the anterior one-third of the vertebral body, the basivertebral veins converge towards the posterior region, where they drain into the anterior part of the internal venous plexus. In the anterior area, these basivertebral veins merge with the external plexus. Positioned on the dorsal surface of the vertebral body, the exit point of the basivertebral vein lies centrally between the pedicles. The anterior component of the internal venous plexus empties into the segmental veins, which exit the spinal canal through the foramen located between the nerve root and the medial aspect of the pedicles. This implies a direct venous link connecting the bone marrow with the foraminal space [20].

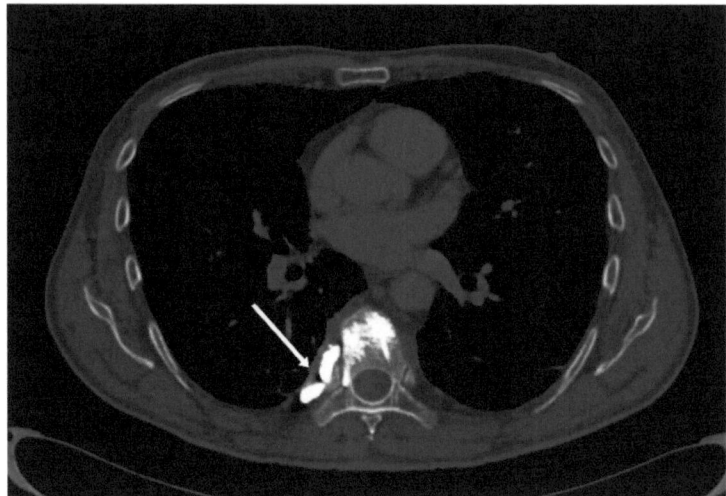

Figure 3. Cement leakage into the right subpleural space following vertebroplasty of Th8 vertebra (arrow).

Three mechanisms are considered responsible for cement embolism following vertebroplasty: insufficient polymerization of the polymethylmethacrylate at the time of its injection, incorrect needle positioning at the time of cement injection, and overfilling of the vertebral body with cement, resulting in cement migration into the venous system [21]. If the cement is inadequately polymerized at the time of injection, it may remain partially liquid or have a semi-solid consistency. This increases the risk of leakage from the vertebral body, allowing cement to enter the surrounding blood vessels leading to potential complications due to emboli. It is important for medical professionals to ensure proper preparation and polymerization of the PMMA bone cement before injection. This may involve thorough mixing of the cement components, appropriate timing to allow for complete polymerization, and adherence to established procedural guidelines to minimize the chances of complications like cement embolisms [22].

The only sign that can predict the development of a pulmonary cement embolism is fluoroscopic evidence of cement leakage to the azygos vein or vena cava during vertebroplasty (Figures 4 and 5). Bone cement extravasates toward the vertebral venous plexus which is connected to the azygos system by which it reaches the inferior vena cava, the right cardiac chamber, and finally the pulmonary arterial system which may lead to a potentially fatal pulmonary embolism [23,24].

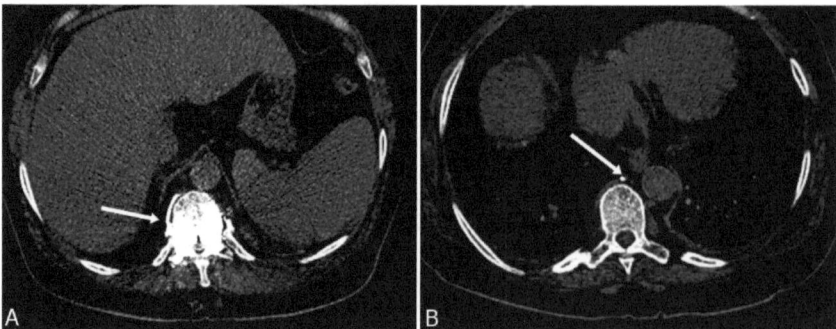

Figure 4. Axial CT scan of a 64-year-old woman following vertebroplasty of Th12 vertebrae with an arrow pointing to a cement leak into the paravertebral venous system (**A**). Cement can be seen in the azygos vein (**B**). Patient remained asymptomatic and late cement migration during follow-up did not occur.

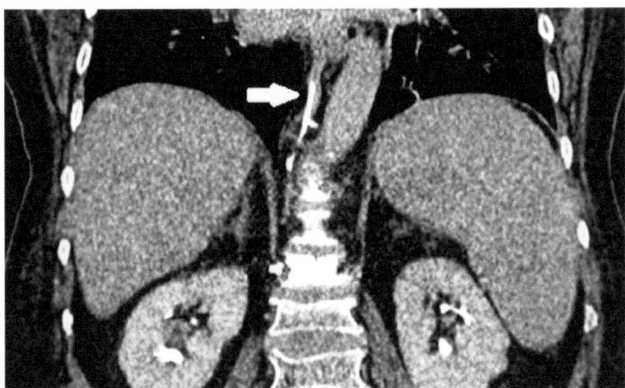

Figure 5. Sagittal CT scan of the same patient. Cement can be seen in the azygos vein (arrow).

A symptomatic pulmonary embolism following vertebroplasty can manifest through either the migration of cement or the migration of fat and bone marrow cells. The majority of instances involving radiologically identified PMMA migration into lung vessels demonstrate no symptoms. In this context, occurrences of fat tissue embolisms tend to surpass those of PMMA embolisms [25]. Clinical indications of a pulmonary cement embolism encompass the abrupt onset of dyspnea, tachypnea, tachycardia, cyanosis, chest pain, cough, hemoptysis, and perspiration following vertebroplasty. Despite the initial lack of symptoms in numerous cases, many cement emboli are fortuitously identified during subsequent imaging assessments [24]. It is imperative to initiate early detection and prompt management even in the absence of clinical signs. Should respiratory symptoms emerge post vertebroplasty, a meticulous evaluation for potential pulmonary cement embolism is warranted [23,24]. In situations where the cement advances into the right ventricle, yet proves too lengthy and rigid to traverse the pulmonary artery, it may lodge in the heart and give rise to cardiac perforation—a truly uncommon complication of vertebroplasty, with only a single case documented in the literature. This particular case was potentially fatal due to hemopericardium and tamponade [2,26]. Instances of cerebral embolus have also been reported, with reports attributing them to fat emboli originating from heightened intramedullary pressure during the cementation process [2,27].

4. Infection

While percutaneous vertebroplasty is a procedure known for its minimal invasiveness, there remains a risk of postprocedural infection, a concern inherent to any percutaneous intervention [28]. Reported infections encompass discitis, osteomyelitis, and potentially epidural infections. The etiology of spondylitis following vertebroplasty can be categorized into three primary groups: preexisting spondylitis, infection triggered by the procedure itself, and infection originating from hematogenous seeding. Infections occurring shortly after the procedure could arise from performing the intervention on an already infected vertebra, perhaps misdiagnosed as an osteoporotic fracture, particularly in cases of conditions like tuberculosis, or on fractured vertebrae coexisting with spondylitis. When an infection occurs within a two-month timeframe, preexisting spondylitis and procedure-induced infection should be considered. In scenarios where the interval between the procedure and the occurrence of infection is brief, the likelihood of preexisting spondylitis is higher than infection caused by the procedure (see Figure 6). Although hematogenous seeding-induced infection can also result in early infection, it predominantly leads to late-onset infections [29,30].

Prevention of infection following vertebroplasty includes preoperative routine checks of inflammatory parameters (C-reactive protein and white blood cell count) and MRI. Enhanced MRI should be performed if inflammatory markers are elevated with suspected infection. For patients with any type of acute infection, the procedure should be delayed until the infection improves and inflammatory parameters decrease. Therefore, a one- to two-weeks window period of conservative management is suggested before the cement augmentation procedure, to exclude infection in patients with an acute compression fracture and elevated inflammatory parameters [29,30].

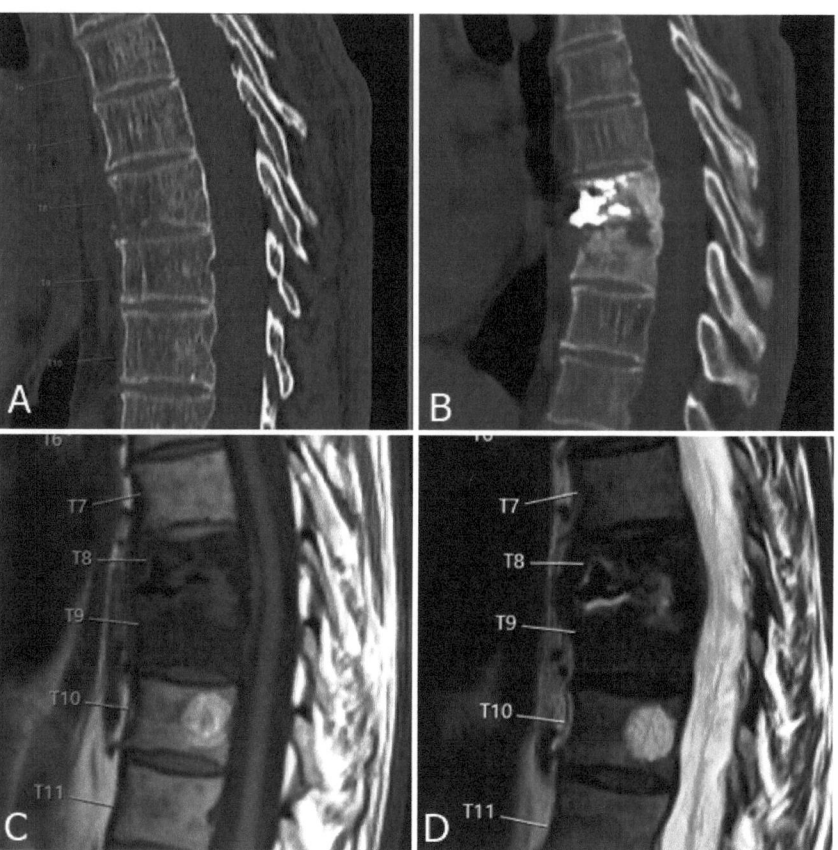

Figure 6. (**A**) CT scan of the thoracic spine of a 59-year-old man shows infiltration of the Th8 vertebral body by a neoplastic process. Biopsy and vertebroplasty were performed. Three months after procedure, the patient was presenting with new severe back pain and high C-reactive protein tests. CT shows the loss of intervertebral disc space height and bony destruction of Th8 and Th9 vertebrae (**B**). Bony destruction and low signal in disc space and adjacent endplates can be seen on T1-weighted images (**C**), as well as high signal in disc space and adjacent endplates on T2-weighted images (**D**), consistent with fluid in disc space and bone marrow oedema, all suggesting advanced spondylodiscitis.

In the case of immunocompromised patients with comorbidities, conservative treatment could lead to better outcomes than cement augmentation. For high-risk patients, some authors recommended the routine addition of tobramycin to the cement, while others suggested usage of perioperative intravenous prophylactic antibiotics. When infection occurred due to vertebroplasty/kyphoplasty surgical debridement, stabilization is the method of choice. However, a considerable number of studies reported that conservative treatment with antibiotics may cure an infection of PMMA in the vertebrae [29].

5. Reducing the Risk and Effects of Complications

In order to avoid complications, procedure technique should allow access through the transpedicular route in the lumbar spine and via the costovertebral junction in the thoracic spine, thereby avoiding a cortical breach when possible. Opacification of cement should be optimized by following the manufacturer recommendations, not exceeding recommended proportions of powder and liquid polymer, and defining the optimal cement viscosity before injection. If cement leakage occurs, termination of the procedure is recommended [11]. A preoperative check of inflammatory parameters and MRI should be mandatory. Persistent severe pain, new severe pain of a different character, signs of spinal canal stenosis, or sudden onset of respiratory symptoms should be sent to emergency diagnostics to exclude complications and start treatment if necessary [1,23,24].

Outpatient clinic follow-up should occur two to four weeks post procedure when the patient should again be assessed for signs of procedural complications. Subsequent follow-up appointments may take place if indicated [1].

6. Discussion

Vertebroplasty is a potentially life-changing procedure for individuals suffering from vertebral compression fractures, osteoporosis, neoplasia, and other bone-structure-weakening conditions. However, complications can arise from the procedure, ranging from mild and temporary side effects to more severe and potentially life-threatening ones. Mild complications may include a temporary increase in pain and hypotension. Moderate complications may involve infection and cement extravasation into the foraminal, epidural, or dural space. Lastly, severe complications include instances of cement extravasation into paravertebral veins and can result in pulmonary embolism, cardiac perforation, and cerebral embolism, which can be fatal [7]. Pulmonary cement embolism is dependent on a number of factors such as affected vertebrae, lesion localization, and puncture method, which are understood as separate risk factors. Surgeons should take these factors into account when devising treatment approaches [31].

7. Conclusions

It is important for clinicians to obtain a clear understanding of the patient's condition before performing the procedure, as well as to be vigilant in following proper protocols during the procedure. Additionally, utilizing a combination of fluoroscopy and CT for needle positioning and injection assessment is also recommended. In conclusion, while vertebroplasty is an effective procedure for treating vertebral compression fractures, it is also important to be aware of the potential complications and take necessary precautions to reduce risks. Percutaneous vertebroplasty is considered a safe and effective option in the management of vertebral fractures. Although the majority of complications following percutaneous vertebroplasty are asymptomatic, serious complications can occur, which is why careful and precise techniques should be executed during the procedure to minimize the risk.

Author Contributions: Conceptualization, M.C. (Mislav Cavka) and M.P.; Methodology, M.C. (Mislav Cavka) and R.R.; Software, R.R.; Formal Analysis, R.R., M.C. (Mislav Cavka) and K.S.D.; Investigation, M.C. (Mislav Cavka), I.D.-C. and M.C. (Mislav Cimic); Resources, D.D.; Data Curation, M.C. (Mislav Cavka), T.Z. and I.D.-C.; Writing—Original Draft Preparation, M.C. (Mislav Cavka), T.Z. and M.C. (Mislav Cimic); Writing—Review and Editing, M.P.; Visualization, D.D.; Supervision, M.P. All authors have read and agreed to the published version of the manuscript.

Funding: This research received no external funding.

Institutional Review Board Statement: This cross-sectional study was granted approval by the institutional review board, which waived the requirement for informed consent due to usage of data from electronic health records without using the patient's identity.

Informed Consent Statement: Not applicable.

Data Availability Statement: Data used for analysis are contained within the article.

Conflicts of Interest: The authors declare no conflict of interest.

References

1. Beall, D.P.; Brook, A.L.; Chambers, M.R.; Hirsch, J.A.; Kelekis, A.; Kim, Y.C.; Kreiner, S.; Murphy, K. Vertebral Augmentation: The Comprehensive Guide to Vertebroplasty, Kyphoplasty and Implant Augmentation. *Thieme* **2020**. [CrossRef]
2. Bai, B.; Yin, Z.; Xu, Q.; Lew, M.; Chen, Y.; Ye, J.; Wu, J.; Chen, D.; Zeng, Y. Histological changes of an injectable rhBMP-2/calcium phosphate cement in vertebroplasty of rhesus monkey. *Spine* **2009**, *34*, 1887–1892. [CrossRef] [PubMed]
3. Vukicevic, S.; Oppermann, H.; Verbanac, D.; Jankolija, M.; Popek, I.; Curak, J.; Brkljacic, J.; Pauk, M.; Erjavec, I.; Francetic, I.; et al. The clinical use of bone morphogenetic proteins revisited: A novel biocompatible carrier device OSTEOGROW for bone healing. *Int. Orthop.* **2014**, *38*, 635–647. [CrossRef] [PubMed]
4. Grgurevic, L.; Erjavec, I.; Gupta, M.; Pecin, M.; Bordukalo-Niksic, T.; Stokovic, N.; Vnuk, D.; Farkas, V.; Capak, H.; Milosevic, M.; et al. Autologous blood coagulum containing rhBMP6 induces new bone formation to promote anterior lumbar interbody fusion (ALIF) and posterolateral lumbar fusion (PLF) of spine in sheep. *Bone* **2020**, *138*, 115448. [CrossRef] [PubMed]
5. Carli, D.; Venmans, A.; Lodder, P.; Donga, E.; van Oudheusden, T.; Boukrab, I.; Schoemaker, K.; Smeets, A.; Schonenberg, C.; Hirsch, J.; et al. Vertebroplasty versus Active Control Intervention for Chronic Osteoporotic Vertebral Compression Fractures: The VERTOS V Randomized Controlled Trial. *Radiology* **2023**, *308*, e222535. [CrossRef]
6. Gu, Y.F.; Li, Y.D.; Wu, C.G.; Sun, Z.K.; He, C.J. Safety and efficacy of percutaneous vertebroplasty and interventional tumor removal for metastatic spinal tumors and malignant vertebral compression fractures. *AJR Am. J. Roentgenol.* **2014**, *202*, W298–W305. [CrossRef]
7. Al-Nakshabandi, N.A. Percutaneous vertebroplasty complications. *Ann. Saudi Med.* **2011**, *31*, 294–297. [CrossRef]
8. Laredo, J.D.; Hamze, B. Complications of percutaneous vertebroplasty and their prevention. *Semin. Ultrasound CT MR* **2005**, *26*, 65–80. [CrossRef]
9. Cotten, A.; Boutry, N.; Cortet, B.; Assaker, R.; Demondion, X.; Leblond, D.; Chastanet, P.; Duquesnoy, B.; Deramond, H. Percutanous Vertebroplasty: State of art. *RadioGraphics* **1998**, *18*, 311–320. [CrossRef]
10. Vasconcelos, C.; Gailloud, P.; Martin, J.B.; Murphy, K.J. Transient arterial hypotension induced by polymethylmethacrylate injection during percutaneous vertebroplasty. *J. Vasc. Interv. Radiol.* **2001**, *12*, 1001–1002. [CrossRef]
11. Heran, M.K.; Legiehn, G.M.; Munk, P.L. Current concepts and techniques in percutaneous vertebroplasty. *Orthop. Clin. N. Am.* **2006**, *37*, 409–434. [CrossRef] [PubMed]
12. Schmidt, R.; Cakir, B.; Mattes, T.; Wegener, M.; Puhl, W.; Richter, M. Cement leakage during vertebroplasty: An underestimated problem? *Eur. Spine J.* **2005**, *14*, 466–473. [CrossRef]
13. Tang, B.; Xu, S.; Chen, X.; Cui, L.; Wang, Y.; Yan, X.; Liu, Y. The impact of intravertebral cleft on cement leakage in percutaneous vertebroplasty for osteoporotic vertebral compression fractures: A case-control study. *BMC Musculoskelet. Disord.* **2021**, *22*, 805. [CrossRef] [PubMed]
14. Jin, Y.J.; Yoon, S.H.; Park, K.W.; Chung, S.K.; Kim, K.J.; Yeom, J.S.; Kim, H.J. The volumetric analysis of cement in vertebroplasty: Relationship with clinical outcome and complications. *Spine* **2011**, *36*, E761–E772. [CrossRef] [PubMed]
15. Chen, Y.; Zhang, H.; Chen, H.; Ou, Z.; Fu, Y.; Zhang, J. Comparison of the effectiveness and safety of unilateral and bilateral percutaneous vertebroplasty for osteoporotic vertebral compression fractures: A protocol for systematic review and meta-analysis. *Medicine* **2021**, *100*, e28453. [CrossRef] [PubMed]
16. Ryu, K.S.; Park, C.K.; Kim, M.C.; Kang, J.K. Dose-dependent epidural leakage of polymethylmethacrylate after percutaneous vertebroplasty in patients with osteoporotic vertebral compression fractures. *J. Neurosurg.* **2002**, *96*, 56–61. [CrossRef]
17. Lador, R.; Dreiangel, N.; Ben-Galim, P.J.; Hipp, J.A. A pictorial classification atlas of cement extravasation with vertebral augmentation. *Spine J.* **2010**, *10*, 1118–1127. [CrossRef]
18. Jing, Z.; Li, L.; Shang, Y. Delayed neurological deficits caused by cement extravasation following vertebroplasty: A case report. *J. Int. Med. Res.* **2021**, *49*, 3000605211019664. [CrossRef]
19. Yeom, J.S.; Kim, W.J.; Choy, W.S.; Lee, C.K.; Chang, B.S.; Kang, J.W. Leakage of cement in percutaneous transpedicular vertebroplasty for painful osteoporotic compression fractures. *J. Bone Jt. Surg. Br.* **2003**, *85*, 83–89. [CrossRef]
20. Venmans, A.; Klazen, C.A.; van Rooij, W.J.; de Vries, J.; Mali, W.P.; Lohle, P.N. Postprocedural CT for perivertebral cement leakage in percutaneous vertebroplasty is not necessary--results from VERTOS II. *Neuroradiology* **2011**, *53*, 19–22. [CrossRef]
21. Kao, F.C.; Tu, Y.K.; Lai, P.L.; Yu, S.W.; Yen, C.Y.; Chou, M.C. Inferior vena cava syndrome following percutaneous vertebroplasty with polymethylmethacrylate. *Spine* **2008**, *33*, E329–E333. [CrossRef] [PubMed]
22. Mo, L.; Wu, Z.; Liang, D.; Cai, Z.; Huang, J.; Lin, S.; Cui, J.; Zhang, S.; Yang, Z.; Yao, Z.; et al. Influence of bone cement distribution on outcomes following percutaneous vertebroplasty: A retrospective matched-cohort study. *J. Int. Med. Res.* **2021**, *49*, 3000605211022287. [CrossRef]
23. Zhao, Z.; Qin, D.; Zhao, W. Asymptomatic cement leakage into inferior vena cava. *QJM* **2022**, *115*, 49–50. [CrossRef] [PubMed]
24. Toru, Ü.; Coşkun, T.; Acat, M.; Onaran, H.; Gül, Ş.; Çetinkaya, E. Pulmonary Cement Embolism following Percutaneous Vertebroplasty. *Case Rep. Pulmonol.* **2014**, *2014*, 851573. [CrossRef] [PubMed]
25. Hsieh, M.K.; Kao, F.C.; Chiu, P.Y.; Chen, L.H.; Yu, C.W.; Niu, C.C.; Lai, P.L.; Tsai, T.T. Risk factors of neurological deficit and pulmonary cement embolism after percutaneous vertebroplasty. *J. Orthop. Surg. Res.* **2019**, *14*, 406. [CrossRef]
26. Kim, S.Y.; Seo, J.B.; Do, K.H.; Lee, J.S.; Song, K.S.; Lim, T.H. Cardiac perforation caused by acrylic cement: A rare complication of percutaneous vertebroplasty. *Am. J. Roentgenol.* **2005**, *185*, 1245–1247. [CrossRef]

27. Edmonds, C.R.; Barbut, D.; Hager, D.; Sharrock, N.E. Intraoperative cerebral arterial embolization during total hip arthroplasty. *Anesthesiology* **2000**, *93*, 315–318. [CrossRef]
28. Kovacevic, L.; Cavka, M.; Marusic, Z.; Kresic, E.; Stajduhar, A.; Grbanovic, L.; Dumic-Cule, I.; Prutki, M. Percutaneous CT-Guided Bone Lesion Biopsy for Confirmation of Bone Metastases in Patients with Breast Cancer. *Diagnostics* **2022**, *12*, 2094. [CrossRef]
29. Park, J.W.; Park, S.M.; Lee, H.J.; Lee, C.K.; Chang, B.S.; Kim, H. Infection following percutaneous vertebral augmentation with polymethylmethacrylate. *Arch. Osteoporos.* **2018**, *13*, 47. [CrossRef]
30. Vats, H.S.; McKiernan, F.E. Infected vertebroplasty: Case report and review of literature. *Spine* **2006**, *31*, E859–E862. [CrossRef]
31. Wang, L.; Lu, M.; Zhang, X.; Zhao, Z.; Li, X.; Liu, T.; Xu, L.; Yu, S. Risk factors for pulmonary cement embolism after percutaneous vertebroplasty and radiofrequency ablation for spinal metastases. *Front. Oncol.* **2023**, *13*, 1129658. [CrossRef] [PubMed]

Disclaimer/Publisher's Note: The statements, opinions and data contained in all publications are solely those of the individual author(s) and contributor(s) and not of MDPI and/or the editor(s). MDPI and/or the editor(s) disclaim responsibility for any injury to people or property resulting from any ideas, methods, instructions or products referred to in the content.

Review

Total Talar Prosthesis, Learning from Experience, Two Reports of Total Talar Prosthesis after Talar Extrusion and Literature Review

Danilo Leonetti [1], Giorgio Carmelo Basile [1,*], Gabriele Giuca [2], Elena Corso [2], Domenico Fenga [1] and Ilaria Sanzarello [1]

[1] Department of Biomedical, Dental and Morphological and Functional Images, University of Messina, 98122 Messina, Italy; d.leonetti@unime.it (D.L.); dfenga@unime.it (D.F.); i.sanzarello@unime.it (I.S.)

[2] Department of Human Pathology of Adult and Developmental Age "Gaetano Barresi", Faculty of Medicine and Surgery, University of Messina, 98122 Messina, Italy; gabgiuca@unime.it (G.G.); elenacorso14@gmail.com (E.C.)

* Correspondence: giorgio.b30397@gmail.com

Abstract: Recently, total talar prosthesis has been proposed to substitute the talus during the management of complex talar lesions such as talar extrusion, comminuted talar fractures, or avascular necrosis. Herein, we report two cases of talar extrusion treated with total talar replacement after a high-intensity trauma. Both cases subsequently required revision surgery due to degenerative changes of the tibial plafond (arthrodesis in the first case, conversion to a total ankle prosthesis in the latter). We report and analyze the literature concerning total talar replacement to discuss strategies that could help improve prosthesis survival and reduce the incidence of osteoarthritis.

Keywords: custom made prosthesis; talar avascular necrosis; talar enucleation; talar extrusion; total talar prosthesis

1. Introduction

In the last three decades, technical and technological advances have allowed surgeons to benefit from a variety of new options to manage complex lesions. Advances such as 3D printing allowed for the re-creation of anatomical structures with custom-made prostheses [1]. In recent years, total talar replacement (TTR) has been proposed as a treatment for complex talar injuries. Talar lesions (such as high-grade avascular necrosis, comminuted fractures, and severe osteoarthritis) represent a challenge for the orthopedic surgeon. Current management options are often burdened by unsatisfactory functional outcomes: Ankle arthrodesis, the most adopted, guarantees pain reduction and stability but can nevertheless lead to dysmetria and secondary osteoarthritis at the adjacent joints. External fixation methods are also associated with a high rate of nonunion and infection, while internal fixation and minimally invasive surgeries account for these complications [2,3].

In 2007, Stevens et al. introduced the so-called third-generation talar prosthesis, reproducing anatomically the talus in its entirety, namely, the TTR [4]. TTR can be isolated or, if the talar prosthesis articulates with a distal tibial component, combined. Combined TTR is conceptually a total ankle replacement with a total talar prosthesis.

Talar extrusion—also known as talar enucleation/missing talus—stands out as one of the rarest and more complex talar injuries. It consists of the complete dislocation of the talus from the tibiotalar, talocalcaneal, and talonavicular joints [5], usually following a forced tibiotalar plantar flexion combined with excessive supination. It is determined by high-energy trauma and has been described 91 times in the literature [6–14]. Due to their peculiar and limited blood supply, talar dislocations are difficult to treat: Re-implantation of the extruded talus is possible but frequently presents fearsome complications such as avascular necrosis, infections, and osteoarthritis [7,8,15]. Historically, primary talectomy or (in selected patients) tibio-calcaneal arthrodesis with the Blair fusion technique was taken into account, although it was burdened by a high rate of complications and reduced functional outcomes, such as loss of function of the peri-talar joints, shortening of the injured leg, and the frequent insurgence of secondary degenerative changes [7,15,16].

As follows, we present, respectively, two cases of talar extrusion treated with custom-made total talar replacement (TTR). Both cases required revision surgery at the 2-year follow-up due to degenerative changes of the tibial plafond (arthrodesis in the first case, conversion to a total ankle prosthesis in the latter). We reviewed the literature regarding TTR. We discussed potential indications of TTR, benefits and drawbacks, and the most common causes of implant failure and surgical revision.

2. Cases Presentation

2.1. Case 1

2.1.1. Talar Extrusion

A 27-year-old male patient suffered a road accident in September 2013, reporting a superficial traumatic head injury and a left fibular fracture with an open wound and complete enucleation of the left talus. The missing talus was collected: It presented minor osteochondral injuries in the medial part and macroscopic contamination but was not fractured. After primary care, the wound on the foot and ankle was washed and debrided, and an antibiotic-coated cement spacer was applied to fill the void left by the talar enucleation (Figure 1). The fibula was stabilized using K-wires, and an external fixator was applied to maintain the stability of the ankle. The talar void was filled by a gentamicin/clindamycin-loaded cement spacer (Figure 1).

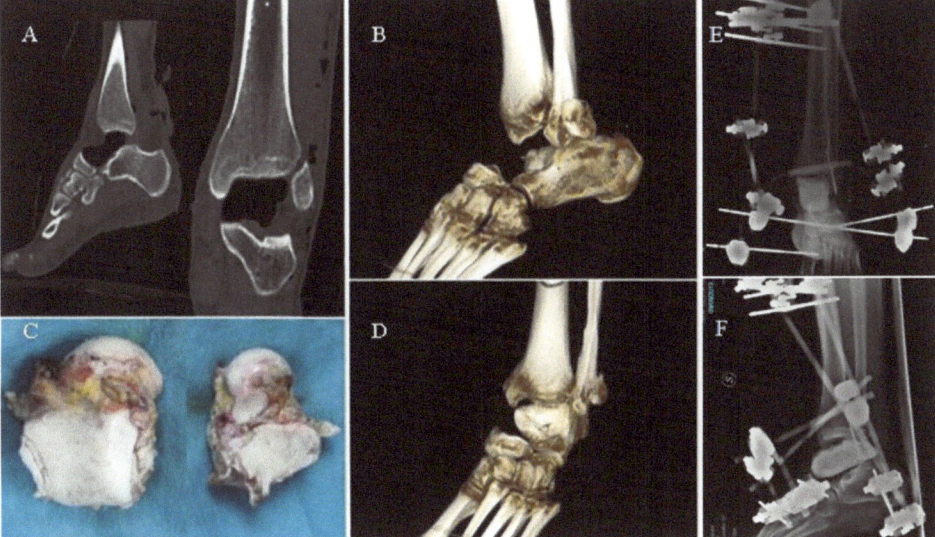

Figure 1. CT images (**A**) and volume rendering (**B**,**D**) showing the gap left by the talus (**C**). External fixation of the ankle joint (**E**,**F**).

2.1.2. Failure of Talar Reimplantation

The extruded talus was sent to the Musculoskeletal Tissue Bank of the Rizzoli Institute (Bologna), where it underwent cleaning and sterilization by gamma irradiation. After 21 days, cement was removed and the original talus was implanted with an anterior approach and a subtalar arthrodesis (Figure 2), as described by Vaienti et al. [15].

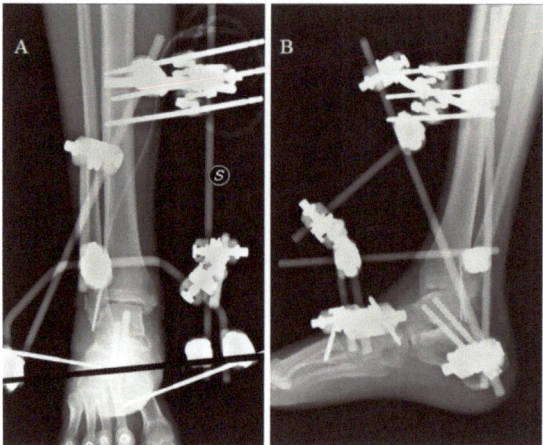

Figure 2. Talar reimplantation with subtalar arthrodesis: anteroposterior (**A**) and latero-lateral (**B**) X-ray.

Post-operative recovery was uneventful. After two months, the patient started to complain of ankle pain and swelling: Single-photon emission computed tomography (SPECT-CT) confirmed the clinical suspicion of a deep tissue infection involving the reimplanted talus (Figure 3). The talus was removed and replaced by a new spacer in antibiotic-coated cement. A negative pressure treatment was applied to facilitate soft tissue healing.

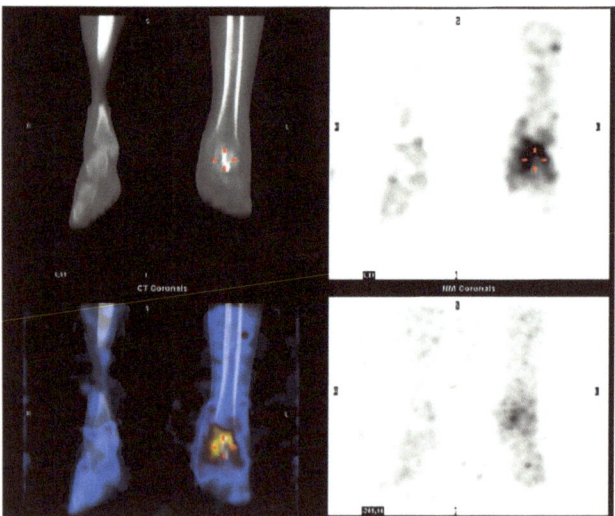

Figure 3. SPECT CT suggesting a deep tissue infection of the reimplanted talus. Red hyphens point out the site of infection.

2.1.3. Total Talar Replacement

After the failure of re-implantation, two therapeutic options (arthrodesis and TTR) were presented to the patient. The patient agreed to undergo the implantation of a talar prosthesis. The prosthesis was made by 3D printing the mirrored CT scan of the contralateral talus. The customized implant was produced by casting a chromium-cobalt alloy (Sintac Srl, Trento, Italy). The talar prosthesis was manufactured using state-of-the-art laser technology by powder melting a cobalt-chromium alloy (nickel, beryllium, and cadmium free, according to standard DIN-EN-ISO 22674:2006) and included porous articular surfaces and a talar-navicular component with two channels to host the lag screws for subtalar fixation. The implant weight was 390 g. In May 2014, after complete healing of the soft tissues, the customized talar prosthesis was implanted: After an anterior-medial approach, the spacer in antibiotic-coated cement was exposed and removed. A thorough soft tissue debridement was performed, and the articular cartilage was removed from the subtalar calcaneal surface. Subsequently, the tailor-made talar prosthesis was implanted and fixed to the calcaneus by two screws (Figure 4).

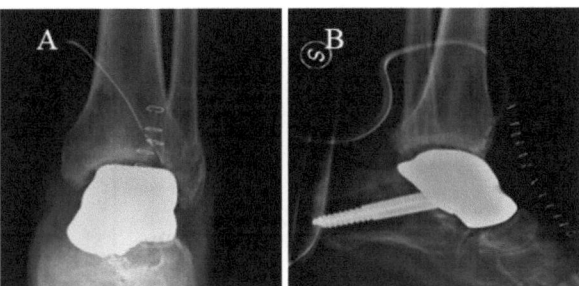

Figure 4. Total talar replacement with subtalar fixation, post-operatory anteroposterior (**A**) and latero-lateral (**B**) X-ray.

Percutaneous Achilles tendon lengthening was performed to improve ankle dorsiflexion. After surgery, a plaster cast was applied for 3 weeks. After 3 weeks, partial weight bearing was allowed, with full weight bearing within 9 weeks of surgery. We decided to examine the patient at 1, 2, 4, 6, and 12 months after surgery, and then once a year (Figure 5). The patient was satisfied with the outcome of the surgery and showed good functional results: At 6 months, he presented an AOFAS (American Orthopedic Foot and Ankle Society Score) of 86 and an NRS (Numeric Rating Scale) of 2. The sagittal range of motion (ROM) was >30°. The patient satisfaction as well as the clinical scores were retained at the 12-month follow-up.

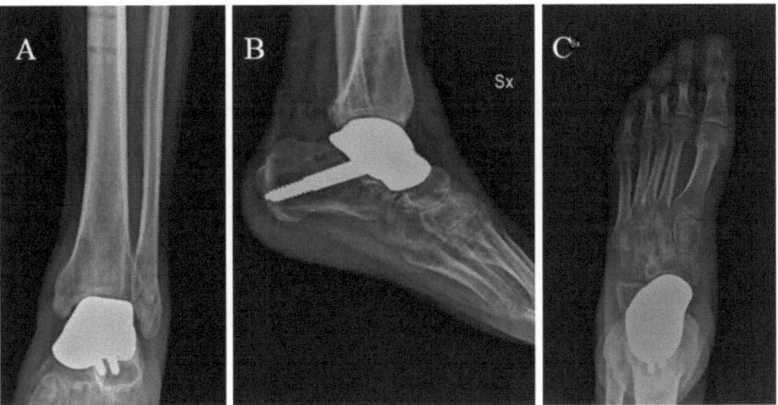

Figure 5. Anterior-posterior (**A**), dorsoplantar (**B**) and latero-lateral (**C**) projections showing the implant at the 6-month follow-up after surgery.

2.1.4. Tibial Osteoarthritis and Arthrodesis

The patient started to complain of pain and functional limitations 24 months after surgery. At the physical exam, the patient presented a limp, and passive ROM on the sagittal plane was reduced to 20°. Ankle X-ray in latero-lateral view revealed osteoarthritic changes with osteophytes and sclerosis of the tibial subchondral bone.

We proposed a tibial resurfacing, but the patient preferred a triple arthrodesis. Via anterior-medial access, the prosthesis was removed, and a fusion of the ankle, subtalar, and talo-navicular joint was performed with the use of a bone graft (Figure 6). At the last follow-up, 5 years after surgery, the patient was pain-free, wore normal shoes, and walked with a very slight limp. The AOFAS score was 81.

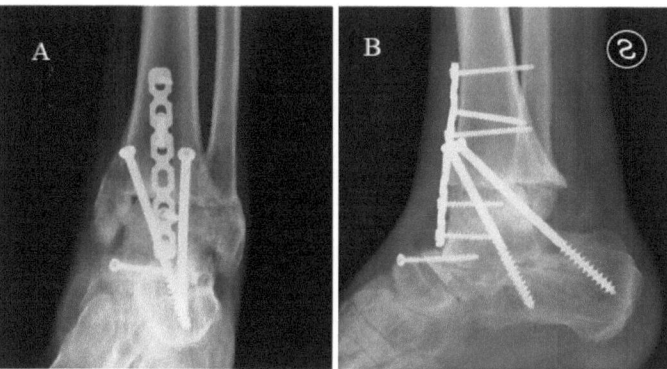

Figure 6. X-ray in anterior posterior (**A**) and latero-lateral (**B**) projections showing the tibio-calcaneal arthrodesis.

2.2. Case 2

2.2.1. Talar Extrusion

In June 2015, a 32-year-old male pilot was the victim of a plane crash, suffering from L2, L3, and L4 amyelic vertebral fractures, a fracture of the right ulna, a comminuted tibial plateau fracture of the right knee, a fracture of the 5th metatarsal bone of the right foot, and a Gustilo Anderson III C open fracture of the right ankle with complete enucleation of the talus, severe capsule-ligamentous lesion, and a tear of the extensor digitorum longus tendon and tibialis anterior artery. The patient underwent primary care, diagnostic investigations, and primary surgery. Approximately 6 h after the admission to the emergency room, the patient underwent surgical lavage and debridement of the ankle injury site with the application of an antibiotic-coated cement spacer. The ankle was stabilized by an external fixator. Meanwhile, the extruded talus was collected and sent to the Musculoskeletal Tissue Bank of the Rizzoli Institute (Bologna) for decontamination. Microbiological analysis revealed severe contamination by filamentous fungi and bacteria; thus, the infective risk for reimplantation was deemed too high (Figure 7).

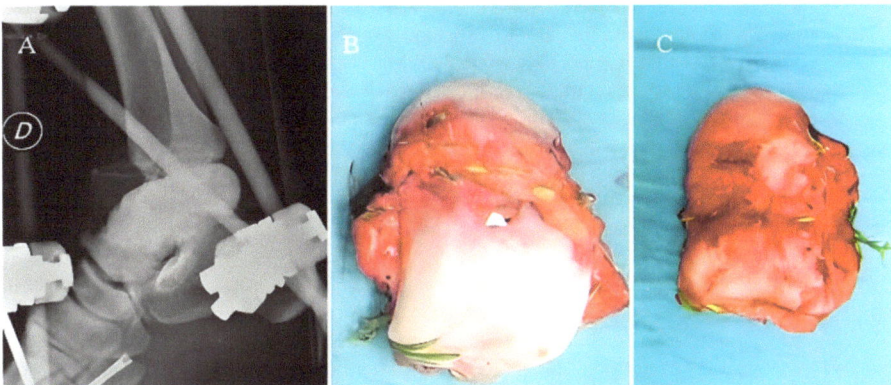

Figure 7. Latero-lateral ankle radiograph (**A**) shows the placement of the cement spacer and the ankle stabilized by external fixation. The talus as it appeared right after being collected from the site of the plane crush: a severe macroscopic contamination can be observed (**B**,**C**).

2.2.2. Total Talar Replacement

A TTR was planned and realized by the Canary Islands Institute of Technology as an exact reproduction of the shape and size of the original talus. A CT scan and volume rendering of the enucleated talus was sent to the institute, where the artificial talus was created by electron beam melting (EBM ARCAM S12, Arcam AB, Mölndal, Sweden). Electron beam melting is a 3D printing process effective and validated for the production of titanium orthopedic implants) [17].

The prosthetic implant was made of trabecular titanium Ti6Al4V, weighing only 78 g, with smooth and chrome-covered tibial, fibular, and navicular joint surfaces. The calcaneal surface was kept porous to ensure the best adhesion of the talo-calcaneal surfaces.

Four channels were carved at the level of the talus neck to fit the screws and allow ligament reconstruction. Two months after the accident, the prosthetic replacement and ligament reconstruction was finally performed by exposing the cement spacer through an anteromedial longitudinal approach. After cement removal, a customized guide was used to prepare the upper surface of the calcaneal bone according to preoperative planning. The talar prosthesis was fixed to the calcaneus by two screws. Antero-medial capsule-ligamentous reconstruction was performed using a peroneus brevis tendon allograft inserted at the level of the talus foramen and stabilized at the tibial level with a transosseous tunnel and Soft Tissue Anchoring System (CONMED) (Figure 8).

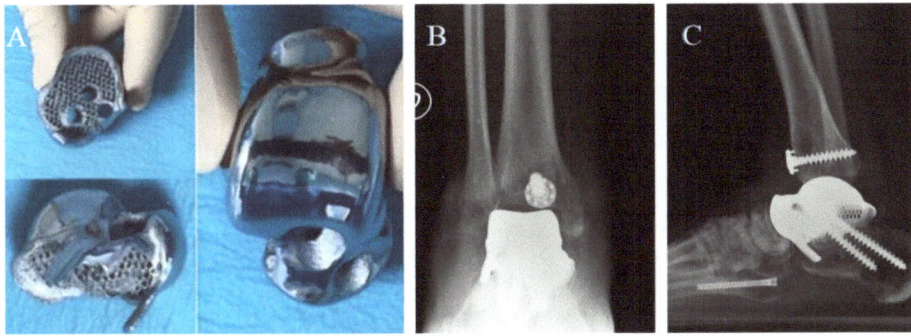

Figure 8. The prosthesis ready to be implanted (**A**). X-ray of the implant from antero-posterior (**B**) and latero-lateral (**C**) projections. Articular space can be observed in figure (**B**).

After surgery, the ankle was immobilized in a plaster cast for 3 weeks. At 6 weeks, the patient started gait re-education with progressive weight bearing and a bivalve brace. In 12 weeks, the patient started walking without any limitations. At 1 year follow-up, good radiographic results and a fair functional outcome were reported (AOFAS = 74; NRS = 2); total ROM was 30° with 10° of dorsiflexion and 20° of plantar flexion.

2.2.3. Secondary Osteoarthritis and Revision to Total Ankle Prosthesis

During the second year of follow-up, the patient experienced a worsening, up to the impossibility of walking without pain. He soon started complaining of painful plantar flexion and morning stiffness. A ROM limitation (ROM = 20°) was observed at the control visit. Two years after surgery, antero-posterior and latero-lateral ankle radiographs suggested a secondary osteoarthritis with articular space narrowing, implying the indication for a prosthesis revision (Figure 9). Either arthrodesis or tibial resurfacing were proposed as management options. In this case, the patient expressed the desire to maintain ankle function: A conversion to total ankle arthroplasty with TTR was performed. The tibial prosthesis consisted of a tibial trabecular titanium (Ti6Al4V) component and 6 mm-thick, high-density polyethylene (Figure 9). The lengthening of the Achilles tendon was performed using a percutaneous technique.

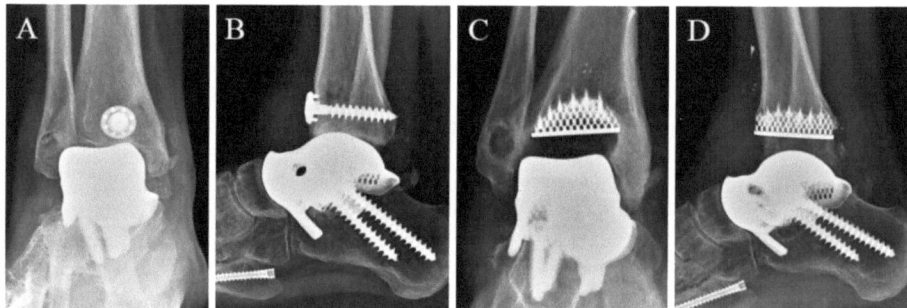

Figure 9. Two-year post-surgery X-ray of the implant from antero-posterior (**A**) and latero-lateral (**B**) projections. Articular space narrowing and osteophyte formation (compared with Figure 7) can be observed (**A**,**B**). The total talar replacement after revision surgery from antero-posterior (**C**) and latero-lateral (**D**) projections. *Image courtesy of Dr. Paola Verde Aerospace Medicine Department, Aerospace Test Division, Pratica di Mare, Rome, Italy.*

After surgery, the patient was enrolled in a rehabilitation program based on continuous passive movement; progressively, partial weight bearing was allowed. Total weight bearing was conceded after 3 months.

Conversion to total ankle arthroplasty achieved a positive outcome: After every 1-year follow-up (up to 5 years), the patient complained of little to no pain and reached 35–40° of total sagittal ROM. After one year, the patient was judged fit to fly, and after two years, he resumed flying on high-performance jets. The outcomes were stationary at the last follow-up, 5 years after surgery. The aforementioned revision surgery and the implications and observations concerning specifically Aerospace and Aviation Medicine have been presented and discussed in detail in the Journal of Aerospace Medicine and Human Performance by Verde and colleagues [18].

3. Materials and Methods

We conducted a literature review to summarize the current knowledge and scientific evidence regarding third-generation TTR. We conducted our search in the following databases from the beginning until November 2021: PubMed, Google Scholar, and MED-

LINE. The search strategy was developed and executed in the mentioned research databases with the following queries:

1. (talus [MeSH Terms]) AND (prosthesis [MeSH Terms])
2. ((total talus) AND (total talar)) AND ((replacement) OR (prosthesis))

Following identification of potential articles, an initial screening of titles and abstracts that addressed the research question of interest was performed before inclusion.

4. Results

The query "(talus [MeSH Terms]) AND (prosthesis [MeSH Terms])" produced 464 results, while "((total talus) AND (total talar)) AND ((replacement) OR (prosthesis))" produced 154 results.

After a thorough literature review, we selected a total of 15 case reports (18 patients), 10 case series (119 patients), and 2 case series (64 patients), for a total of 201 cases.

In the studies analyzed, the average follow-up was 36.06 months (4.7–132 months, SD ± 16.16). Follow-up was reported in a heterogeneous manner, with several studies not reporting the follow-up time for every single patient but only as an average value.

Outcomes were measured by evaluation of post-operative total ROM, ROM in dorsiflexion, and ROM in plantar flexion: Often, studies did not specify if the evaluation was limited to active ROM or included both passive and active ROM. ROM was reported in 3 case reports and in 5 case series, with an average total ROM of 43.1°: an average dorsiflexion ROM of 11.7°, and an average plantar-flexion ROM of 34.0°.

To evaluate functional outcomes, a wide variety of scoring systems were adopted: The only two validated outcome measures adopted in >2 studies at the last follow-up were AOFAS (81.94 points; 23 patients) [10,19–26] and the Japanese Society for Surgery of the Foot scale (JSSF) (mean 89.68 points, 98 patients) [27–31]. Due to the diversity of the results obtained by the literature review, a statistical analysis was deemed not feasible. Results are therefore presented and discussed in narrative form.

5. Discussion

A customized talar prosthesis tends to reproduce as much as possible the tridimensional shape of the native talus. CT images of the original talus or 3D mirroring of the contralateral talus are often used as references. By reproducing the anatomic structure of the native talus, this prosthesis aims to overcome the main drawbacks of ankle arthrodesis (limb shortening, decreased shock absorption, and ROM limitation).

5.1. Case Reports

In the two cases discussed, the TTR showed satisfactory functional outcomes in the short term. Nevertheless, after approximately two years, the functional outcome was impaired by secondary arthritic degeneration of the tibial plafond, requiring secondary surgical revision. This is the first paper to report and discuss the failure of TTR and management strategies: In the first case, the patient preferred ankle arthrodesis, while in the second case, due to higher functional needs (high-performance aircraft pilot), a distal tibial resurfacing was performed. Ankle arthrodesis, the most adopted approach to treat complex talar injuries, guarantees pain reduction and stability of the ankle joint but often leads to unsatisfying functional outcomes, rigidity, dysmetria, and secondary osteoarthritis, commonly at the subtalar, talonavicular, calcaneocuboid, navicular-cuneiform, tarso metatarsal, and first metatarsophalangeal joints [2]. In the first case, the patient expressed the main desire to achieve ankle stability and pain reduction with a definitive solution, minimizing the risk for supplemental surgeries: ankle arthrodesis presents lower failure, complication, and reoperation rates when compared to total ankle arthroplasty [32].

The second patient needed optimal ankle functionality (with physiological ROM) to keep working as a military jet pilot. To avoid limb dysmetria and guarantee satisfactory sagittal ROM, there was a need to keep the talar prosthesis and create a tibial surface able to slide on the titanium without erosion. The material of the tibial prosthesis, Ti6A4V, exhibits tolerance to mechanical load and enhances maintenance and regulation of bone mass density due to its porous gyroid structure. This material guarantees good osteoconductive potential. A 6 mm-thick mobile ultra-high molecular weight polyethylene, such as in standard ankle replacements [33], was adopted with the aim of achieving approximately 40° of total sagittal ROM, necessary to resume flight activity. To prevent retraction after Achilles tendon lengthening, the continued passive motion of the operated ankle was programmed up to two months after surgery.

5.2. Literature Revision

5.2.1. Main Indications

In managing patients with severe talar lesions, loss of the original bone, or poor bone stock, such as avascular necrosis, advanced osteoarthritis, rheumatoid arthritis, or bone tumors, TTR could be part of a total ankle replacement [27–29]. In 2020, Morita and colleagues presented a case series of 10 total ankle arthroplasties revised for subtalar subsidence with the implant of a TTR. All patients significantly improved their ROM and NRS scores and returned to activities of daily living at a long-term follow-up [29]. The authors suggested that TTR could be an option to address unfavorable but common complications of total ankle replacements, such as talar component subsidence, in selected patients with large bone defects. Studies comparing the long-term outcomes of total ankle replacement with those of combined TTR are still missing.

TTR has been used to treat severe ankle injuries with loss or irreversible damage to the talar bone. In severe comminuted fractures, where simple open or closed reduction is burdened by the risk of aseptic necrosis, arthritis, and pseudarthrosis postoperatively [19]. TTR guarantees good congruency with adjacent joints and preserves leg length and ankle mobility. In a 2015 case report, Giannini and colleagues provided a remarkable example of TTR adopted to achieve valid functional outcomes in a 27-year-old rock climber with high functional requirements and poor bone quality: The patient was suffering severe osteoarthritis and talar osteonecrosis following an open reduction and internal fixation of a talonavicular fracture. The implant of a TTR (including the navicular bone) achieved optimal results: He resumed alpine skiing, climbing, running, and even became a climbing instructor. In this case, specifically, these functional results were otherwise impossible to achieve: insufficient bone support for implant integration contraindicated a typical total ankle arthroplasty [22].

Katsui and colleagues described a series of six severely comminuted talar fractures; again, TTR allowed to avoid arthrodesis: in this case, three patients resumed sports activities (golf, aerobics, and even jogging) [19].

Gadkari et al. and Stevens et al. reported the case of a 14-year-old female who suffered a talar extrusion and underwent a talectomy after a failed talar reimplantation. A TTR was the only option to avoid arthrodesis: In this case, the patient achieved a good ROM and was capable of walking on uneven terrain [4,21]. Finally, as previously reported, in the second of our cases, the combined implant was necessary to resume high-performance jet driving.

5.2.2. Clinical Outcomes

As mentioned in the results, TTR demonstrates favorable functional outcomes. The mean AOFAS and JSSF scores at the last follow-up were comparable to or better than those achieved with ankle arthrodesis or total ankle replacement [34,35]. The attained range of motion (ROM) enables patients to perform daily activities and successfully resume sports participation in many cases [18,28,31].

5.2.3. Cartilage Degeneration and Secondary Osteoarthritis

Like the two cases reported, the majority of TTR described worldwide are isolated. In 2015, Taniguchi and colleagues published a series of 55 isolated TTR with a minimum follow-up of 24 months (follow-up range: 24–96 months): 24 patients (44%) total presented tibial plafond osteoarthritis at the last follow-up. Additionally, 5 patients (9%) presented osteosclerosis of the navicular bone, and 19 patients (35%) had osteosclerosis of the calcaneus [36].

Among 42 combined TTR (with a follow-up >24 months), only 2 cases of degenerative changes were reported: specifically, in the work by Morita et al., 1 case of osteosclerosis at the talonavicular joint was reported, while 1 out of 3 patients described by West and colleagues presented loosening of the tibial component [29,37].

It is well known that the contact of native cartilage with prosthetic material could lead to degeneration and revision surgery. In total knee arthroplasty, direct metal contact on cartilage leads to long-term degeneration and suffering of the subchondral bone [38]. Several meta-analyses state that the risk of reoperation for hip hemiarthroplasty is higher than the one for total hip arthroplasty at long-term follow-up (over 24 months), often because of thigh pain and loss of function determined by acetabular cartilage degeneration [39–41]. Being the tibial plafond the most common site of osteoarthritis, we may speculate that choosing combined over isolated TTR (preventing tibial plafond osteosclerosis) could decrease the incidence of prosthesis revisions. In our second case (and in the one reported by Katsui et al.), a combined TTR could have eventually avoided a secondary surgery [19]. It is worth noting that the only study that compares total ankle arthroplasty with combined TTR showed that the latter achieves equivalent pain reduction, and significantly superior functional outcomes showed in Table 1 [27].

Table 1. Mean American Orthopedic Foot and Ankle Society Score (AOFAS) and Japanese Society for Surgery of the Foot scale (JSSF) mean scores at the last follow-up as reported in the cited papers. N.R. = not reported.

Author and Year	Number of Cases	Follow-Up (Months)	AOFAS	JSSF
Taniguchi et al., 2015, [25]	54	52.8	N.R.	89.1
Katsui et al., 2019, [11]	6	46	78.8	N.R.
Kanzaki et al., 2019, [10]	22	34.9	N.R.	91.5
Morita et al., 2020, [16]	10	49	N.R.	88.5
Tonogai et al., 2017, [28]	2	18	N.R.	95
Kurokawa et al., 2019, [13]	10	58	N.R.	89
Mu et al., 2021, [18]	9	23.17	79.67	N.R.
Gadkari et al., 2013, [6]	1	48	97	N.R.
Ando et al., 2015, [1]	1	24	90	N.R.
Giannini et al., 2015, [7]	1	30	81	N.R.
Ruatti et al., 2017, [21]	2	24	77	N.R.
Fang et al., 2018, [5]	1	6	91	N.R.
Chinzei et al., 2017, [3]	1	48	88	N.R.
Hussain et al., 2020, [8]	1	12	94	N.R.
Mean value (total patients)			81.94 (23)	89.68 (98)

5.3. Limitations

The knowledge concerning TTR, particularly combined design, is still preliminary. A limited number of non-comparative, retrospective studies (namely, case series/reports) have been published, providing a scarce level of evidence with a high risk of publication bias. Furthermore, the current literature is characterized by heterogeneity of reporting regarding outcome measures and follow-up length; therefore, synthesizing results from different studies could be complex and, to some extent, misleading.

Further studies are needed to describe the potential advantages of TTR, for example, compared with TAA in patients with poor bone stock. Long-term outcomes of TTR are scarcely described, with current studies focusing on limited follow-up times that do not allow estimating the survival of these implants. The case series/report design exposes it to a high risk of publication bias compared to prospective studies.

Our manuscript should be considered a narrative overview of the state of the art concerning TTR, but a systematic and pooled approach will be needed in the future, considering the growing body of literature on this topic.

6. Conclusions

Due to the limited number of cases described, the approach towards severe damage and talar bone loss is diverse and, to some extent, empirical. To date, only case report/series have been published.

In our experience, custom-made TTR could find indication as a component of a total ankle replacement, in particular, if the talar bone is lacking in quality, such as in severe avascular necrosis or osteoarthritis, and could reduce the risk of talar component and subtalar subsidence. It represents a management option when the integrity of the talar bone is compromised, for example, in high-grade ankle injuries with severely comminuted talar fractures, extrusion (a minor risk of failure over reimplantation), or bone tumors. TTR maintains congruency with the adjacent joints to achieve ankle stability, a functional ROM, and prevent dysmetria.

Osteoarthritic changes in the adjacent joints (most frequently at the tibial plafond) represent one of the main drawbacks of TTR and the main cause of long-term (>2 years) failure of the implants.

This is the first article to present two cases of failed isolated TTR and to specifically discuss the reasons behind the need for secondary surgery and the pros and cons of the two main revision options (arthrodesis and tibial plafond resurfacing).

Comparing the data reported in several case reports and series in the literature, a combined TTR could prevent tibial degenerative changes, reducing the incidence of osteoarthritis and the need for secondary surgery.

In conclusion, although talar replacement is a growing and challenging topic in orthopedic research, standardized and reproducible research is still missing. Further research, with systematically collected data and a follow-up of at least 24 months, is needed to allow direct comparison with other surgical options and to provide the scientific basis for a cost–benefit analysis.

Author Contributions: Conceptualization, E.C. and G.C.B.; methodology, G.C.B.; validation, D.L., I.S.; formal analysis, D.F.; investigation, G.G.; resources, D.F.; data curation, D.F.; writing—original draft preparation, G.C.B.; writing—review and editing, I.S.; supervision, D.L. All authors have read and agreed to the published version of the manuscript.

Funding: This research received no external funding.

Data Availability Statement: Not applicable.

Acknowledgments: The authors would like to express their gratitude to Paola Verde for the contribution.

Conflicts of Interest: The authors declare no conflict of interest.

References

1. Tack, P.; Victor, J.; Gemmel, P.; Annemans, L. 3D-printing techniques in a medical setting: A systematic literature review. *Biomed. Eng. Online* **2016**, *15*, 115. [CrossRef]
2. Ling, J.S.; Smyth, N.A.; Fraser, E.J.; Hogan, M.V.; Seaworth, C.M.; Ross, K.A.; Kennedy, J.G. Investigating the relationship between ankle arthrodesis and adjacent-joint arthritis in the hindfoot a systematic review a systematic review. *J. Bone Jt. Surg.* **2015**, *97*, 513–519. [CrossRef]
3. Biz, C.; Hoxhaj, B.; Aldegheri, R.; Iacobellis, C. Minimally Invasive Surgery for Tibiotalocalcaneal Arthrodesis Using a Retrograde Intramedullary Nail: Preliminary Results of an Innovative Modified Technique. *J. Foot Ankle Surg.* **2016**, *55*, 1130–1138. [CrossRef]

4. Stevens, B.W.; Dolan, C.M.; Anderson, J.G.; Bukrey, C.D. Custom talar prosthesis after open talar extrusion in a pediatric patient. *Foot Ankle Int.* **2007**, *28*, 933–938. [CrossRef] [PubMed]
5. Moussa, M.K.; Bou Raad, R.; Ghanem, I.; Mansour, O. Complete Extrusion of Talar Body Associated with Ipsilateral Floating Knee. *Cureus* **2020**, *12*, e10346. [CrossRef] [PubMed]
6. Magnan, B.; Facci, E.; Bartolozzi, P. Traumatic loss of the talus treated with a talar body prosthesis and total ankle arthroplasty: A case report. *J. Bone Jt. Surg-Ser. A* **2004**, *86*, 1778–1782. [CrossRef] [PubMed]
7. Weston, J.T.; Liu, X.; Wandtke, M.E.; Liu, J.; Ebrahim, N.E. A Systematic Review of Total Dislocation of the Talus. *Orthop. Surg.* **2015**, *7*, 97–101. [CrossRef] [PubMed]
8. Ortiz-Cruz, J.R.; Ojeda Boscana, I.L. Talar extrusion, a very rare sequela of trauma: A case report. *Am. J. Case Rep.* **2019**, *20*, 575–579. [CrossRef]
9. Lalchandani, G.R.; Hung, N.J.; Janghala, A.; Terry, M.; Morshed, S. Total Talar and Navicular Extrusions A Case Report. *JBJS Case Connect.* **2022**, *12*, e20. [CrossRef]
10. Ruatti, S.; Corbet, C.; Boudissa, M.; Kerschbaumer, G.; Milaire, M.; Merloz, P.; Tonetti, J. Total Talar Prosthesis Replacement after Talar Extrusion. *J. Foot Ankle Surg.* **2017**, *56*, 905–909. [CrossRef]
11. Genena, A.; Abouelela, A. A Case Report of an Open Pan-Talar Dislocation Case Presentation. *Cureus* **2020**, *12*, e9274. [CrossRef]
12. Stirling, P.; MacKenzie, S.P.; Maempel, J.F.; McCann, C.; Ray, R.; Clement, N.D.; White, T.O.; Keating, J.F. Patient-reported functional outcomes and health-related quality of life following fractures of the talus. *Ann. R. Coll. Surg. Engl.* **2019**, *101*, 399–404. [CrossRef] [PubMed]
13. Almaeen, B.N.; Elmaghrby, I.S.; Alnour, M.K.; Alrefeidi, T.A.; Adas, S.M.A. Complete Revascularization of Reimplanted Talus After Isolated Total Talar Extrusion: A Case Report. *Cureus* **2020**, *12*, e7947. [CrossRef] [PubMed]
14. Kwak, J.; Heo, S.; Jung, G. Six-year survival of reimplanted talus after isolated total talar extrusion: A case report. *J. Med. Case Rep.* **2017**, *11*, 348. [CrossRef] [PubMed]
15. Vaienti, L.; Maggi, F.; Gazzola, R.; Lanzani, E. Therapeutic management of complicated talar extrusion: Literature review and case report. *J. Orthop. Traumatol.* **2011**, *12*, 61–64. [CrossRef]
16. Joshi, A.K.; Joshi, C.; Singh, S.; Singh, V. Traumatic loss of talus: A rare injury. *Foot* **2012**, *22*, 319–321. [CrossRef]
17. Tamayo, J.A.; Riascos, M.; Vargas, C.A.; Baena, L.M. Additive manufacturing of Ti6Al4V alloy via electron beam melting for the development of implants for the biomedical industry. *Heliyon* **2021**, *7*, e06892. [CrossRef]
18. Verde, P.; Guardigli, S.; Morgagni, F.; Roberts, S.; Monopoli, D.; Scala, A. Total Ankle Replacement in a Military Jet Pilot. *Aerosp. Med. Hum. Perform.* **2020**, *91*, 597–603. [CrossRef]
19. Katsui, R.; Takakura, Y.; Taniguchi, A.; Tanaka, Y. Ceramic Artificial Talus as the Initial Treatment for Comminuted Talar Fractures. *Foot Ankle Int.* **2020**, *41*, 79–83. [CrossRef]
20. Ando, Y.; Yasui, T.; Isawa, K.; Tanaka, S.; Tanaka, Y.; Takakura, Y. Total Talar Replacement for Idiopathic Necrosis of the Talus: A Case Report. *J. Foot Ankle Surg.* **2016**, *55*, 1292–1296. [CrossRef]
21. Gadkari, K.P.; Anderson, J.G.; Bohay, D.R.; Maskill, J.D.; Padley, M.A.; Behrend, L.A. An Eleven-Year Follow-up of a Custom Talar Prosthesis After Open Talar Extrusion in an Adolescent Patient. *JBJS Case Connect.* **2013**, *3*, e118. [CrossRef]
22. Giannini, S.; Cadossi, M.; Mazzotti, A.; Ramponi, L.; Belvedere, C.; Leardini, A. Custom-Made Total Talonavicular Replacement in a Professional Rock Climber. *J. Foot Ankle Surg.* **2016**, *55*, 1271–1275. [CrossRef] [PubMed]
23. Fang, G.; Wang, C.; Piao, Y.; Zhang, L. Chondro-osseous respiratory epithelial adenomatoid hamartoma of the nasal cavity. *Pediatr. Int.* **2016**, *58*, 229–231. [CrossRef]
24. Hussain, R.M. Metallic 3D Printed Total Talus Replacement: A Case Study. *J. Foot Ankle Surg.* **2021**, *60*, 634–641. [CrossRef]
25. Mu, M.D.; Yang, Q.D.; Chen, W.; Tao, X.; Zhang, C.K.; Zhang, X.; Xie, M.M.; Tang, K.L. Three dimension printing talar prostheses for total replacement in talar necrosis and collapse. *Int. Orthop.* **2021**, *45*, 2313–2321. [CrossRef]
26. Chinzei, N.; Kanzaki, N.; Matsushita, T.; Matsumoto, T.; Hayashi, S.; Hoshino, Y.; Hashimoto, S.; Takayama, K.; Araki, D.; Kuroda, R. Total ankle arthroplasty with total talar prosthesis for talar osteonecrosis with ankle osteoarthritis: A case report. *J. Orthop. Sci.* **2018**, *26*, 725–730. [CrossRef] [PubMed]
27. Kurokawa, H.; Taniguchi, A.; Morita, S.; Takakura, Y.; Tanaka, Y. Total ankle arthroplasty incorporating a total talar prosthesis a comparative study against the standard total ankle arthroplasty. *Bone Jt. J.* **2019**, *101*, 443–446. [CrossRef]
28. Kanzaki, N.; Chinzei, N.; Yamamoto, T.; Yamashita, T.; Ibaraki, K.; Kuroda, R. Clinical Outcomes of Total Ankle Arthroplasty With Total Talar Prosthesis. *Foot Ankle Int.* **2019**, *40*, 948–954. [CrossRef]
29. Morita, S.; Taniguchi, A.; Miyamoto, T.; Kurokawa, H.; Tanaka, Y. Application of a Customized Total Talar Prosthesis for Revision Total Ankle Arthroplasty. *JBJS Open Access* **2020**, *5*, e20.00034. [CrossRef]
30. Tonogai, I.; Hamada, D.; Yamasaki, Y.; Wada, K.; Takasago, T.; Tsutsui, T.; Goto, T.; Sairyo, K. Custom-Made Alumina Ceramic Total Talar Prosthesis for Idiopathic Aseptic Necrosis of the Talus: Report of Two Cases. *Case Rep. Orthop.* **2017**, *2017*, 8290804. [CrossRef]
31. Taniguchi, A.; Tanaka, Y. An Alumina Ceramic Total Talar Prosthesis for Avascular Necrosis of the Talus. *Foot Ankle Clin.* **2019**, *24*, 163–171. [CrossRef]
32. Lawton, C.D.; Butler, B.A.; Ii, R.G.D.; Prescott, A.; Kadakia, A.R. Total ankle arthroplasty versus ankle arthrodesis—A comparison of outcomes over the last decade. *J. Orthop. Surg. Res.* **2017**, *12*, 76. [CrossRef]

33. Daras-ballester, A.; Vicent-carsi, V.; Ramirez-fuentes, C. Polyethylene Fractures in Mobile-Bearing Total Ankle Arthroplasty: Report of 2 Cases. *Foot Ankle Orthop.* **2022**, *7*, 1–6. [CrossRef] [PubMed]
34. Teramoto, A.; Nozaka, K.; Kamiya, T.; Kashiwagura, T.; Shoji, H.; Watanabe, K.; Shimada, Y.; Yamashita, T. The Journal of Foot & Ankle Surgery Screw Internal Fixation and Ilizarov External Fixation: A Comparison of Outcomes in Ankle Arthrodesis. *J. Foot Ankle Surg.* **2020**, *59*, 343–346. [CrossRef]
35. Shih, C.; Chen, S.; Huang, P. Clinical Outcomes of Total Ankle Arthroplasty Versus Ankle Arthrodesis for the Treatment of End-Stage Ankle Arthritis in the Last Decade: A Systematic Review and Meta-analysis. *J. Foot Ankle Surg.* **2020**, *59*, 1032–1039. [CrossRef] [PubMed]
36. Taniguchi, A.; Takakura, Y.; Tanaka, Y.; Kurokawa, H. An Alumina Ceramic Total Talar Prosthesis for Osteonecrosis of the Talus. *J. Bone Jt. Surg.* **2015**, *97*, 1348–1353. [CrossRef]
37. West, T.A.; Rush, S.M. Total Talus Replacement: Case Series and Literature Review. *J. Foot Ankle Surg.* **2021**, *60*, 187–193. [CrossRef]
38. Khatod, M.; Inacio, M.C.S.; Bini, S. Short-Term Outcomes of Unresurfaced Patellas in Total Knee Arthroplasty. *J. Knee Surg.* **2013**, *26*, 105–108. [PubMed]
39. The Health Investigators. Total Hip Arthroplasty or Hemiarthroplasty for Hip Fracture. *N. Engl. J. Med.* **2019**, *381*, 2199–2208. [CrossRef]
40. Burgers, P.T.P.W.; Geene, A.R. Van Total hip arthroplasty versus hemiarthroplasty for displaced femoral neck fractures in the healthy elderly: A meta-analysis and systematic review of randomized trials. *Int. Orthop.* **2012**, *36*, 1549–1560. [CrossRef]
41. Hopley, C.; Stengel, D.; Ekkernkamp, A.; Wich, M. Primary total hip arthroplasty versus hemiarthroplasty for displaced intracapsular hip fractures in older patients: Systematic review. *BMJ* **2010**, *340*, c2332. [CrossRef] [PubMed]

Disclaimer/Publisher's Note: The statements, opinions and data contained in all publications are solely those of the individual author(s) and contributor(s) and not of MDPI and/or the editor(s). MDPI and/or the editor(s) disclaim responsibility for any injury to people or property resulting from any ideas, methods, instructions or products referred to in the content.

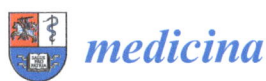 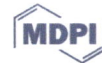

Review

Application of Virtual Reality Systems in Bone Trauma Procedures

Chiedozie Kenneth Ugwoke [1,*], Domenico Albano [2], Nejc Umek [1], Ivo Dumić-Čule [3,4] and Žiga Snoj [5,6,*]

1. Institute of Anatomy, Faculty of Medicine, University of Ljubljana, Korytkova Ulica 2, 1000 Ljubljana, Slovenia; nejc.umek@mf.uni-lj.si
2. Unità Operativa di Radiologia Diagnostica ed Interventistica, IRCCS Istituto Ortopedico Galeazzi, Via Riccardo Galeazzi 4, 20161 Milano, Italy
3. Department of Nursing, University North, 104. Brigade 3, 42000 Varaždin, Croatia
4. Department of Diagnostic and Interventional Radiology, University Hospital Center Zagreb, Kišpatićeva Ulica 12, 10000 Zagreb, Croatia
5. Department of Radiology, Faculty of Medicine, University of Ljubljana, Vrazov trg 2, 1000 Ljubljana, Slovenia
6. Clinical Institute of Radiology, University Medical Centre Ljubljana, Zaloška 7, 1000 Ljubljana, Slovenia
* Correspondence: chiedozie.ugwoke@mf.uni-lj.si (C.K.U.); ziga.snoj@gmail.com (Ž.S.); Tel.: +386-6976-1436 (C.K.U.)

Abstract: *Background and Objectives*: Bone fractures contribute significantly to the global disease and disability burden and are associated with a high and escalating incidence and tremendous economic consequences. The increasingly challenging climate of orthopaedic training and practice re-echoes the established potential of leveraging computer-based reality technologies to support patient-specific simulations for procedural teaching and surgical precision. Unfortunately, despite the recognised potential of virtual reality technologies in orthopaedic surgery, its adoption and integration, particularly in fracture procedures, have lagged behind other surgical specialities. We aimed to review the available virtual reality systems adapted for orthopaedic trauma procedures. *Materials and Methods*: We performed an extensive literature search in Medline (PubMed), Science Direct, SpringerLink, and Google Scholar and presented a narrative synthesis of the state of the art on virtual reality systems for bone trauma procedures. *Results*: We categorised existing simulation modalities into those for fracture fixation techniques, drilling procedures, and prosthetic design and implantation and described the important technical features, as well as their clinical validity and applications. *Conclusions*: Over the past decade, an increasing number of high- and low-fidelity virtual reality systems for bone trauma procedures have been introduced, demonstrating important benefits with regard to improving procedural teaching and learning, preoperative planning and rehearsal, intraoperative precision and efficiency, and postoperative outcomes. However, further technical developments in line with industry benchmarks and metrics are needed in addition to more standardised and rigorous clinical validation.

Keywords: virtual reality; simulation; fracture; bone trauma; orthopaedics; preoperative planning

Citation: Ugwoke, C.K.; Albano, D.; Umek, N.; Dumić-Čule, I.; Snoj, Ž. Application of Virtual Reality Systems in Bone Trauma Procedures. *Medicina* **2023**, *59*, 562. https://doi.org/10.3390/medicina59030562

Academic Editors: Cory Xian and Vassilios S. Nikolaou

Received: 13 February 2023
Revised: 2 March 2023
Accepted: 10 March 2023
Published: 14 March 2023

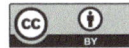

Copyright: © 2023 by the authors. Licensee MDPI, Basel, Switzerland. This article is an open access article distributed under the terms and conditions of the Creative Commons Attribution (CC BY) license (https:// creativecommons.org/licenses/by/ 4.0/).

1. Introduction

1.1. The Burden of Bone Trauma

Traumatic bone conditions are an important contributor to global disease and disability burden. A worldwide incidence estimate using the framework of the Global Burden of Diseases, Injuries, and Risk Factors Study showed that there were 178 million new fractures in 2019, representing an increase of 33.4% since 1990 [1]. At 11.58%, the global incidence of imminent fracture is also worrisome [2]. In the United States, about 340,000 hip fractures are reported annually among elderly patients, and across Europe, about 600,000 hip fractures were reported in 2010 [3–6]. The incidence of musculoskeletal injuries in low- and middle-income countries is estimated to be between 779 and 1574 per 100,000 person years [7]. In developed countries with an ageing population, the bulk of the fracture burden is related to degenerative bone conditions such as osteoporosis, while in developing countries, traumatic injuries such as road traffic accidents account for the vast majority of fractures [5,7]. Although the COVID-19 pandemic has contributed to a global decline in the overall fracture burden, the rate of fragility fractures remained unchanged [8–10]. Refractures occur in approximately 50% of index fragility fractures within two years [2], and in the United States, post-traumatic osteoarthritis accounts for about 12% of symptomatic osteoarthritis [11]. Traumatic orthopaedic conditions are further associated with a considerable economic burden. In 2017, the annual cost of fragility fractures was estimated at EUR 37.5 billion in the five largest European Union states plus Sweden, with an additional loss of 1.0 million quality-adjusted life years [12].

1.2. Rationale and Fundamentals of Virtual Reality in Bone Trauma

Coexisting with the escalating burden of traumatic bone conditions is an increasingly challenging climate of orthopaedic training and practice. The changing trends in clinical work hours, healthcare budgets, legislative frameworks, patient safety considerations, and public expectations significantly impact surgical training and practice in the current era [13–15]. A worrisome decline in the volume of orthopaedic and trauma specialists has been well-documented over the past few decades [16–19]. Compounding the existing workforce shortages, the disturbances to global healthcare systems due to the COVID-19 pandemic caused further negative disruptions to orthopaedic and trauma care and education [20–23]. These realities have further re-echoed the established potential of leveraging computer-based technologies to enhance the efficiency of orthopaedic training and practice. Among other benefits, the diverse developments in computer-assisted surgery and simulation technologies are expected to foster improvements in surgical precision, safety, and outcomes [24–27].

Driven by the rapid evolution of computing power and imaging capabilities over the past few decades, several reality technologies have been developed for clinical and pedagogical applications. In orthopaedic trauma surgery, different modalities of reality technologies are currently available to support procedural teaching, practice, and patient-specific simulations, namely, virtual reality (VR), augmented reality, and mixed reality. These three reality modalities may sometimes be collectively described with the umbrella term *extended reality* [28] (Figure 1). VR systems provide total visual immersion, movements, and interactions in an artificial, computer-generated environment that may incorporate artificial stimuli such as sounds or hand-operated controllers to improve the interactive experience [29]. VR systems increasingly combine haptic feedback to simulate touch, vibration, and motion, in addition to standard components such as a 3D-capable computer, head-mounted display, and controllers with position sensors [25]. While VR employs an entirely artificial computer-generated environment, augmented reality superimposes digital images onto physical environments in real-time. The term *augmented virtual reality* is also used distinctively in some literature to describe the real-time representation of physical world events in a virtual environment [28]. On the other hand, mixed reality utilises a digital display overlay in conjunction with interactive projected holograms, allowing the operator to explore the physical environment while simultaneously interacting with and controlling the digital material provided by the device. [29,30]. Table 1 summarises the important features of virtual, augmented, and mixed reality surgical systems.

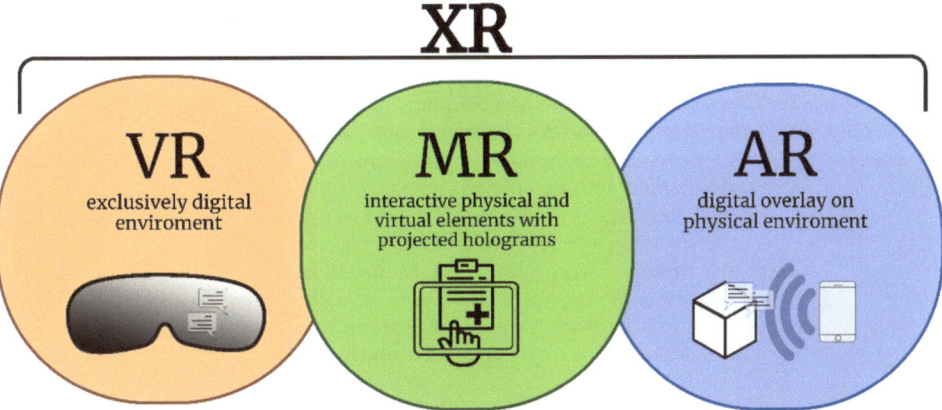

Figure 1. The spectrum of surgical reality systems. VR = virtual reality; MR = mixed reality; AR = augmented reality; and XR = extended reality (umbrella term encompassing all three modalities).

Table 1. Essential features of virtual, augmented, and mixed reality surgical systems [29,31].

Virtual Reality	Augmented Reality	Mixed Reality
• Complete visual immersion in an artificial digital (computer-generated) environment. • Uses 2D/3D graphic software for reconstructing clinical CT/MRI images. • Visual experience may be complemented by incorporating haptic devices, artificial sounds, and other stimuli. • Current hardware support systems include the Touch 3D Systems, W5D Enact Robotics, Ascension trakSTAR, Optotrak optical tracking camera, smartphones, tablets (e.g., Google Cardboard or Samsung Gear VR), mice, etc. • Suitable for preoperative planning/rehearsal, patient education, and surgical training/assessment.	• Digital images superimposed on real-world physical surfaces. • Uses 3D graphic software for reconstructing clinical CT/MRI images. • Enhances the operator's perception of depth. • Current hardware supports systems include smartphones, tablets, and both optical and video see-through-based head-mounted displays such as the Google Glass or Microsoft HoloLens. • Possibility of remote training experience. • Suitable for pre-op planning, intra-op surgical navigation, and surgical training/assessment.	• Most functionally advanced surgical reality technology combining an interactive digital display overlay and projected holograms. • Uses 3D graphic software for reconstructing clinical CT/MRI images. • Requires less preoperative calibration and allows a greater degree of freedom for preoperative image reconstruction. • Better control of intraoperative visualisation and the possibility of remote communication, e.g., via Skype. • The most adapted hardware support system currently is the Microsoft HoloLens. • Suitable for pre-op planning, intra-op surgical navigation, and surgical training/assessment.

The arguments for integrating VR technologies into orthopaedic practice are compelling, especially considering the widening spectrum of technically challenging procedures in the field. Unfortunately, despite the recognised potential, the adoption of VR and other reality technologies in orthopaedics has lagged behind other surgical specialities [31–33]. While there have been notable advancements in the integration of VR for arthroscopic surgeries [34–37], the evolution of VR technologies for bone fracture procedures has followed a more modest course [31]. The present review aims to describe the state of the art on VR systems for orthopaedic trauma procedures.

2. Methodology

2.1. Search Strategy

An extensive literature search was performed on Medline (PubMed), Science Direct, SpringerLink, and Google Scholar databases to identify original reports and relevant reviews focusing on the review subject. The following medical subject headings (MeSH) terms were used in various combinations using the Boolean operators "AND" and "OR" in accordance with the advanced search algorithms of the searched databases: "virtual reality" with 'fracture' or 'bone' or 'trauma surgery' 'orthopaedics' or 'orthopaedic surgery'. The terms were tested on the platforms to obtain the best search strategy. The following search criteria were applied: full-text-accessible articles, articles in English, peer-reviewed original research papers or relevant systematic reviews, without restriction to the year of publication. Additional literature was sourced by reviewing the reference lists of all the studies identified from the database search.

2.2. Literature Selection and Analysis

Two researchers (C.K.U. and N.U.) independently assessed the search results and screened the studies for relevance. The eligibility of the studies was evaluated in a stepwise approach: screening by title, followed by a critical reading of the abstracts and the full texts of potentially relevant studies. Differences between the two independent researchers were settled by a joint discussion with the other authors. We included only studies that specifically focussed on the application of VR systems in orthopaedic trauma procedures and performed a narrative synthesis of the extracted data using a thematic approach. Reports describing VR systems primarily developed for elective arthroscopy or arthroplasty procedures were excluded from the synthesis and discussion, but those adaptable for trauma procedures are highlighted in the appropriate contexts. Each author independently re-evaluated the extracted data and the initial narrative synthesis during the manuscript preparation process and the final draft were critically reviewed by two orthopaedic surgeons experienced with VR tools.

3. VR Systems for Bone Trauma Procedures

3.1. Background

Based on technical features and capabilities, VR platforms may be loosely categorised into low- and high-fidelity systems. High-fidelity VR modalities enhance immersion by simulating clinical and surgical environments and procedures with increased interactivity, visual accuracy and appeal, and content specificity. They allow the replication of most or all aspects of a procedure or technique, closely emulating the operating room environment [24,38,39]. Conversely, low-fidelity VR systems replicate single or multiple tasks with restrictions on interactivity, visual presentation, available content, and commands. Such modalities permit the demonstration of specific aspects of procedures or techniques, enabling the rapid and repetitive simulation of a skill to attain proficiency, and are therefore suitable as a basic learning platform for junior trainees. Compared to low-fidelity modalities, high-fidelity systems are more expensive and require more complex logistical considerations for set-up [24,38,40]. Most clinically available orthopaedic trauma VR systems fall into the high-fidelity category. Patient-specific VR simulations are enabled by the incorporation and conversion of MRI or CT data into 3D models using image processing and visualisation software. Examples of such software for quantitative analysis and visualisation of medical images include MIPAV (Medical Image Processing, Analysis, and Visualization) [41], Medical Imaging Interaction Toolkit (MITK) [42], 3D Slicer [43], Simpleware [44], 3D-DOCTOR [45], and Osirix [46].

While there is currently no formal classification system for VR modalities in orthopaedic trauma, for convenience, we have categorised existing simulation modalities into those for fracture fixation techniques, drilling procedures, and prosthetic design and implantation. Table 2 summarises the essential features of the described categories of orthopaedic trauma VR systems. It should be understood, however, that some multimodal simulators encompass diverse procedural modules and may not technically be restricted to a specific category.

3.2. Fracture Fixation VR Simulators

Surgical repair of bone fractures involves the reduction and fixation of the fracture fragments by means of screws, plates, or implants as appropriate for the nature and complexity of the fracture. Procedural accuracy is imperative for creating optimal mechanical and biological conditions for bone healing and restoration of bone anatomy and function. In addition, when an articulating joint like the hip, knee, or ankle is affected, it is essential to repair the bone joint surface precisely to prevent post-traumatic osteoarthritis. Enhanced surgical precision in orthopaedic trauma improves procedural safety, promotes proper anatomic healing, and reduces post-operative morbidity and long-term complications such as delayed, mal- or non-union, and post-traumatic osteoarthritis [38,47–49]. Five procedural phases of preoperative VR planning of fracture fixation have been described, namely, the generation of patient-specific geometrical models, fracture reduction, fixation, analysis of surgical planning, and intra-operative guidance [50]. A number of experimental and clinically applicable VR systems have been developed to accomplish one or more of the fracture fixation procedure phases.

The TraumaVision software developed by Swemac, Melerit, and Simulution Inc. (Burnsville, MN, USA) simulates a variety of orthopaedic trauma scenarios, including femoral neck fracture, trochanteric fracture, subtrochanteric fracture, femoral shaft fracture, pelvis fracture, spinal surgery, slipped capital femoral epiphysis, and Motec® wrist prosthesis [51,52]. The software contains several preloaded training modules such as drill skills, cannulated screws, dynamic hip screws, and fluoroscopy training. A conventional A-P and lateral radiograph records fluoroscopy, which is provided by pushing a foot-controlled paddle. Phantom Omni, a computer-connected robot arm controllable with either of the operator's hands, mimics operating tools and provides haptic feedback [52]. A Geomagic Touch X (Geomagic, Cary, NC, USA) haptic device may also be employed for positional sensing and precise force-feedback output, enabling the operator to appreciate tissue and bone resistance and even differentiate cortical and cancellous bone [53]. During a simulated operation, the software tracks a variety of performance parameters and reliably discriminates between novices and experts [52].

The BoneDoc DHS simulator is a web-browser-based non-haptic VR platform that operates on a regular PC and mouse and simulates screw and plate fixation of hip fractures [54]. Two-dimensional radiographic images facilitate fracture reduction and 3D implant placement on a virtual hip model. The simulated decision-making steps in the program include placing the C-arm to examine the fracture, reduction of the fracture using the virtual fracture table, skin incision, determination of entry location, guide wire angulation and depth of entry, and installation of the lag screw and cortical screws supporting the side plate [54,55]. The simulator also includes an assessment feedback component, and despite the lack of haptic function, the simulator was shown to have good face validity (closely mimics the actual procedure) [54]. Besides the lack of haptic/somatosensory feedback, the other remarkable limitation of this method is the absence of the psychomotor movements performed in surgery.

The first patient-specific biomechanical model developed by Boudissa et al. could replicate success or failure in the virtual reduction of an acetabular fracture depending on the selected surgical reduction strategy and sequence [56]. To recreate intraoperative bone fragment behaviour and reduction quality, the model simulated the impact of forces on the fragments and soft tissue–bone interactions. The model demonstrated clinical feasibility and favourable intraoperative outcomes [57]. Buschbaum et al. developed and evaluated a VR system based on preoperative CT scans for the automated repositioning and planning of the optimal reduction approach for femoral fractures [58,59]. Using a reference-coordinate system for calculating reduction parameters allowed for effective planning of reduction approaches. Adjustments to the reduction parameters are applied progressively until the fracture target position is attained.

The SQ Pelvis software, a PC-based preoperative planning VR program with 3D visualisation and surgical simulation tools for pelvic and acetabular fracture, was developed by clinicians at the University Clinical Centre, Ljubljana, in collaboration with computer engineers from Sekvenca Inc. [60]. The program provides a virtual comprehensive procedural simulation, including osteosynthesis and C-arm simulations, based on actual patient information (patient CT data is in DICOM format). The software permits the movement and rotation of bone fragments in all three planes to enable reduction and subsequent fixation. In addition, it allows for selecting the appropriate reconstruction plate, automatic contouring of the plate to the reduced pelvis, control of the direction and length of screws, and comprehensive C-arm imaging during surgery. All procedure steps are recorded in a printable format for surgical documentation, patient education, or research. Preliminary studies of the SQ Pelvis software in clinical settings demonstrated good practical utility for preoperative planning and facilitation of actual surgical experience, and it is currently routinely used at the traumatology department of the University Medical Centre in Ljubljana.

A system that employs a novel blend of cutting-edge 2D/3D image processing and surface processing algorithms to virtually recreate shattered bone pieces for severity classification or preoperative planning in complex bone fractures was proposed by Liu et al. [61]. A number of cutting-edge algorithms for identifying, extracting, and reassembling virtual pieces are integrated into a single system to facilitate reconstruction. To aid surgeons in classifying the clinical severity of comminuted bone fractures, the approach allows for the extraction of quantitative information not previously accessible from fracture cases in terms of bone fragment data. Tibial plafond fractures, which are difficult-to-treat, complex fractures typically resulting from high-energy trauma such as a gunshot wound or road traffic accidents, were used as a model for the system. Similarly, Fürnstahl et al. developed a semiautomated virtual environment to reconstruct complex proximal humerus fractures. A contralateral matching algorithm showed the efficacy of contralateral bone modelling for this type of fracture and permitted precise and efficient fragment alignment. On cadaver specimens, the fracture reduction approach was associated with decreased procedural time and minimal translational displacement and rotational errors in the reconstructed bone geometries [62].

A volume-based orthopaedic surgery simulator for complex orthopaedic surgeries, including arthroplasty, corrective or open osteotomy, open reduction of fractures and amputation, was developed by Tsai et al. [63]. The system comprises multiple modules, including an interface module, a volume conversion module, an isosurface reconstruction module, a rendering module, and a simulation module. The software can simulate different orthopaedic procedures and provide stereographic images of the simulated geometric and topologic alterations to bones, prostheses, and bone grafts and is adaptable for both preoperative verification/rehearsal of surgical modality and surgical training.

The innovative minimally invasive plate osteosynthesis (MIPO) approach in orthopaedic trauma surgery requires substantial training for adequate skill acquisition. A VR platform was developed by Negrillo-Cárdenas et al. for training in the MIPO technique for surgical reduction of humeral supracondylar fractures [64]. It was shown that the common malrotation of MIPO-treated fractures might be avoided by enhancing the motor skills and expertise of surgeons via an emphasis on the mobility of bone fragments. By using high-quality lighting, post-processing effects, and comprehensive medical assets, the planned setting provides a genuine experience throughout the procedure.

VR systems have also been developed for procedures in non-appendicular bones. A surgical planning VR system for the evaluation and reconstruction of severe atrophic mandibular fractures was described by Castro-Núñez et al. [65]. The tool enabled mirror imaging, facilitating the alignment of pieces and the restoration of incomplete segments, and was found to be clinically beneficial in reducing surgical time and delivering predictable outcomes. Rambani et al. developed a desktop-based simulation for the training of pedicle screw insertion in the lumbar spine and a Computer-Assisted Orthopaedic Training System for fracture fixation with Polaris optical tracking-based haptic functions and demonstrated a significant improvement in procedural time, accuracy, and the number of exposures after the training on the simulator systems [66,67].

3.3. Orthopaedic Drilling Simulators

Precision drilling is an integral skill in orthopaedic surgery. Nonetheless, bone drilling is a delicate procedure that demands a high degree of dexterity and expertise. The associated high drilling resistance and intense vibrations make it difficult to grip the handpiece and escalate the risk of damage to the drill. An assessment of the impact of haptic feedback in VR simulation of cortical bone drilling using changes in drill plunge depth as an evaluative metric suggests that bone drilling simulation with haptic feedback is effective in simulating the required motor skill dexterity and control and leads to a decrease in soft tissue injury [68].

To simulate and predict the hip drilling process, Tsai et al. developed a volume-based surgical simulator with haptic functions utilising a force and torque computation model and demonstrated its practical application in screw and plate surgery for hip trochanter fracture positioning [69]. The force and torque computation model is employed to simulate haptic reactions in the drilling procedure based on patient-specific volumetric data harnessed to simulate the dynamics of the bone geometry during the surgical process. The calculated torques are used to evaluate the required work for drilling, the drill bend, and the handpiece oscillation during the drilling process [69].

Vankipuram et al. developed a realistic drilling software deploying a Geomagic Touch X haptic device for visiohaptic interaction with virtual bones. The program permits horizontal drilling into the femoral body with simulated targets for precision and tracks and analyses the surgeon's movements to assess surgical proficiency. The simulator was confirmed to have a learning effect that is transferable to actual drilling, and its surgical performance indicators could distinguish the hierarchy of expertise from senior surgeons, residents, and medical students [70]. Similarly, Sang-Won Han et al. demonstrated the clinical and educational effects of a VR simulation system designed to perform a high tibial osteotomy [71]. The system uses a morphable haptic controller that provides geometric and tactile feedback facilitating interaction between the surgical instruments and surgical sites.

The Haptic Orthopaedic Training (HOOT) simulator developed at the Imperial College London focuses on dynamic hip screw (DHS) operations for certain hip fractures [72]. Drilling a pilot hole through the outside border of the femur into the femoral head is a critical initial step in DHS surgery that determines its trajectory and ultimate outcome. However, precise positioning of the pilot hole is difficult to achieve since the surgeon cannot visually monitor the location of the guide wire's tip and must rely on several X-ray images to track its progress (with obvious problems including repeated radiation exposures and extended procedure time). Accordingly, the HOOT project aimed to develop and validate a haptically enabled simulator for training guide wire placement in DHS surgery. Unlike other haptic applications, the HOOT simulator is unique in its use of W5D from Entact Robotics to produce both linear forces (x,y,z) and rotational forces (torques: roll, pitch, yaw) [73]. The researchers plan to enhance the realism of the haptic feedback and perform validation studies in the next phase of the project.

Pettersson et al. developed a surgical simulator for the drilling procedure in cervical hip fracture surgery. The volumetric dataset obtained from the patient's CT scan is used to produce visuohaptic feedback by replicating fluoroscopic images and the drilling procedure. Prior to simulation, the bone must be relocated into the correct position. An automatic segmentation based on nonrigid registration with the Morphon method is deployed to identify the fracture's constituent pieces and estimate the link between the fracture elements [74].

3.4. Prosthesis Development and Implantation VR Modalities

This category of VR systems is mostly applied to elective orthopaedic procedures but is nevertheless highlighted for potential relevance in certain contexts related to orthopaedic trauma.

The Virtual Operation Planning in Orthopaedic Surgery (VIRTOPS) software is a VR system for 3D planning and simulation of hip and pelvic surgeries, including endoprosthetic hip reconstruction with hemipelvic replacement [75]. The software also facilitates the personalised design of anatomically flexible, modular prostheses for bone tumour surgery [76]. A patient-specific 3D hip model is created from CT images, and an ROI-based segmentation separates the bone tumour in multispectral MRI sequences; CT and MRI data are then fused by a segmentation-based registration approach enabling visualisation of the tumour position. Texture mapping, quantitative parameter colour coding, and transparency aid in optimal prosthesis positioning and geometry. Virtual models can interact in 3D using stereoscopic visualisation tools and 3D input devices. The virtual planning environment eliminates the need for expensive solid 3D models and permits the comparison of different surgical approaches. The generated 3D images and videos can be utilised for patient preoperative educational counselling and surgical planning documentation [75,76].

Another prosthetic placement VR modality is HipNav, an image-guided surgical navigation system. It combines a 3D preoperative planner, a simulator, and an intraoperative surgical navigator to precisely measure and direct the placement of prosthetic components during total hip arthroplasty [77]. The use of virtual surgical planning to fabricate the required hardware in preparation for open reduction and internal fixation of atrophic edentulous mandible fractures was reported by Maloney et al. [78]. As already noted, multimodal VR systems such as the SQ Pelvis [60] and TraumaVision software [51,52] also consist of prosthetic design and implantation modules.

Table 2. Summary of bone trauma virtual reality (VR) systems.

Category	Examples	Procedures	Remarkable Features
Fracture fixation/ Bone drilling/ prosthesis design	TraumaVision software [51,52].	Femoral, pelvic, and wrist fracture repair	Preloaded training modules such as drill skills, cannulated screws, dynamic hip screws, and fluoroscopy training
Fracture fixation	BoneDoc Dynamic hip screw (DHS) simulator [54,55].	Screw and plate fixation of hip fractures	Simulates several procedural decision steps and enables feedback assessment; non-haptic
Fracture fixation	Boudissa et al. [56].	Virtual reduction of an acetabular fracture	Patient-specific biomechanical model
Fracture fixation	Buschbaum et al. [58,59].	Reduction of femoral fracture	Uses a reference-coordinate system for the calculation of reduction parameters
Fracture fixation/ prosthesis design	SQ Pelvis software [60].	Pelvic and acetabular fracture repair	Comprehensive procedural simulation, including osteosynthesis and C-arm simulations
Fracture fixation	Liu et al. [61].	Complex fracture repair	Preoperative planning and severity classification
Fracture fixation	Fürnstahl et al. [62].	Reconstruct complex proximal humerus fractures	Semiautomated virtual environment; contralateral bone modelling
Fracture fixation	Tsai et al. [63].	Open reduction of fractures and other complex surgeries like arthroplasty, corrective or open osteotomy, and amputation	Volume-based orthopaedic simulator

Table 2. Cont.

Category	Examples	Procedures	Remarkable Features
Fracture fixation	Negrillo-Cárdenas et al. [64].	Minimally invasive plate osteosynthesis (MIPO) technique for surgical reduction of humeral supracondylar fractures	Uses high-quality lighting, post-processing effects, and comprehensive medical assets
Fracture fixation	Castro-Núñez et al. [65].	Evaluation and reconstruction of severe atrophic mandibular fractures	
Fracture fixation	Rambani et al. [66,67].	Pedicle screw insertion in the lumbar spine	Polaris optical tracking-based haptic functions
Bone drilling	Tsai et al. [69].	Screw and plate surgery for hip trochanter fracture positioning	Uses a force and torque computation model
Bone drilling	Vankipuram et al. [70].	Horizontal drilling into the femoral body	Geomagic Touch X haptic device
Bone drilling	Sang-Won Han et al. [71].	High tibial osteotomy	Uses a morphable haptic controller that provides geometric and tactile feedback
Bone drilling	Haptic Orthopaedic Training (HOOT) simulator [72].	Dynamic hip screw (DHS) operations	For training guide wire placement in DHS surgery, uses W5D from Entact Robotics to produce both linear forces and rotational forces.
Bone drilling	Pettersson et al. [74].	Cervical hip fracture surgery	Automatic segmentation based on nonrigid registration with the Morphon method
Prosthesis design/ implantation	VIRTOPS [75].	Endoprosthetic hip reconstruction with hemipelvic replacement	Facilitates the personalised design of anatomically flexible, modular prostheses
Prosthesis design/ implantation	HipNav [77].	Placement of prosthetic components during total hip arthroplasty	Combines a 3D preoperative planner, a simulator, and an intraoperative surgical navigator
Prosthesis design/ implantation	Maloney et al. [78].	Preparation for open reduction and internal fixation of atrophic edentulous mandible fractures	

4. Clinical Translation and Efficacy of Orthopaedic Trauma VR Modalities

Several studies have reported the advantages of both high- and low-fidelity VR over conventional surgical training modalities [34,79–85]. In the current era of surgical training, it has become increasingly clear that the required skill sets in specialist orthopaedics training cannot be solely realised in the clinical setting. Indeed, in recent decades, practical teaching and learning outside the operating room have become a compelling necessity in orthopaedic surgery, mostly due to rising training costs and ethical concerns over traditional pedagogical approaches [32,33]. VR simulation systems are well-adapted to meet the current training gaps in orthopaedic residency programmes. Table 3 summarises the potential advantages of VR-based modalities in orthopaedic trauma surgery. In addition, different studies have also assessed the reliability and clinical validity of existing VR systems applicable to orthopaedic trauma procedures. Reliability refers to the repeatability and accuracy of the modality, while validity assesses if the simulator is teaching or assessing the intended objective [86]. Different concepts of validity are applied in assessing the validity of VR simulation systems. Face validity evaluates how realistic a simulator is; content validity evaluates how appropriate it is as a training tool; concurrent validity measures how well it corresponds with the gold standard; predictive validity assesses how well it forecasts future performance; construct validity measures its ability to differentiate between a skilled and unskilled user; and transfer validity assesses whether training on the simulator results in skill transfer to a realistic environment [86,87].

Table 3. Potential benefits of bone trauma virtual reality systems.

Enhanced procedural teaching and learning efficiency
• Decreased use of animal models, cadavers, and patients for procedural teaching and practice • Avoidance of ethical issues associated with traditional procedural teaching and learning • Faster knowledge acquisition and visuospatial appreciation of surgical anatomy • Improved psychomotor skill acquisition and appreciation of complex surgical manoeuvres • Better knowledge and skill retention and clinical transfer • Improved procedural accuracy • Reduced number of procedural learning attempts • Increased procedural completion rate • Objective assessment of surgical proficiency and tracking of learning progression
Enhanced preoperative planning
• Enhanced preoperative patient counselling and education • Low-risk environment for preoperative procedural rehearsal/practice • Objective and comprehensive procedural documentation • Objective analysis and evaluation of different surgical approaches • Objective prediction of intraoperative complications • Design and analysis of patient-specific prosthetic models
Enhanced intraoperative efficiency
• Decreased procedural time (intraoperative duration) • Decreased radiation exposure (e.g., fluoroscopy frequency) • Decreased intraoperative blood loss • Reduced surgical invasiveness • Improved clinical and radiographic quality of fracture reduction
Improved postoperative outcomes
• Decreased rehabilitation and fracture healing time • Improved return of functional capacity • Decreased postoperative complications • Decreased incidence of hospital readmissions • Decreased fracture repair revisions

Validity assessments of bone trauma VR simulators show wide methodological variability, and no formal evaluation protocol currently exists. Twenty-two orthopaedic surgery residents participated in a stratified, randomised, controlled study that evaluated their performance on a virtual haptic-enabled ulnar fracture fixation simulator compared to the conventional synthetic manikin simulator (Sawbones simulator). It was noted that both methods demonstrated evidence of construct validity (capacity to evaluate trainees' technical skills), but although the virtual simulator showed potential value as a surgical educational tool, it failed to attain similar standards as the Sawbones simulator [88,89]. Compared to a conventional learning method, an immersive VR system was shown to efficiently teach a complex surgical procedure (optimum glenoid exposure in shoulder arthroplasty) and demonstrated face, content, construct, and transfer validity [90].

When compared with a technique guide, VR was shown to improve both the procedural accuracy and completion rate in intramedullary tibial nail insertion in a recent randomised control trial, demonstrating its capacity to assist trainees in understanding surgical processes and manoeuvres [91]. A similar randomised control study found that training novice medical students to perform a simulated tibial intramedullary tibial nail operation using an interactive VR simulation had superior results than training with a passive standard guide [92]. Clinically relevant objective performance indicators of inexperienced surgical trainees, including total procedural time, fluoroscopy time, number of radiographs, tip–apex distance, attempts at guide wire insertion, and probability of cut-out, were significantly improved following exposure to a VR DHS simulation with the TraumaVision (SveMac, Sweden) haptic- and fluoroscopy-enabled VR simulator [93].

A recent randomised, controlled, double-blinded trial assessed the educational value of integrated haptic feedback in a VR bone drilling simulation comparing the performance (assessed by plunge gap distance, drilling time, and objective structured assessment of technical skills) of 31 junior surgeons randomly allocated to a haptic or non-haptic group. The trainee doctors experienced a VR training module for drilling bicortical holes for screw insertion on a VR tibia bone model with either haptic or no haptic feedback, followed by an ex vivo identical test on a tibial sawbone model. The authors proved the higher performance of participants included in the haptic group, highlighting the potential educational role of haptic feedback in orthopaedic training simulation models [94].

For training in the distal interlocking of intramedullary nails, the Digitally Enhanced Hands-On Surgical Training (DEHST) concept and technology scored highly in terms of training capability and realism and reliably differentiated between experts and novices [95]. DEHST is a novel modular surgical skills training and evaluation system incorporating digital tools with haptic stations for hands-on learning. Position and orientation may be tracked in six directions from a single plane of the projected image using a specialised optical tracking technique [96].

In a slipped capital femoral epiphysis model, orthopaedic trainees rated VR training as more valuable than reading/video methods despite similar performance outcomes (surgical time, Global Rating Scale score, radiographic or physical accuracy of screw position, or articular surface breaching) to training with physical simulations [97]. Following training with immersive VR to revise a failed percutaneous pinning of a slipped capital femoral epiphysis, Lohre et al. reported an immediate skill acquisition and transfer to a real operating setting by a senior orthopaedic trainee [98]. Similarly, superior learning efficiency, knowledge acquisition, and skill transfer were found among senior orthopaedic surgery residents who underwent surgical training with an immersive VR training platform offering a case-based module for reverse shoulder arthroplasty for advanced rotator cuff tear arthropathy [99].

Virtual preoperative planning enables the precise evaluation of fracture features and simulation of fracture reduction and internal fixation prior to surgery. Several studies have also evaluated surgical outcomes with virtual preoperative planning compared to traditional preprocedural planning. A range of intraoperative and postoperative indices have been applied for comparison, including surgical duration, intraoperative blood loss, radiation exposure frequency, clinical and radiographic quality of fracture reduction, and postoperative complications. Overall, compared to conventional planning, VR-based preoperative planning for fracture fixation was shown to be associated with enhanced intra-operative efficiency (decreased operating length, bleeding, and fluoroscopy frequency, and better fracture reduction quality) and superior postoperative outcomes (improved functional outcomes, quicker fracture healing, fewer postoperative morbidities, hospital readmissions, and reoperations) [48,50,57,100–105].

Immersive VR has also been exploited as a form of distraction therapy and adjunct to surgical anaesthesia to alleviate pain and anxiety and promote patient relaxation [106–108]. However, Peuchot et al. reported that the use of VR for immersive distraction during total knee arthroplasty under spinal anaesthesia did not seem to reduce patient anxiety or alter patient satisfaction, although improvements in postoperative comfort and reductions in intraoperative complications were achieved [109]. In addition, as a rehabilitation tool, VR training, compared to sensory–motor training, was found to have a more favourable impact on pain, functional disability, and the modification of inflammatory biomarkers in post-traumatic osteoarthritis after an anterior cruciate ligament injury, although a negligible effect on bone morphogenic proteins expression was reported [110].

5. Drawbacks of VR in Bone Trauma

While several advantages and benefits of VR simulation systems in bone trauma surgery have been highlighted, some important drawbacks and limitations should be equally understood. Currently, most immersive VR technologies suffer remarkable limitations with regard to image quality, degree of immersion, haptic accuracy, and other technical issues (e.g., battery life and wireless technologies) [111]. The distressing phenomenon of cybersickness (signs and symptoms related to VR experience) is another important drawback of immersive VR systems [112]. Many of the available bone trauma VR systems lack the requisite computing power and high-performance software architecture to provide optimally reliable audio–visual and haptic output. Further developments in haptic technology are specifically required to overcome the current limitations of haptic devices for VR simulation of fracture procedures, including challenges in a high-fidelity virtual recreation of sensations of density and palpability of convex surfaces, the limitations in maximum force, multi–modal telepresence, and teleaction in conventional haptic devices, and the high-bandwidth requirement barrier for an online haptic system [31,113]. In addition, a wide variability currently exists among the different VR tools in terms of technical quality and functional value [99]. This is partly due to the lack of regulatory standards and metrics in the design and manufacture of clinical VR systems and the lack of uniform protocols for clinical validation. Furthermore, although VR technology represents a well-adapted option to meet the current needs of orthopaedic training programmes, few studies have examined the long-term implications of orthopaedic simulation training on the retention of new skills [114]. Meanwhile, cost remains a prohibitive barrier for high-fidelity bone trauma VR systems, especially in resource-limited settings. Nevertheless, future VR tools are expected to be cheaper, more user-friendly, and in tandem with technological advancements [38,109].

6. Conclusions and Future Perspectives

Over the past two decades, an increasing number of VR systems for orthopaedic trauma surgeries have been introduced, although a considerable number are still in the experimental phases. The use of VR simulation modalities minimises the reliance on patients, cadavers, and animals for surgical training and skill practice. VR training simulators aid in developing a visuospatial appreciation of anatomy and provide learners with a controlled, low-risk environment to practise techniques before attempting them on a real patient [31]. Besides facilitated procedural learning and enhanced preoperative planning, VR systems have been shown to improve a broad range of intraoperative and postoperative outcomes. Nevertheless, clinical outcomes may be further enhanced by including biomechanical analysis within the framework of VR preoperative planning for fracture repair [50]. Rigorous validation of existing orthopaedic trauma VR systems in relation to the face, content, concurrent, and transfer validity is crucial, in addition to further development of orthopaedic VR systems in line with industry standards and metrics of immersion, multisensory realism, and versatility. The design and reporting guidelines proposed by the European Association of Endoscopic Surgeons Work Group for Evaluation and Implementation of Simulators and Skills Training Programmes represents an important step for harmonizing and standardising the appraisal of simulation studies [115]. Additional research is also warranted to demonstrate the cognitive simulation validity of immersive VR platforms, skill retention and decay with VR, translation to patient-derived outcomes, as well as the security, privacy, and cost-effectiveness of current orthopaedic trauma VR systems [38,114].

Author Contributions: Conceptualization, Ž.S., C.K.U. and N.U.; writing—original draft preparation, C.K.U.; writing—review and editing, C.K.U., D.A., Ž.S., I.D.-Č. and N.U.; visualisation, C.K.U., D.A., I.D.-Č. and Ž.S.; supervision, Ž.S., N.U. and I.D.-Č. All authors have read and agreed to the published version of the manuscript.

Funding: C.K.U. and N.U. gratefully acknowledge financial support from the Slovenian Research Agency (ARRS), Slovenia, through the research core funding No. P3-0043.

Institutional Review Board Statement: Not applicable.

Informed Consent Statement: Not applicable.

Data Availability Statement: Not applicable.

Acknowledgments: We are grateful to our orthopaedic colleagues, Rihard Trebše and Urban Slokar, for many stimulating discussions and critical insights, and to Nejc Petrišič for assistance with the graphics.

Conflicts of Interest: The authors declare no conflict of interest.

References

1. Wu, A.M.; Bisignano, C.; James, S.L.; Abady, G.G.; Abedi, A.; Abu-Gharbieh, E.; Alhassan, R.K.; Alipour, V.; Arabloo, J.; Asaad, M.; et al. Global, Regional, and National Burden of Bone Fractures in 204 Countries and Territories, 1990–2019: A Systematic Analysis from the Global Burden of Disease Study 2019. *Lancet Healthy Longev.* **2021**, *2*, e580–e592. [CrossRef] [PubMed]
2. Wong, R.M.Y.; Wong, P.Y.; Liu, C.; Wong, H.W.; Chung, Y.L.; Chow, S.K.H.; Law, S.W.; Cheung, W.H. The Imminent Risk of a Fracture-Existing Worldwide Data: A Systematic Review and Meta-Analysis. *Osteoporos. Int.* **2022**, *33*, 2453–2466. [CrossRef] [PubMed]
3. Sterling, R.S. Gender and Race/Ethnicity Differences in Hip Fracture Incidence, Morbidity, Mortality, and Function. *Clin. Orthop. Relat. Res.* **2011**, *469*, 1913–1918. [CrossRef] [PubMed]
4. Gullberg, B.; Johnell, O.; Kanis, J.A. World-Wide Projections for Hip Fracture. *Osteoporos. Int.* **1997**, *7*, 407–413. [CrossRef]
5. Hernlund, E.; Svedbom, A.; Ivergård, M.; Compston, J.; Cooper, C.; Stenmark, J.; McCloskey, E.V.; Jönsson, B.; Kanis, J.A. Osteoporosis in the European Union: Medical Management, Epidemiology and Economic Burden. A Report Prepared in Collaboration with the International Osteoporosis Foundation (IOF) and the European Federation of Pharmaceutical Industry Associations (EFPIA). *Arch. Osteoporos.* **2013**, *8*, 136. [CrossRef]
6. Werner, M.; Macke, C.; Gogol, M.; Krettek, C.; Liodakis, E. Differences in Hip Fracture Care in Europe: A Systematic Review of Recent Annual Reports of Hip Fracture Registries. *Eur. J. Trauma Emerg. Surg.* **2022**, *48*, 1625. [CrossRef]
7. Cordero, D.M.; Miclau, T.A.; Paul, A.V.; Morshed, S.; Theodore Miclau, I.; Martin, C.; Shearer, D.W. The Global Burden of Musculoskeletal Injury in Low and Lower-Middle Income Countries: A Systematic Literature Review. *OTA Int.* **2020**, *3*, e062. [CrossRef]
8. Lopez Gavilanez, E.; Navarro Chávez, M.; Gavilanes, A.W.D.; Cedeño German, R.; Chedraui, P. Decreasing Incidence Rates of Osteoporotic Hip Fractures in Ecuador during the COVID-19 Pandemic. *Arch. Osteoporos.* **2022**, *18*, 15. [CrossRef]
9. Oulianski, M.; Rosinsky, P.J.; Fuhrmann, A.; Sokolov, R.; Arriola, R.; Lubovsky, O. Decrease in Incidence of Proximal Femur Fractures in the Elderly Population during the COVID-19 Pandemic: A Case–Control Study. *BMC Musculoskelet. Disord.* **2022**, *23*, 61. [CrossRef]
10. Kumar Jain, V.; Lal, H.; Kumar Patralekh, M.; Vaishya, R. Fracture Management during COVID-19 Pandemic: A Systematic Review. *J. Clin. Orthop. Trauma* **2020**, *11*, S431–S441. [CrossRef]
11. Brown, T.D.; Johnston, R.C.; Saltzman, C.L.; Marsh, J.L.; Buckwalter, J.A. Posttraumatic Osteoarthritis: A First Estimate of Incidence, Prevalence, and Burden of Disease. *J. Orthop. Trauma* **2006**, *20*, 739–744. [CrossRef] [PubMed]
12. Borgström, F.; Karlsson, L.; Ortsäter, G.; Norton, N.; Halbout, P.; Cooper, C.; Lorentzon, M.; McCloskey, E.V.; Harvey, N.C.; Javaid, M.K.; et al. Fragility Fractures in Europe: Burden, Management and Opportunities. *Arch. Osteoporos.* **2020**, *15*, 59. [CrossRef] [PubMed]
13. Sakorafas, G.H.; Tsiotos, G.G. New Legislative Regulations, Problems, and Future Perspectives, with a Particular Emphasis on Surgical Education. *J. Postgrad. Med.* **2004**, *50*, 274–277. [PubMed]
14. Waurick, R.; Weber, T.; Bröking, K.; van Aken, H. The European Working Time Directive: Effect on Education and Clinical Care. *Curr. Opin. Anaesthesiol.* **2007**, *20*, 576–579. [CrossRef]
15. Benes, V. The European Working Time Directive and the Effects on Training of Surgical Specialists (Doctors in Training): A Position Paper of the Surgical Disciplines of the Countries of the EU. *Acta Neurochir.* **2006**, *148*, 1227–1233. [CrossRef]
16. Napolitano, L.M.; Fulda, G.J.; Davis, K.A.; Ashley, D.W.; Friese, R.; van Way, C.W.; Meredith, J.W.; Fabian, T.C.; Jurkovich, G.J.; Peitzman, A.B. Challenging Issues in Surgical Critical Care, Trauma, and Acute Care Surgery: A Report from the Critical Care Committee of the American Association for the Surgery of Trauma. *J. Trauma* **2010**, *69*, 1619–1633. [CrossRef]
17. Elkbuli, A.; Sutherland, M.; Sanchez, C.; Liu, H.; Ang, D.; McKenney, M. The Shortage of Trauma Surgeons in the US. *Am. Surg.* **2022**, *88*, 280–288. [CrossRef]
18. Cohn, S.M.; Price, M.A.; Villarreal, C.L. Trauma and Surgical Critical Care Workforce in the United States: A Severe Surgeon Shortage Appears Imminent. *J. Am. Coll. Surg.* **2009**, *209*, 446–452.e4. [CrossRef]
19. Comeau, P. Waiting Times: Crisis in Orthopedic Care: Surgeon and Resource Shortage. *CMAJ Can. Med. Assoc. J.* **2004**, *171*, 223. [CrossRef]

20. Barahona, M.; Infante, C.A.; Palet, M.J.; Barahona, M.A.; Barrientos, C.; Martinez, A. Impact of the COVID-19 Outbreak on Orthopedic Surgery: A Nationwide Analysis of the First Pandemic Year. *Cureus* **2021**, *13*, e17252. [CrossRef]
21. Ding, B.T.K.; Tan, K.G.; Oh, J.Y.L.; Lee, K.T. Orthopaedic Surgery after COVID-19—A Blueprint for Resuming Elective Surgery after a Pandemic. *Int. J. Surg.* **2020**, *80*, 162–167. [CrossRef] [PubMed]
22. Kamacı, S.; Göker, B.; Çağlar, Ö.; Atilla, B.; Mazhar Tokgözoğlu, A. The Effect of the COVID-19 Pandemic on Orthopedic Surgeries in a Tertiary Referral Center. *Jt. Dis. Relat. Surg.* **2021**, *32*, 333–339. [CrossRef]
23. Vaishya, R.; Vaish, A.; Kumar, A. Impact of COVID-19 on the Practice of Orthopaedics and Trauma—An Epidemiological Study of the Full Pandemic Year of a Tertiary Care Centre of New Delhi. *Int. Orthop.* **2021**, *45*, 1391–1397. [CrossRef] [PubMed]
24. Morgan, M.; Aydin, A.; Salih, A.; Robati, S.; Ahmed, K. Current Status of Simulation-Based Training Tools in Orthopedic Surgery: A Systematic Review. *J. Surg. Educ.* **2017**, *74*, 698–716. [CrossRef]
25. Kalun, P.; Wagner, N.; Yan, J.; Nousiainen, M.T.; Sonnadara, R.R. Surgical Simulation Training in Orthopedics: Current Insights. *Adv. Med. Educ. Pract.* **2018**, *9*, 125–131. [CrossRef]
26. Jerman, A.; Janáček, J.; Snoj, Ž.; Umek, N. Quantification of the Interventional Approaches Into the Pterygopalatine Fossa by Solid Angles Using Virtual Reality. *Image Anal. Stereol.* **2021**, *40*, 63–69. [CrossRef]
27. Jerman, A.; Umek, N.; Cvetko, E.; Snoj, Ž. Comparison of the Feasibility and Safety of Infrazygomatic and Suprazygomatic Approaches to Pterygopalatine Fossa Using Virtual Reality. *Reg. Anesth. Pain Med.* **2023**, rapm-2022-104068. [CrossRef]
28. Zhang, J.; Lu, V.; Khanduja, V. The Impact of Extended Reality on Surgery: A Scoping Review. *Int. Orthop.* **2023**, *47*, 611–621. [CrossRef]
29. Verhey, J.T.; Haglin, J.M.; Verhey, E.M.; Hartigan, D.E. Virtual, Augmented, and Mixed Reality Applications in Orthopedic Surgery. *Int. J. Med. Robot. Comput. Assist. Surg.* **2020**, *16*, e2067. [CrossRef]
30. Azuma, R.; Baillot, Y.; Behringer, R.; Feiner, S.; Julier, S.; MacIntyre, B. Recent Advances in Augmented Reality. *IEEE Comput. Graph. Appl.* **2001**, *21*, 34–47. [CrossRef]
31. Vaughan, N.; Dubey, V.N.; Wainwright, T.W.; Middleton, R.G. A Review of Virtual Reality Based Training Simulators for Orthopaedic Surgery. *Med. Eng. Phys.* **2016**, *38*, 59–71. [CrossRef] [PubMed]
32. Atesok, K.; Hurwitz, S.; Anderson, D.D.; Satava, R.; Thomas, G.W.; Tufescu, T.; Heffernan, M.J.; Papavassiliou, E.; Theiss, S.; Marsh, J.L. Advancing Simulation-Based Orthopaedic Surgical Skills Training: An Analysis of the Challenges to Implementation. *Adv. Orthop.* **2019**, *2019*, 2586034. [CrossRef] [PubMed]
33. Atesok, K.; MacDonald, P.; Leiter, J.; Dubberley, J.; Satava, R.; van Heest, A.; Hurwitz, S.; Marsh, J.L. Orthopaedic Education in the Era of Surgical Simulation: Still at the Crawling Stage. *World J. Orthop.* **2017**, *8*, 290–294. [CrossRef] [PubMed]
34. Rahm, S.; Wieser, K.; Bauer, D.E.; Waibel, F.W.; Meyer, D.C.; Gerber, C.; Fucentese, S.F. Efficacy of Standardized Training on a Virtual Reality Simulator to Advance Knee and Shoulder Arthroscopic Motor Skills. *BMC Musculoskelet. Disord.* **2018**, *19*, 150. [CrossRef]
35. Frank, R.M.; Erickson, B.; Frank, J.M.; Bush-Joseph, C.A.; Bach, B.R.; Cole, B.J.; Romeo, A.A.; Provencher, M.T.; Verma, N.N. Utility of Modern Arthroscopic Simulator Training Models. *Arthrosc.-J. Arthrosc. Relat. Surg.* **2014**, *30*, 121–133. [CrossRef]
36. Slade Shantz, J.A.; Leiter, J.R.S.; Gottschalk, T.; MacDonald, P.B. The Internal Validity of Arthroscopic Simulators and Their Effectiveness in Arthroscopic Education. *Knee Surg. Sports Traumatol. Arthrosc.* **2014**, *22*, 33–40. [CrossRef]
37. Vaghela, K.R.; Trockels, A.; Lee, J.; Akhtar, K. Is the Virtual Reality Fundamentals of Arthroscopic Surgery Training Program a Valid Platform for Resident Arthroscopy Training? *Clin. Orthop. Relat. Res.* **2022**, *480*, 807–815. [CrossRef]
38. Lohre, R.; Warner, J.J.P.; Athwal, G.S.; Goel, D.P. The Evolution of Virtual Reality in Shoulder and Elbow Surgery. *JSES Int.* **2020**, *4*, 215–223. [CrossRef]
39. Sarker, S.K.; Patel, B. Simulation and Surgical Training. *Int. J. Clin. Pract.* **2007**, *61*, 2120–2125. [CrossRef]
40. Srivastava, A.; Gibson, M.; Patel, A. Low-Fidelity Arthroscopic Simulation Training in Trauma and Orthopaedic Surgery: A Systematic Review of Experimental Studies. *Arthrosc. J. Arthrosc. Relat. Surg.* **2022**, *38*, 190–199.e1. [CrossRef]
41. Medical Image Processing, Analysis and Visualization. Available online: https://mipav.cit.nih.gov/ (accessed on 11 November 2022).
42. The Medical Imaging Interaction Toolkit (MITK)—Mitk.Org. Available online: https://www.mitk.org/wiki/The_Medical_Imaging_Interaction_Toolkit_(MITK) (accessed on 11 November 2022).
43. 3D Slicer Image Computing Platform | 3D Slicer. Available online: https://www.slicer.org/ (accessed on 11 November 2022).
44. 3D Image Processing Solutions—Simpleware | Synopsys. Available online: https://www.synopsys.com/simpleware.html (accessed on 1 January 2023).
45. 3D-DOCTOR, Medical Modeling, 3D Medical Imaging. Available online: http://www.ablesw.com/3d-doctor/ (accessed on 1 January 2023).
46. OsiriX DICOM Viewer | The World Famous Medical Imaging Viewer. Available online: https://www.osirix-viewer.com/ (accessed on 1 January 2023).
47. Phen, H.M.; Schenker, M.L. Minimizing Posttraumatic Osteoarthritis After High-Energy Intra-Articular Fracture. *Orthop. Clin. N. Am.* **2019**, *50*, 433–443. [CrossRef] [PubMed]
48. Jia, X.; Zhang, K.; Qiang, M.; Wu, Y.; Chen, Y. Association of Computer-Assisted Virtual Preoperative Planning With Postoperative Mortality and Complications in Older Patients With Intertrochanteric Hip Fracture. *JAMA Netw. Open* **2020**, *3*, e205830. [CrossRef] [PubMed]

49. Maini, L.; Verma, T.; Sharma, A.; Sharma, A.; Mishra, A.; Jha, S. Evaluation of Accuracy of Virtual Surgical Planning for Patient-Specific Pre-Contoured Plate in Acetabular Fracture Fixation. *Arch. Orthop. Trauma Surg.* **2018**, *138*, 495–504. [CrossRef] [PubMed]
50. Moolenaar, J.Z.; Tümer, N.; Checa, S. Computer-Assisted Preoperative Planning of Bone Fracture Fixation Surgery: A State-of-the-Art Review. *Front. Bioeng. Biotechnol.* **2022**, *10*, 1037048. [CrossRef]
51. Simulation—Swemac. Available online: https://swemac.com/simulation/ (accessed on 20 December 2022).
52. Pedersen, P.; Palm, H.; Ringsted, C.; Konge, L. Virtual-Reality Simulation to Assess Performance in Hip Fracture Surgery. *Acta Orthop.* **2014**, *85*, 403–407. [CrossRef]
53. Akhtar, K.; Sugand, K.; Sperrin, M.; Cobb, J.; Standfield, N.; Gupte, C. Training Safer Orthopedic Surgeons. Construct Validation of a Virtual-Reality Simulator for Hip Fracture Surgery. *Acta Orthop.* **2015**, *86*, 616–621. [CrossRef]
54. Blyth, P.; Stott, N.S.; Anderson, I.A. A Simulation-Based Training System for Hip Fracture Fixation for Use within the Hospital Environment. *Injury* **2007**, *38*, 1197–1203. [CrossRef]
55. Blyth, P.; Stott, N.S.; Anderson, I.A. Virtual Reality Assessment of Technical Skill Using the Bonedoc DHS Simulator. *Injury* **2008**, *39*, 1127–1133. [CrossRef]
56. Boudissa, M.; Oliveri, H.; Chabanas, M.; Tonetti, J. Computer-Assisted Surgery in Acetabular Fractures: Virtual Reduction of Acetabular Fracture Using the First Patient-Specific Biomechanical Model Simulator. *Orthop. Traumatol. Surg. Res.* **2018**, *104*, 359–362. [CrossRef]
57. Boudissa, M.; Bahl, G.; Oliveri, H.; Chabanas, M.; Tonetti, J. Virtual Preoperative Planning of Acetabular Fractures Using Patient-Specific Biomechanical Simulation: A Case-Control Study. *Orthop. Traumatol. Surg. Res.* **2021**, *107*, 103004. [CrossRef]
58. Buschbaum, J.; Fremd, R.; Pohlemann, T.; Kristen, A. Computer-Assisted Fracture Reduction: A New Approach for Repositioning Femoral Fractures and Planning Reduction Paths. *Int. J. Comput. Assist. Radiol. Surg.* **2015**, *10*, 149–159. [CrossRef] [PubMed]
59. Buschbaum, J.; Fremd, R.; Pohlemann, T.; Kristen, A. Introduction of a Computer-Based Method for Automated Planning of Reduction Paths under Consideration of Simulated Muscular Forces. *Int. J. Comput. Assist. Radiol. Surg.* **2017**, *12*, 1369–1381. [CrossRef] [PubMed]
60. Cimerman, M.; Kristan, A. Preoperative Planning in Pelvic and Acetabular Surgery: The Value of Advanced Computerised Planning Modules. *Injury* **2007**, *38*, 442–449. [CrossRef]
61. Liu, P.; Hewitt, N.; Shadid, W.; Willis, A. A System for 3D Reconstruction of Comminuted Tibial Plafond Bone Fractures. *Comput. Med. Imaging Graph.* **2021**, *89*, 101884. [CrossRef]
62. Fürnstahl, P.; Székely, G.; Gerber, C.; Hodler, J.; Snedeker, J.G.; Harders, M. Computer Assisted Reconstruction of Complex Proximal Humerus Fractures for Preoperative Planning. *Med. Image Anal.* **2012**, *16*, 704–720. [CrossRef] [PubMed]
63. Tsai, M.D.; Hsieh, M.S.; Jou, S.-B. Virtual Reality Orthopedic Surgery Simulator. *Comput. Biol. Med.* **2001**, *31*, 333–351. [CrossRef]
64. Negrillo-Cárdenas, J.; Jiménez-Pérez, J.R.; Madeira, J.; Feito, F.R. A Virtual Reality Simulator for Training the Surgical Reduction of Patient-Specific Supracondylar Humerus Fractures. *Int. J. Comput. Assist. Radiol. Surg.* **2022**, *17*, 65–73. [CrossRef]
65. Castro-Núñez, J.; Shelton, J.M.; Snyder, S.; Sickels, J. Virtual Surgical Planning for the Management of Severe Atrophic Mandible Fractures. *Craniomaxillofac Trauma Reconstr.* **2018**, *11*, 150–156. [CrossRef]
66. Rambani, R.; Ward, J.; Viant, W. Desktop-Based Computer-Assisted Orthopedic Training System for Spinal Surgery. *J. Surg. Educ.* **2014**, *71*, 805–809. [CrossRef]
67. Rambani, R.; Viant, W.; Ward, J.; Mohsen, A. Computer-Assisted Orthopedic Training System for Fracture Fixation. *J. Surg. Educ.* **2013**, *70*, 304–308. [CrossRef]
68. Benjamin, M.W.; Sabri, O. Using Haptic Feedback in a Virtual Reality Bone Drilling Simulation to Reduce Plunge Distance. *Cureus* **2021**, *13*, e18315. [CrossRef] [PubMed]
69. Tsai, M.D.; Hsieh, M.S.; Tsai, C.H. Bone Drilling Haptic Interaction for Orthopedic Surgical Simulator. *Comput. Biol. Med.* **2007**, *37*, 1709–1718. [CrossRef] [PubMed]
70. Vankipuram, M.; Kahol, K.; McLaren, A.; Panchanathan, S. A Virtual Reality Simulator for Orthopedic Basic Skills: A Design and Validation Study. *J. Biomed. Inform.* **2010**, *43*, 661–668. [CrossRef] [PubMed]
71. Han, S.W.; Sung, S.K.; Shin, B.S. Virtual Reality Simulation of High Tibial Osteotomy for Medical Training. *Mob. Inf. Syst.* **2022**, *2022*, 3055898. [CrossRef]
72. Procedure Modelling and Simulation | Faculty of Medicine | Imperial College London. Available online: https://www.imperial.ac.uk/simms/research/procedure-modelling-and-simulation/ (accessed on 21 December 2022).
73. Barrow, A.; Akhtar, K.; Gupte, C.; Bello, F. Requirements Analysis of a 5 Degree of Freedom Haptic Simulator for Orthopedic Trauma Surgery. *Stud. Health Technol. Inform.* **2013**, *184*, 43–47. [CrossRef]
74. Pettersson, J.; Palmerius, K.L.; Knutsson, H.; Wahlström, O.; Tillander, B.; Borga, M. Simulation of Patient Specific Cervical Hip Fracture Surgery with a Volume Haptic Interface. *IEEE Trans. Biomed. Eng.* **2008**, *55*, 1255–1265. [CrossRef]
75. Handels, H.; Ehrhardt, J.; Plötz, W.; Pöppl, S.J. Virtual Planning of Hip Operations and Individual Adaption of Endoprostheses in Orthopaedic Surgery. *Int. J. Med. Inform.* **2000**, *58–59*, 21–28. [CrossRef]
76. Handels, H.; Ehrhardt, J.; Plötz, W.; Pöppl, S.J. Three-Dimensional Planning and Simulation of Hip Operations and Computer-Assisted Construction of Endoprostheses in Bone Tumor Surgery. *Comput. Aided Surg.* **2001**, *6*, 65–76. [CrossRef]
77. Digioia, A.M.; Jaramaz, B.; Nikou, C.; Labarca, R.S.; Moody, J.E.; Colgan, B.D. Surgical Navigation for Total Hip Replacement with the Use of Hipnav. *Oper. Tech. Orthop.* **2000**, *10*, 3–8. [CrossRef]

78. Maloney, K.; Rutner, T. Virtual Surgical Planning and Hardware Fabrication Prior to Open Reduction and Internal Fixation of Atrophic Edentulous Mandible Fractures. *Craniomaxillofac Trauma Reconstr.* **2019**, *12*, 156–162. [CrossRef]
79. Seymour, N.E.; Gallagher, A.G.; Roman, S.A.; O'Brien, M.K.; Bansal, V.K.; Andersen, D.K.; Satava, R.M.; Pellegrini, C.A.; Sachdeva, A.K.; Meakins, J.L.; et al. Virtual Reality Training Improves Operating Room Performance: Results of a Randomized, Double-Blinded Study. *Ann. Surg.* **2002**, *236*, 458–464. [CrossRef] [PubMed]
80. Palter, V.N.; Grantcharov, T.P. Individualized Deliberate Practice on a Virtual Reality Simulator Improves Technical Performance of Surgical Novices in the Operating Room: A Randomized Controlled Trial. *Ann. Surg.* **2014**, *259*, 443–448. [CrossRef] [PubMed]
81. Rebolledo, B.J.; Hammann-Scala, J.; Leali, A.; Ranawat, A.S. Arthroscopy Skills Development with a Surgical Simulator: A Comparative Study in Orthopaedic Surgery Residents. *Am. J. Sports Med.* **2015**, *43*, 1526–1529. [CrossRef] [PubMed]
82. Aïm, F.; Lonjon, G.; Hannouche, D.; Nizard, R. Effectiveness of Virtual Reality Training in Orthopaedic Surgery. *Arthrosc.—J. Arthrosc. Relat. Surg.* **2016**, *32*, 224–232. [CrossRef]
83. Banaszek, D.; You, D.; Chang, J.; Pickell, M.; Hesse, D.; Hopman, W.M.; Borschneck, D.; Bardana, D. Virtual Reality Compared with Bench-Top Simulation in the Acquisition of Arthroscopic Skill: A Randomized Controlled Trial. *J. Bone Jt. Surg.—Am. Vol.* **2017**, *99*, e34.1–e34.8. [CrossRef]
84. Logishetty, K.; Rudran, B.; Cobb, J.P. Virtual Reality Training Improves Trainee Performance in Total Hip Arthroplasty: A Randomized Controlled Trial. *Bone Jt. J.* **2019**, *101-B*, 1585–1592. [CrossRef]
85. Cevallos, N.; Zukotynski, B.; Greig, D.; Silva, M.; Thompson, R.M. The Utility of Virtual Reality in Orthopedic Surgical Training. *J. Surg. Educ.* **2022**, *79*, 1516–1525. [CrossRef]
86. McDougall, E.M. Validation of Surgical Simulators. *J. Endourol.* **2007**, *21*, 244–247. [CrossRef]
87. van Nortwick, S.S.; Lendvay, T.S.; Jensen, A.R.; Wright, A.S.; Horvath, K.D.; Kim, S. Methodologies for Establishing Validity in Surgical Simulation Studies. *Surgery* **2010**, *147*, 622–630. [CrossRef]
88. LeBlanc, J.; Hutchison, C.; Hu, Y.; Donnon, T. A Comparison of Orthopaedic Resident Performance on Surgical Fixation of an Ulnar Fracture Using Virtual Reality and Synthetic Models. *J. Bone Jt. Surg. Am.* **2013**, *95*, e60–e65. [CrossRef]
89. LeBlanc, J.; Hutchison, C.; Hu, Y.; Donnon, T. Feasibility and Fidelity of Practising Surgical Fixation on a Virtual Ulna Bone. *Can. J. Surg.* **2013**, *56*, E91–E97. [CrossRef] [PubMed]
90. Lohre, R.; Bois, A.J.; Athwal, G.S.; Goel, D.P. Improved Complex Skill Acquisition by Immersive Virtual Reality Training: A Randomized Controlled Trial. *J. Bone Jt. Surg. Am.* **2020**, *102*, e26. [CrossRef]
91. Orland, M.D.; Patetta, M.J.; Wieser, M.; Kayupov, E.; Gonzalez, M.H. Does Virtual Reality Improve Procedural Completion and Accuracy in an Intramedullary Tibial Nail Procedure? A Randomized Control Trial. *Clin. Orthop. Relat. Res.* **2020**, *478*, 2170. [CrossRef] [PubMed]
92. Blumstein, G.; Zukotynski, B.; Cevallos, N.; Ishmael, C.; Zoller, S.; Burke, Z.; Clarkson, S.; Park, H.; Bernthal, N.; SooHoo, N.F. Randomized Trial of a Virtual Reality Tool to Teach Surgical Technique for Tibial Shaft Fracture Intramedullary Nailing. *J. Surg. Educ.* **2020**, *77*, 969–977. [CrossRef] [PubMed]
93. Sugand, K.; Akhtar, K.; Khatri, C.; Cobb, J.; Gupte, C. Training Effect of a Virtual Reality Haptics-Enabled Dynamic Hip Screw Simulator. *Acta Orthop.* **2015**, *86*, 695–701. [CrossRef]
94. Gani, A.; Pickering, O.; Ellis, C.; Sabri, O.; Pucher, P. Impact of Haptic Feedback on Surgical Training Outcomes: A Randomised Controlled Trial of Haptic versus Non-Haptic Immersive Virtual Reality Training. *Ann. Med. Surg.* **2022**, *83*, 104734. [CrossRef]
95. Pastor, T.; Pastor, T.; Kastner, P.; Souleiman, F.; Knobe, M.; Gueorguiev, B.; Windolf, M.; Buschbaum, J. Validity of a Novel Digitally Enhanced Skills Training Station for Freehand Distal Interlocking. *Medicina* **2022**, *58*, 773. [CrossRef]
96. Windolf, M.; Richards, R.G. Generic Implant Positioning Technology Based on Hole Projections in X-Ray Images. *J. Med. Device* **2021**, *15*, 025002. [CrossRef]
97. Margalit, A.; Suresh, K.v.; Marrache, M.; Lentz, J.M.; Lee, R.; Tis, J.; Varghese, R.; Hayashi, B.; Jain, A.; Laporte, D. Evaluation of a Slipped Capital Femoral Epiphysis Virtual Reality Surgical Simulation for the Orthopaedic Trainee. *J. Am. Acad. Orthop. Surg. Glob. Res. Rev.* **2022**, *6*, e22.00028. [CrossRef]
98. Lohre, R.; Leveille, L.; Goel, D.P. Novel Application of Immersive Virtual Reality Simulation Training: A Case Report. *JAAOS Glob. Res. Rev.* **2021**, *5*, e21.00114. [CrossRef]
99. Lohre, R.; Bois, A.J.; Pollock, J.W.; Lapner, P.; McIlquham, K.; Athwal, G.S.; Goel, D.P. Effectiveness of Immersive Virtual Reality on Orthopedic Surgical Skills and Knowledge Acquisition Among Senior Surgical Residents: A Randomized Clinical Trial. *JAMA Netw. Open* **2020**, *3*, e2031217. [CrossRef] [PubMed]
100. Wang, D.; Zhang, K.; Qiang, M.; Jia, X.; Chen, Y. Computer-Assisted Preoperative Planning Improves the Learning Curve of PFNA-II in the Treatment of Intertrochanteric Femoral Fractures. *BMC Musculoskelet. Disord.* **2020**, *21*, 34. [CrossRef] [PubMed]
101. Chen, S.; Zhang, K.; Jia, X.; Qiang, M.; Chen, Y. Evaluation of the Computer-Assisted Virtual Surgical Technology in Preoperative Planning for Distal Femoral Fracture. *Injury* **2020**, *51*, 443–451. [CrossRef] [PubMed]
102. Qiang, M.; Zhang, K.; Chen, Y.; Jia, X.; Wang, X.; Chen, S.; Wang, S. Computer-Assisted Virtual Surgical Technology in Pre-Operative Design for the Reconstruction of Calcaneal Fracture Malunion. *Int. Orthop.* **2019**, *43*, 1669–1677. [CrossRef]
103. Chen, Y.; Qiang, M.; Zhang, K.; Li, H.; Dai, H. Novel Computer-Assisted Preoperative Planning System for Humeral Shaft Fractures: Report of 43 Cases. *Int. J. Med. Robot* **2015**, *11*, 109–119. [CrossRef]
104. Zheng, Y.; Chen, J.; Yang, S.; Ke, X.; Xu, D.; Wang, G.; Cai, X.; Liu, X. Application of Computerized Virtual Preoperative Planning Procedures in Comminuted Posterior Wall Acetabular Fractures Surgery. *J. Orthop. Surg. Res.* **2022**, *17*, 51. [CrossRef]

105. Assink, N.; Reininga, I.H.F.; ten Duis, K.; Doornberg, J.N.; Hoekstra, H.; Kraeima, J.; Witjes, M.J.H.; de Vries, J.P.P.M.; IJpma, F.F.A. Does 3D-Assisted Surgery of Tibial Plateau Fractures Improve Surgical and Patient Outcome? A Systematic Review of 1074 Patients. *Eur. J. Trauma Emerg. Surg.* **2022**, *48*, 1737–1749. [CrossRef]
106. Faruki, A.A.; Nguyen, T.B.; Gasangwa, D.V.; Levy, N.; Proeschel, S.; Yu, J.; Ip, V.; McGourty, M.; Korsunsky, G.; Novack, V.; et al. Virtual Reality Immersion Compared to Monitored Anesthesia Care for Hand Surgery: A Randomized Controlled Trial. *PLoS ONE* **2022**, *17*, e0272030. [CrossRef]
107. Faruki, A.; Nguyen, T.; Proeschel, S.; Levy, N.; Yu, J.; Ip, V.; Mueller, A.; Banner-Goodspeed, V.; O'Gara, B. Virtual Reality as an Adjunct to Anesthesia in the Operating Room. *Trials* **2019**, *20*, 782. [CrossRef]
108. Huang, M.Y.; Scharf, S.; Chan, P.Y. Effects of Immersive Virtual Reality Therapy on Intravenous Patient-Controlled Sedation during Orthopaedic Surgery under Regional Anesthesia: A Randomized Controlled Trial. *PLoS ONE* **2020**, *15*, e0229320. [CrossRef]
109. Peuchot, H.; Khakha, R.; Riera, V.; Ollivier, M.; Argenson, J.N. Intraoperative Virtual Reality Distraction in TKA under Spinal Anesthesia: A Preliminary Study. *Arch. Orthop. Trauma Surg.* **2021**, *141*, 2323–2328. [CrossRef] [PubMed]
110. Nambi, G.; Abdelbasset, W.K.; Elsayed, S.H.; Khalil, M.A.; Alrawaili, S.M.; Alsubaie, S.F. Comparative Effects of Virtual Reality Training and Sensory Motor Training on Bone Morphogenic Proteins and Inflammatory Biomarkers in Post-Traumatic Osteoarthritis. *Sci. Rep.* **2020**, *10*, 15864. [CrossRef] [PubMed]
111. Logishetty, K.; Gofton, W.T.; Rudran, B.; Beaulé, P.E.; Cobb, J.P. Fully Immersive Virtual Reality for Total Hip Arthroplasty: Objective Measurement of Skills and Transfer of Visuospatial Performance After a Competency-Based Simulation Curriculum. *J. Bone Jt. Surg. Am.* **2020**, *102*, e27. [CrossRef]
112. Weech, S.; Kenny, S.; Barnett-Cowan, M. Presence and Cybersickness in Virtual Reality Are Negatively Related: A Review. *Front. Psychol.* **2019**, *10*, 158. [CrossRef] [PubMed]
113. Motaharifar, M.; Norouzzadeh, A.; Abdi, P.; Iranfar, A.; Lotfi, F.; Moshiri, B.; Lashay, A.; Mohammadi, S.F.; Taghirad, H.D. Applications of Haptic Technology, Virtual Reality, and Artificial Intelligence in Medical Training During the COVID-19 Pandemic. *Front. Robot. AI* **2021**, *8*, 258. [CrossRef]
114. Atesok, K.; Satava, R.M.; van Heest, A.; Hogan, M.V.; Pedowitz, R.A.; Fu, F.H.; Sitnikov, I.; Marsh, J.L.; Hurwitz, S.R. Retention of Skills After Simulation-Based Training in Orthopaedic Surgery. *J. Am. Acad. Orthop. Surg.* **2016**, *24*, 505–514. [CrossRef]
115. Carter, F.J.; Schijven, M.P.; Aggarwal, R.; Grantcharov, T.; Francis, N.K.; Hanna, G.B.; Jakimowicz, J.J. Consensus Guidelines for Validation of Virtual Reality Surgical Simulators. *Surg. Endosc. Other Interv. Tech.* **2005**, *19*, 1523–1532. [CrossRef]

Disclaimer/Publisher's Note: The statements, opinions and data contained in all publications are solely those of the individual author(s) and contributor(s) and not of MDPI and/or the editor(s). MDPI and/or the editor(s) disclaim responsibility for any injury to people or property resulting from any ideas, methods, instructions or products referred to in the content.

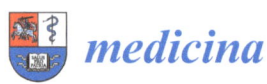

Case Report

Conservative Treatment for Spontaneous Resolution of Postoperative Symptomatic Thoracic Spinal Epidural Hematoma—A Case Report

Stjepan Dokuzović [1,2], Mario Španić [2], Sathish Muthu [3,4,5], Jure Pavešić [1], Stjepan Ivandić [6], Gregor Eder [6], Bogdan Bošnjak [7], Ksenija Prodan [8], Zoran Lončar [9] and Stipe Ćorluka [1,10,11,*]

1. Spinal Surgery Division, Department of Traumatology, University Hospital Center Sestre Milosrdnice, 10000 Zagreb, Croatia; stjepan.dokuzovic@kbcsm.hr (S.D.); jure.pavesic@kbcsm.hr (J.P.)
2. Akromion Special Hospital for Orthopaedic Surgery, 49217 Krapinske Toplice, Croatia; mario.spanic@hotmail.com
3. Orthopaedic Research Group, Coimbatore 641045, Tamil Nadu, India; drsathishmuthu@gmail.com
4. Department of Biotechnology, Faculty of Engineering, Karpagam Academy of Higher Education, Coimbatore 641021, Tamil Nadu, India
5. Department of Orthopaedics, Government Medical College, Karur 639004, Tamil Nadu, India
6. Traumatology Department, University Hospital Centre Sestre Milosrdnice, 10000 Zagreb, Croatia; stjepan.ivandic@kbcsm.hr (S.I.); gregor.eder@kbcsm.hr (G.E.)
7. General Hospital, Croatian Veterans, 49210 Zabok, Croatia; bosnjak.bogdan@gmail.com
8. Clinical Department of Diagnostic and Interventional Radiology, Department of Traumatology, University Hospital Center Sestre Milosrdnice, 10000 Zagreb, Croatia; ksenija.prodan@kbcsm.hr
9. Anesthesiology, Intensive Care and Pain Management Division, Traumatology Department, University Hospital Centre Sestre Milosrdnice, 10000 Zagreb, Croatia; zoran.loncar@kbcsm.hr
10. St. Catherine Specialty Hospital, 10000 Zagreb, Croatia
11. Department of Anatomy and Physiology, University of Applied Health Sciences, 10000 Zagreb, Croatia
* Correspondence: stipe@corluka.hr

Abstract: *Introduction*: Postoperative epidural hematomas of the cervical and thoracic spine can pose a great risk of rapid neurological impairment and sometimes require immediate decompressive surgery. *Case Report*: We present the case of a young patient operated on for stabilization of a two-level thoracic vertebra fracture who developed total paralysis due to an epidural hematoma postoperatively. The course of epidural hematoma was quickly reversed with the help of a conservative technique that prevented revision surgery. The patient regained complete neurologic function very rapidly, and has been well on every follow-up to date. *Conclusion*: There is a role of similar maneuvers as described in this case to be employed in the management of postoperative epidural hematomas. However, prolonged watchful waiting should still be discouraged, and patients should remain ready for revision surgery if there are no early signs of rapid recovery.

Keywords: thoracic; spine; trauma; fracture; hematoma

1. Introduction

An epidural hematoma can rapidly lead to neurological impairment [1]. Even though spinal surgeries are the most common cause, epidural hematomas can also arise spontaneously due to injury, blood thinning medication, bleeding from abnormal blood vessels in the spinal cord (such as an arteriovenous malformation), epidural steroid injections, or spinal or epidural anesthesia [2–4]. Given their potentially disastrous long-term effects, epidural hematomas warrant the attention of all spinal surgeons.

Epidural hematomas, although rare, can be a severe postoperative complication after spinal surgery. The reported incidence of a symptomatic epidural hematoma is less than 1% ranging from 0.10% to 0.69% [5,6]. While asymptomatic epidural hematomas are relatively more common postoperatively, symptomatic epidural hematoma mandates immediate attention and appropriate management to avoid untoward long-term complications. Various studies looking into the pharmacological prophylaxis for deep vein thrombosis and pulmonary embolism have reported epidural hematoma rates of less than 1% [7]. Although commonly employed, wound drains cannot be fully relied upon to eliminate the occurrence of epidural hematomas [8].

The diagnosis of symptomatic postoperative epidural hematoma necessitates a high index of suspicion and is made based on clinical symptoms such as evolving sudden postoperative axial pain in the area of surgery with neurological deficit and urinary retention [9]. In such cases, an emergency magnetic resonance imaging (MRI) is carried out to confirm the diagnosis, followed by emergency evacuation of the hematoma within 6–12 h [10]. Here, we present a case of post-operative epidural hematoma that was quickly reversed with the help of a conservative technique that prevented revision surgery.

2. Case Report

A 36-year-old male patient was admitted to our emergency trauma department with compressive Th6 and Th12 fractures, as shown in Figure 1 sustained from a fall on the head and upper spine. The initial examination ruled out accompanying head or any organ injury. There were no rib fractures or injuries to the extremities. The patient was neurologically normal upon admission.

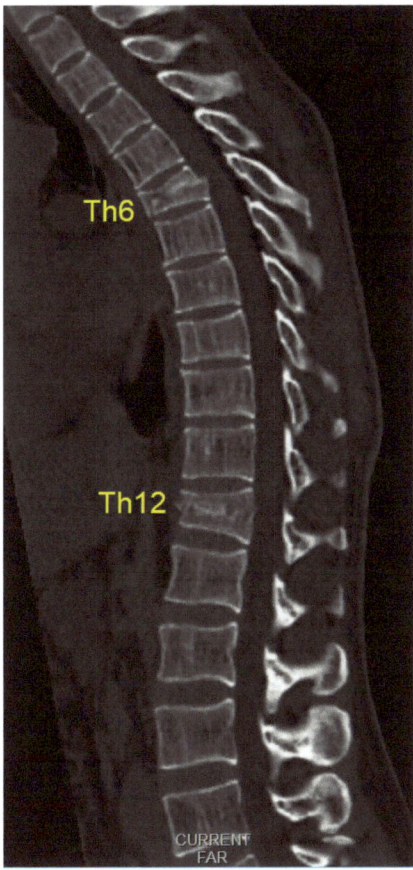

Figure 1. Initial multi-slice computerized tomography scans (midsagittal view) of compression fractures (Th6 A3 type fracture, and an Th12 A1 type fracture, classified according to the AO system).

There were no fracture lines through the posterior elements or indirect signs of rupture of the posterior tension band. Low-molecular-weight heparin was routinely applied the evening before surgery. Spinal stabilization surgery was performed the day after admission after a brief period of preoperative preparation. Intraoperatively, no disturbance of the posterior tension band was observed (interspinous ligaments were intact, and the laminar bone showed no subtle fractures). All transpedicular screws were placed under fluoroscopic guidance in two planes, as shown in Figure 2. There was no breach of the medial pedicular walls, and no laminectomy was performed, since there was no need initially. Intraoperatively, there was minimal blood loss, and the anesthesiologist did not report any significant changes in blood pressure or pulse.

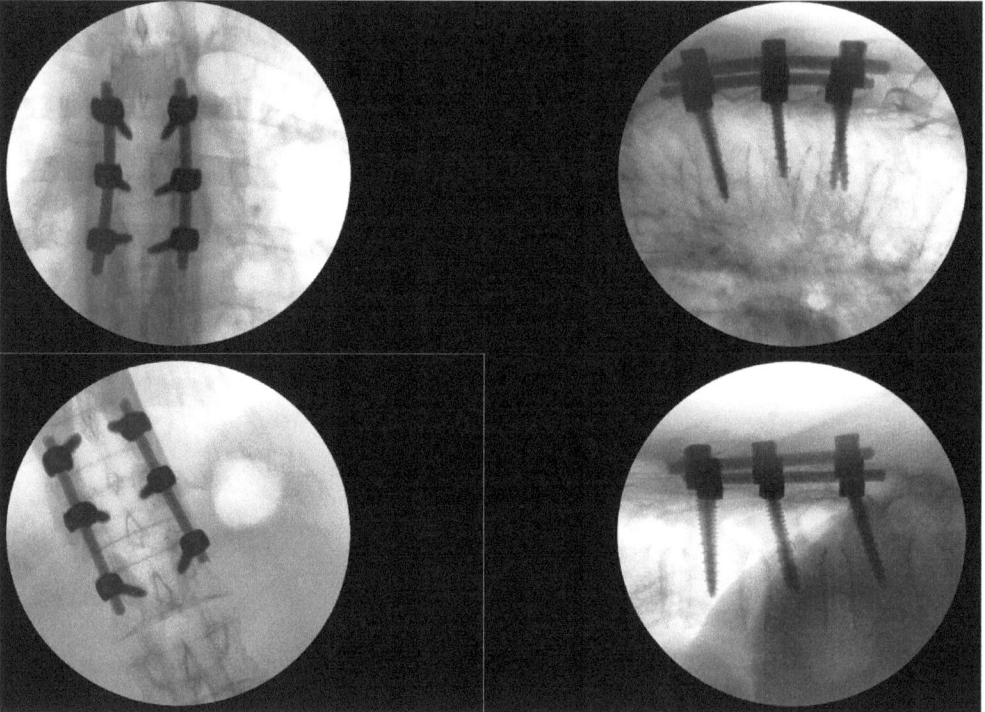

Figure 2. Intraoperative fluoroscopy images of the two short stabilizations performed; the upper images show the Th5–Th7 fixation that includes the fractured vertebra, and the lower images show the Th11–L1 fixation, the height of the fractured Th12 having been restored using postural reduction on the operating table.

Upon awakening from general anesthesia, the initial postoperative neurological state was without any impairment, and the patient was able to urinate spontaneously. Approximately 45 min after surgery, he began to develop signs of hypesthesia in the lower extremities, weakness in the legs, an unsettling sensation in the abdomen, and was covered with cold sweat. Due to neurological worsening, an emergency MRI of the thoracic spine was performed, which revealed a hyperacute epidural hematoma that developed at the level of the Th6 fracture and spread cranially to Th4, as shown in Figure 3. The width was measured 7 mm, and compressed the spinal cord against the laminae, as shown in Figure 4.

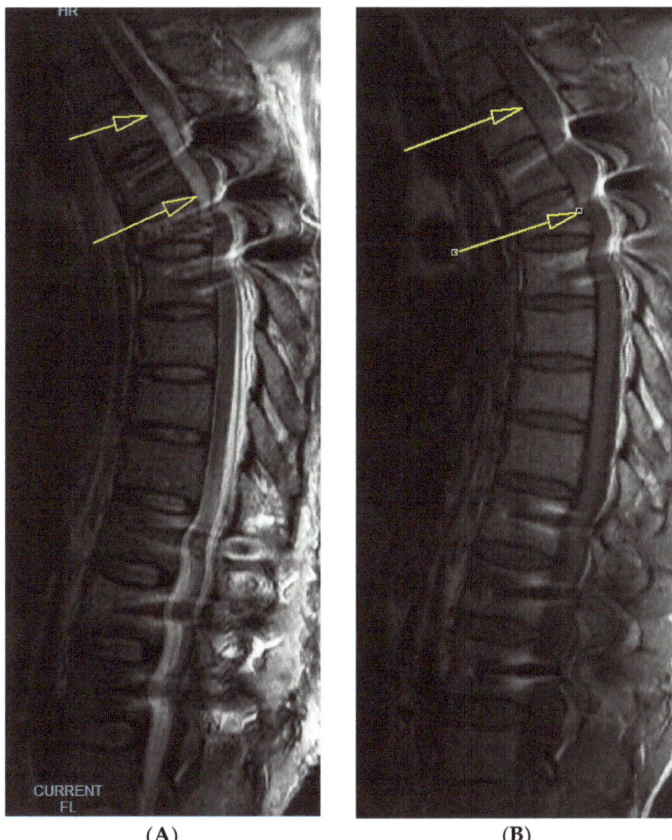

Figure 3. Emergency T2- (**A**) and T1 (**B**)-weighted MRI images, midsagittal views of the thoracic spine, show a hyperacute hematoma developing anterior to the spinal cord and spreading cranially to Th4, measuring 7 mm at its thickest. The yellow arrows in both the iamges depict the hematoma that is visible despite interference from implant artifacts.

Upon completion of the MRI, total paralysis was observed in the legs, as well as skin anesthesia up to the level of the lower ribcage (roughly corresponding to the Th7 dermatome). Emergency revision surgery was immediately planned, and the patient was placed in a semi-seated position while awaiting entry into the operating room. There was a roughly 45 min wait for the operating theatre to be ready, during which time rapid and complete resolution of the sensory and motor deficit was observed. The need for emergency surgery was revised and postponed due to the observation of spontaneous neurological recovery.

Serial neurological exams were conducted every 30 min, during which there was no worsening of neurological status. The daily dose of low-molecular-weight heparin was skipped on the day of the incident to avoid any potential ongoing minor epidural bleeding, and the patient was encouraged to frequently test his muscle strength by isometric contractions of the groups of the leg muscle while recovering in bed.

Normal bladder function was restored 2 days after surgery. Repeat MRI evaluation was done on third postoperative day, demonstrating significant resolution of the hematoma, as shown in Figures 5 and 6. The subsequent hospital stay was uneventful. The patient was mobilized the day after surgery, with pain medication tapered in 2 days; the wound healed primarily without signs of inflammation or dehiscence, and the patient is now fully independent in daily tasks that do not require much stress on the spine.

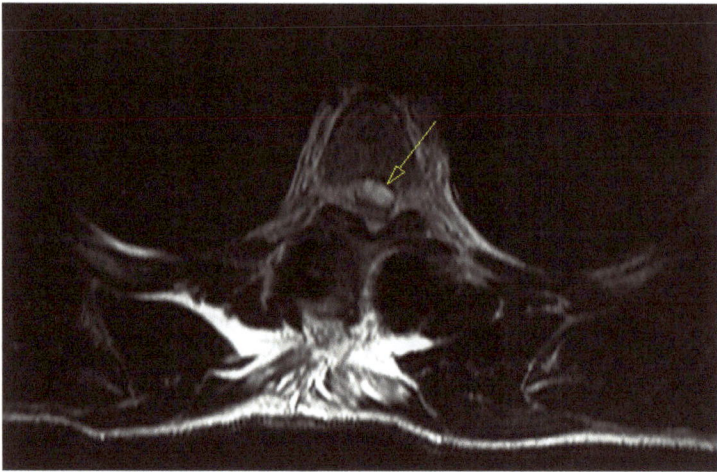

Figure 4. Emergency T2-weighted MRI image, an axial view at the Th5 level, revealing hyperacute hematoma development anterior to the spinal cord and causing significant dorsal displacement and compression.

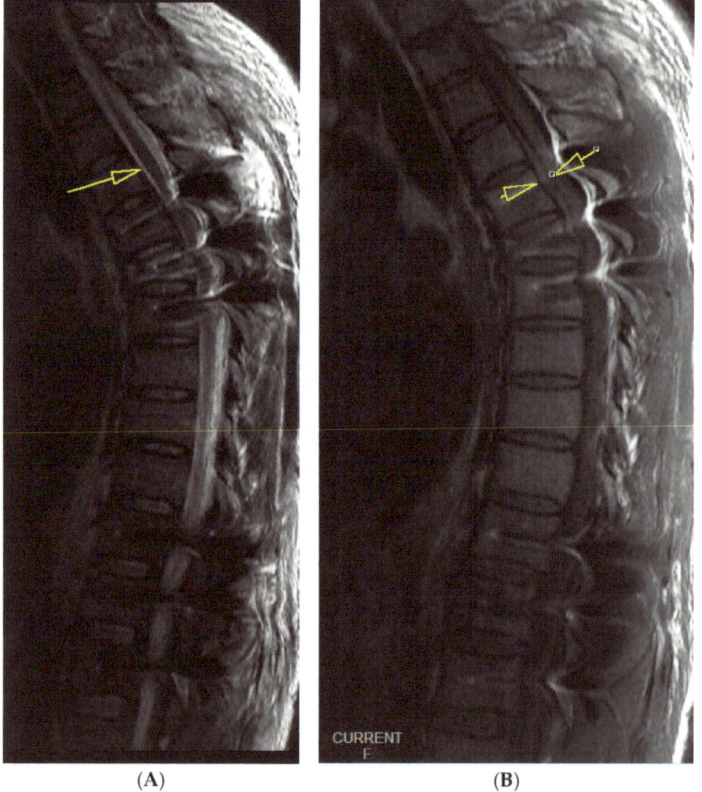

Figure 5. Follow-up midsagittal views of T2-weighted (**A**) and T1-weighted (**B**) MRI images taken 3 days after the initial emergency MRI showing near complete resolution of the hematoma, measuring 2 mm at its thickest.

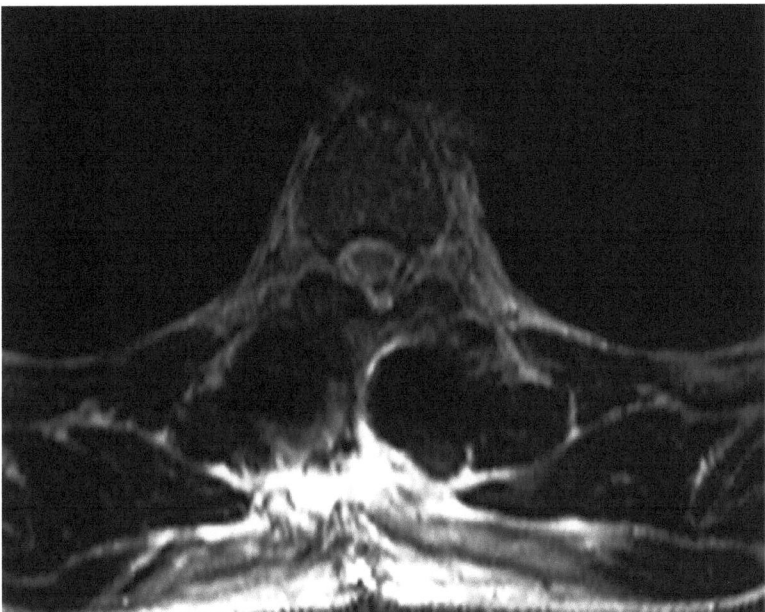

Figure 6. Follow-up axial view of an MRI taken 3 days after the initial emergency MRI, showing significant resolution of the hematoma. The view is at the level of Th4.

3. Discussion

A symptomatic epidural hematoma can occur post-surgery, since decompressive methods expose the dura to pressure from bleeding [11]. The bleeding can come from various places, such as epidural veins, muscle surfaces, or bone surfaces disrupted during fusion. Particularly, the Batson's plexus, a vein network, can bleed profusely, especially during posterior interbody fusion procedures. Visualization of the bleeding source, hemostasis, and hematoma evacuation may be quite challenging to manage, especially in obese patients [12]. Small arteries near facet joints that are injured during surgical dissection may also contribute. Injuries in paraspinal blood vessels can become active post-retraction. It is crucial to achieve hemostasis throughout and reassess before wound closure. Addressing a significant bleed during the initial surgery is preferable to needing to return to the operative room due to hematoma-induced symptoms.

An epidural hematoma that presents with symptoms following spine surgery is an uncommon occurrence, yet it has the potential to cause irreversible nerve damage and lasting serious disability. Factors that increase the likelihood of developing an epidural hematoma are older age, the use of blood-thinning medication before or after surgery, or a procedure involving the removal of multiple laminae [13]. If clinical symptoms suggest a hematoma, an urgent MRI is essential. An MRI helps confirm the diagnosis, showing fluid causing thecal sac compression. While some compression is normal and accepted, severe compression demands attention. The differential diagnosis for postoperative weakness includes tumor, infection, epidural hematoma, and disc herniation. An MRI serves as a confirmatory test, and it is crucial to correlate its findings with patient symptoms.

Sokolowski and colleagues created a "critical ratio" for evaluating thecal sac compression severity, but it is not an absolute criterion to decide on the method of management [14]. After diagnosing a symptomatic epidural hematoma, immediate evacuation is necessary to prevent permanent ischemic damage to the spinal cord. The existing incision can be used or extended for access. Potential bleeding sources need to be identified and eliminated using techniques such as coagulation and bone wax. Subfascial drains are typically employed during wound closure. Coagulation profiles should be conducted, and anticoagulants are paused if used as in our case. The time delay to evacuation and pre-evacuation neurologic impairment are key factors in prognosis. Neurologic recovery is maximized when deficits occur gradually, are incomplete, and when evacuation is undertaken within the first 12 h of onset [15]. After diagnosis, prompt surgical intervention should be prioritized.

In the case presented, due to the spontaneous resolution of the hematoma over a short time period, emergency revision surgery was avoided. Emergency revision is no guarantee of neurological recovery, as the procedure may require extensive decompression, costo-transversectomy, and slight cord manipulation to access the anteriorly located hematoma; these are maneuvers that can cause further injury to the fragile mid-thoracic spinal cord. The bleeding most likely occurred from the fracture line itself. The assumption is that the slight elevation of the upper part of the body to a semi-seated position of approximately 20° (initially conducted to avoid further cranial migration of the hematoma) allowed caudal diversion (under gravity alone) of the hyperacute hematoma to the lumbar epidural space, where there is significantly more space to accommodate the few milliliters of blood.

To date, literature on such simple spontaneous resolutions of an otherwise potentially devastating complication is scarce. The reported cases are mostly cervical spinal epidural hematomas with spontaneous resolution without any known identifiable reason for the spontaneous resolution [16,17]. To the authors' knowledge, this is the first case report of the spontaneous resolution of a thoracic postoperative spinal epidural hematoma with a simple conservative measure following thoracic stabilization surgery.

Continued passive observation for an extended period is not recommended, and patients should be prepared for the possibility of a follow-up surgical intervention if early indications of swift recovery are not apparent. This is to suggest that while it is crucial to give the body some time to heal and show signs of improvement after initial surgery, an excessively long period of inaction or "watchful waiting" may not be in the patient's best interest. If the patient does not show signs of rapid recovery in the initial stages following the procedure, they should be mentally and physically prepared for a potential secondary surgery or revision surgery. This secondary surgery aims to rectify issues that have not been resolved with the initial operation.

4. Conclusions

Although in our case, this was sudden and most unexpected, there may be a rationale to attempt similar simple elevation maneuvers when spontaneous or postoperative epidural hematomas are encountered as a cause of acute neurological deterioration. Prolonged watchful waiting should still be discouraged, and patients should remain ready for revision surgery if there are no early signs of rapid recovery.

Author Contributions: Conceptualization, S.D. and S.Ć.; methodology, J.P. and Z.L.; writing—original draft preparation, M.Š., G.E., B.B. and S.I.; writing—review and editing, S.D., S.Ć. and S.M.; visualization, S.D., K.P. and S.I.; supervision, S.M., S.D. and S.Ć. All authors have read and agreed to the published version of the manuscript.

Funding: This research received no external funding.

Institutional Review Board Statement: Not applicable.

Informed Consent Statement: Informed consent was obtained from the patient.

Data Availability Statement: No new data were created or analyzed in this study. Data sharing is not applicable to this article.

Conflicts of Interest: The authors declare no conflict of interest.

References

1. Glotzbecker, M.; Bono, C.; Wood, K.; Harris, M. Postoperative Spinal Epidural Hematoma: A Systematic Review. *Spine* **2010**, *35*, E413–E420. [CrossRef] [PubMed]
2. Bhosle, R.; Raju, D.; Patel, S.S.; Aditya, G.; Shukla, J.; Ghosh, N.; Krishnan, P. Spinal Subdural Hematoma Following Epidural Anesthesia. *Asian J. Neurosurg.* **2023**, *18*, 347–351. [CrossRef] [PubMed]

3. Brown, M.W.; Yilmaz, T.S.; Kasper, E.M. Iatrogenic Spinal Hematoma as a Complication of Lumbar Puncture: What Is the Risk and Best Management Plan? *Surg. Neurol. Int.* **2016**, *7*, S581–S589. [CrossRef] [PubMed]
4. Benyaich, Z.; Laghmari, M.; Lmejjati, M.; Aniba, K.; Ghannane, H.; Ait Benali, S. Acute Lumbar Spinal Subdural Hematoma Inducing Paraplegia After Lumbar Spinal Manipulation: Case Report and Literature Review. *World Neurosurg.* **2019**, *128*, 182–185. [CrossRef] [PubMed]
5. Amiri, A.R.; Fouyas, I.P.; Cro, S.; Casey, A.T.H. Postoperative Spinal Epidural Hematoma (SEH): Incidence, Risk Factors, Onset, and Management. *Spine J.* **2013**, *13*, 134–140. [CrossRef] [PubMed]
6. Aono, H.; Ohwada, T.; Hosono, N.; Tobimatsu, H.; Ariga, K.; Fuji, T.; Iwasaki, M. Incidence of Postoperative Symptomatic Epidural Hematoma in Spinal Decompression Surgery. *J. Neurosurg. Spine* **2011**, *15*, 202–205. [CrossRef] [PubMed]
7. Alvarado, A.M.; Porto, G.B.F.; Wessell, J.; Buchholz, A.L.; Arnold, P.M. Venous Thromboprophylaxis in Spine Surgery. *Glob. Spine J.* **2020**, *10*, 65S–70S. [CrossRef] [PubMed]
8. Muthu, S.; Ramakrishnan, E.; Natarajan, K.K.; Chellamuthu, G. Risk-Benefit Analysis of Wound Drain Usage in Spine Surgery: A Systematic Review and Meta-Analysis with Evidence Summary. *Eur. Spine J.* **2020**, *29*, 2111–2128. [CrossRef] [PubMed]
9. Modi, H.N.; Lee, D.Y.; Lee, S.-H. Postoperative Spinal Epidural Hematoma after Microscopic Lumbar Decompression: A Prospective Magnetic Resonance Imaging Study in 89 Patients. *J. Spinal Disord. Tech.* **2011**, *24*, 146–150. [CrossRef] [PubMed]
10. Domenicucci, M.; Mancarella, C.; Santoro, G.; Dugoni, D.E.; Ramieri, A.; Arezzo, M.F.; Missori, P. Spinal Epidural Hematomas: Personal Experience and Literature Review of More than 1000 Cases. *J. Neurosurg. Spine* **2017**, *27*, 198–208. [CrossRef] [PubMed]
11. Butler, A.J.; Mohile, N.; Phillips, F.M. Postoperative Spinal Hematoma and Seroma. *J. Am. Acad. Orthop. Surg.* **2023**, *31*, 908–913. [CrossRef] [PubMed]
12. Kao, F.-C.; Tsai, T.-T.; Chen, L.-H.; Lai, P.-L.; Fu, T.-S.; Niu, C.-C.; Ho, N.Y.-J.; Chen, W.-J.; Chang, C.-J. Symptomatic Epidural Hematoma after Lumbar Decompression Surgery. *Eur. Spine J.* **2015**, *24*, 348–357. [CrossRef] [PubMed]
13. Djurasovic, M.; Campion, C.; Dimar, J.R.; Glassman, S.D.; Gum, J.L. Postoperative Epidural Hematoma. *Orthop. Clin. N. Am.* **2022**, *53*, 113–121. [CrossRef] [PubMed]
14. Sokolowski, M.J.; Garvey, T.A.; Perl, J.; Sokolowski, M.S.; Akesen, B.; Mehbod, A.A.; Mullaney, K.J.; Dykes, D.C.; Transfeldt, E.E. Postoperative Lumbar Epidural Hematoma: Does Size Really Matter? *Spine* **2008**, *33*, 114–119. [CrossRef] [PubMed]
15. Mukerji, N.; Todd, N. Spinal Epidural Haematoma; Factors Influencing Outcome. *Br. J. Neurosurg.* **2013**, *27*, 712–717. [CrossRef] [PubMed]
16. Fattahi, A.; Taheri, M. Spontaneous Resolved Cervical Spine Epidural Hematoma: A Case Report. *Surg. Neurol. Int.* **2017**, *8*, 183. [CrossRef] [PubMed]
17. Jang, J.-W.; Lee, J.-K.; Seo, B.-R.; Kim, S.-H. Spontaneous Resolution of Tetraparesis Because of Postoperative Cervical Epidural Hematoma. *Spine J.* **2010**, *10*, e1–e5. [CrossRef] [PubMed]

Disclaimer/Publisher's Note: The statements, opinions and data contained in all publications are solely those of the individual author(s) and contributor(s) and not of MDPI and/or the editor(s). MDPI and/or the editor(s) disclaim responsibility for any injury to people or property resulting from any ideas, methods, instructions or products referred to in the content.

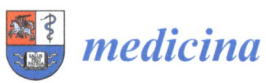 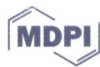

Case Report

A Combination of Ilizarov Frame, Externalized Locking Plate and Tibia Bridging for an Adult with Large Tibial Defect and Severe Varus Deformity Due to Chronic Osteomyelitis in Childhood: A Case Report

Pan Hong [1,†], Yuhong Ding [2,†], Ruijing Xu [1,†], Saroj Rai [3], Ruikang Liu [4,*] and Jin Li [1,*]

1. Department of Orthopaedic Surgery, Union Hospital, Tongji Medical College, Huazhong University of Science and Technology, Wuhan 430022, China
2. Second Clinical School, Tongji Medical College, Huazhong University of Science and Technology, Wuhan 430030, China
3. Department of Orthopedics, Al Ahalia Hospital, Mussafah, Abu Dhabi P.O. Box 2419, United Arab Emirates
4. Department of Endocrinology, Union Hospital, Tongji Medical College, Huazhong University of Science and Technology, Wuhan 430022, China

* Correspondence: rickylrk@163.com (R.L.); lijin2003whxh@foxmail.com (J.L.)
† These authors contributed equally to this work.

Abstract: *Background*: Various techniques have been reported to treat large, segmental tibial defects, such as autogenous bone graft, vascularized free fibula transfer and bone transport. We present a case of a 24-year-old male with a 17-year history of chronic osteomyelitis with obvious lower limb length discrepancy and severe varus deformity of the tibia secondary to osteomyelitis in childhood. *Aim*: The aim of this work is to provide an alternative choice for treating patients in developing countries with severe lower limb deformity caused by chronic osteomyelitis. *Case Presentations*: Without surgical intervention for a prolonged period of time, the patient was admitted in our institute for corrective surgery. Corrective surgery consisted of three stages: lengthening with Ilizarov frame, removal of Ilizarov frame and fixation with externalized locking plate, and removal of externalized locking plate. Tibia bridging was achieved at the distal and proximal junction. The range of motion (ROM) of the knee joint was nearly normal, but the stiffness of the ankle joint was noticeable. The remaining leg discrepancy of 0.1 cm required no application of a shoe lift. Moreover, the patient could engage in daily activities without noted limping. *Conclusions*: Distraction–compression osteogenesis using the Ilizarov apparatus is a powerful tool to lengthen the shortened long bone and adjust the deformity of the lower limbs. Externalized locking plates provide an alternative to the traditional bulky external fixator, as its low profile makes it more acceptable to patients without compromising axial and torsional stiffness. In all, a combination of Ilizarov frame, externalized locking plate and tibia bridging is an alternative for patients in similar conditions.

Keywords: bone defect; Ilizarov frame; locking plate; chronic osteomyelitis; varus deformity

Citation: Hong, P.; Ding, Y.; Xu, R.; Rai, S.; Liu, R.; Li, J. A Combination of Ilizarov Frame, Externalized Locking Plate and Tibia Bridging for an Adult with Large Tibial Defect and Severe Varus Deformity Due to Chronic Osteomyelitis in Childhood: A Case Report. *Medicina* **2023**, *59*, 262. https://doi.org/10.3390/medicina59020262

Academic Editors: Johannes Mayr, Ivo Dumić-Čule and Tomislav Čengić

Received: 15 December 2022
Revised: 11 January 2023
Accepted: 19 January 2023
Published: 29 January 2023

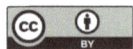

Copyright: © 2023 by the authors. Licensee MDPI, Basel, Switzerland. This article is an open access article distributed under the terms and conditions of the Creative Commons Attribution (CC BY) license (https://creativecommons.org/licenses/by/4.0/).

1. Introduction

Chronic osteomyelitis usually results from poorly treated or untreated acute osteomyelitis, open fractures and severe surgical complications [1]. It is seen more frequently in developing countries [2]. Several factors contribute to this situation, including virulence of bacteria, delayed presentation, poor nutritional and immune status and low social-economic status with limited access to antimicrobial agents [3].

Without proper treatment, osteomyelitis in childhood might lead to severe complications, including growth disturbance, severe leg length discrepancy (LLD) and varus or valgus malalignment [4]. The treatment strategy could be quite challenging if the residual deformity remains untreated till adulthood. With underlying osteomyelitis, staged treatment might be appropriate. As for the massive segmental bone defect in the tibia, various techniques have been proposed, including simple autogenous bone graft, allograft reconstruction, vascularized free fibula transfer, Masquelet technique and bone transport [5–10].

Here, we present a case of a 24-year-old male with residual deformity from chronic osteomyelitis in childhood. Severe LLD (cm), varus deformity (35 degrees), recurvatum deformity (33 degrees), internal rotational deformity (12 degrees), segmental tibial defect and hypertrophy of fibula was noteworthy. The patient was limping at presentation. Unlike the typical case of segmental defect of the tibia with the normal fibula, the long medical history and compensation mechanism resulted in a massive defect in the middle of the tibia, the hypertrophy of the fibula and the spontaneous bony fusion of proximal tibiofibular joint and distal tibiofibular syndesmosis. The compensatory hypertrophic fibula connected the tibial stump proximally as a *bridge*. Therefore, we distracted the fibula and strengthened the fusion between the stumps and *bridge*. We hope to provide an alternative choice for treating patients in developing countries with severe lower limb deformity caused by chronic osteomyelitis.

2. Case Presentation

All procedures performed in this study were in accordance with the ethical standards of the national research committee and the 1964 Helsinki declaration and its later amendments or comparable ethical standards. The patient provided informed consent for publication of this case.

A 24-year-old male was diagnosed with suppurative osteomyelitis and treated at a local hospital 17 years ago. The treatment details were unknown, and the osteomyelitis did not relapse in the past decade. At the outpatient clinic visit, he demonstrated limping with obvious lower limb length discrepancy (14 cm) and severe varus deformity of the tibia. Pelvic tilt was noticeable, and pseudoarthrosis of the tibia was formed. His ankle function was assessed by American Orthopedics Foot and Ankle Score (AOFAS) in the outpatient clinic and resulted in a score of 55 points (pain: 20, function: 25, alignment: 10) [11]. The muscle strength of the ankle assessed by the Lovett scale was level III in all directions. No active infection was detected.

3. Surgical Technique

The treatment strategy consisted of three staged surgeries.

Stage 1. Correction of the varus deformity and the shortening: In October 2016, the mid-section of the tibia was exposed to excise the necrotic and fibrous tissue, and synthetic bone with vancomycin was placed after copious irrigation with normal saline. Osteotomy was performed by drilling multiple holes beneath the proximal tibial fibular joint. Distal tibiofibular syndesmosis was explored, and osseous fusion was found. The Ilizarov frame was installed with 2 rings in the proximal tibia and fibula and 2 rings in the distal tibia. Seven days after the operation, the adjustment of the Ilizarov frame began (see Figures 1 and 2). Distraction was performed as 1 mm per day. After 4 months of distractions, the operated leg was lengthened from 31 cm to 45 cm (total distraction index: 1.17 mm/d).

Stage 2. Removal of Ilizarov apparatus and fixation of the tibia with externalized locking plate: After the length of the operated leg was adjusted to the same as the contralateral leg and mineralization was continued for eight months, the bulky Ilizarov apparatus was removed in October 2017. However, the union between the proximal tibia and fibula was not fully consolidated based on the radiological manifestation. In order to maintain the axis and stability of the lower extremity, a 5.0 mm locking plate was used to fixate the tibia and fibula. Autologous bone was harvested at the ipsilateral iliac crest and placed at the proximal interface between the tibia and fibula (see Figure 3).

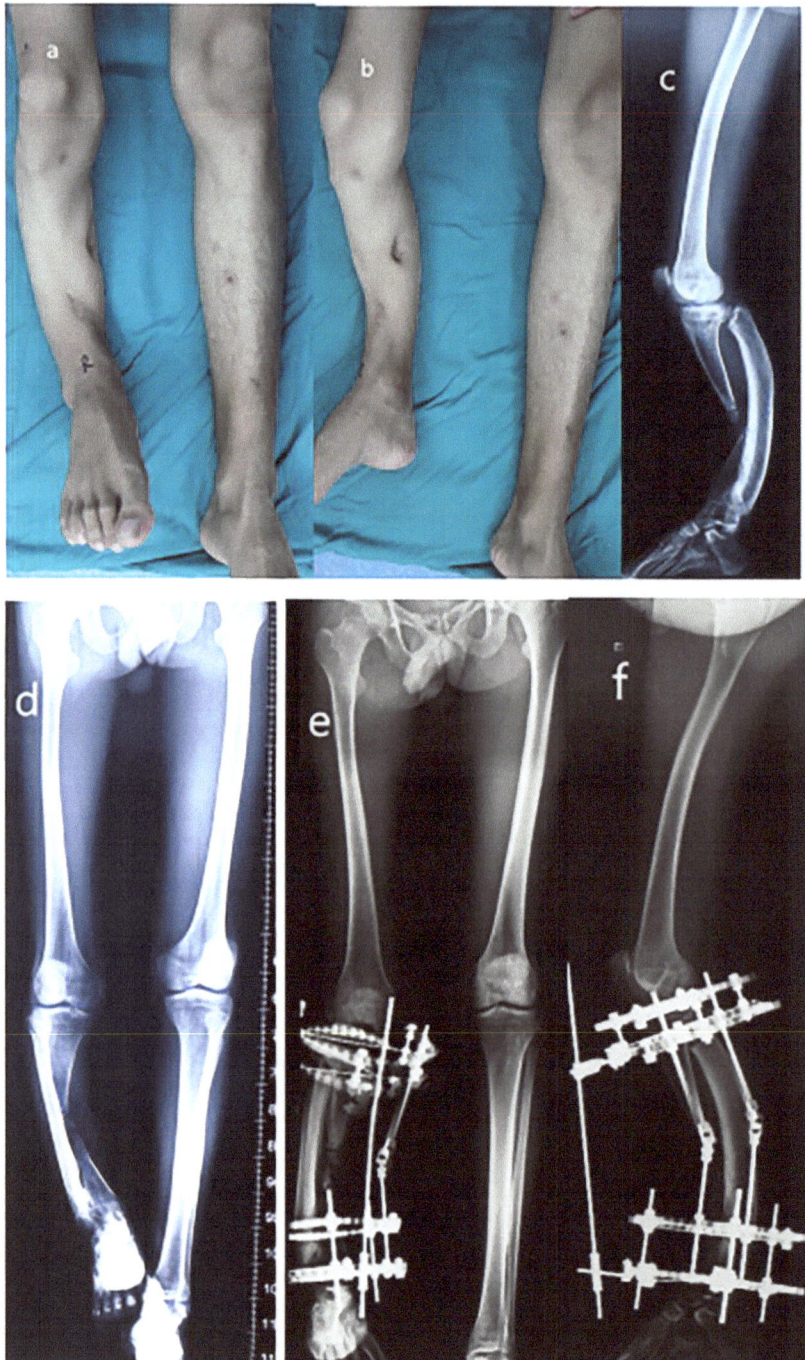

Figure 1. Radiograph of a 24-year-old male of severe limb length discrepancy and tibia varus. (**a**) Appearance (AP view); (**b**) Appearance (lateral view); (**c**) Preoperative later view radiograph; (**d**) Preoperative AP view radiograph; (**e**) Postoperative AP view radiograph; (**f**) Postoperative lateral view radiograph.

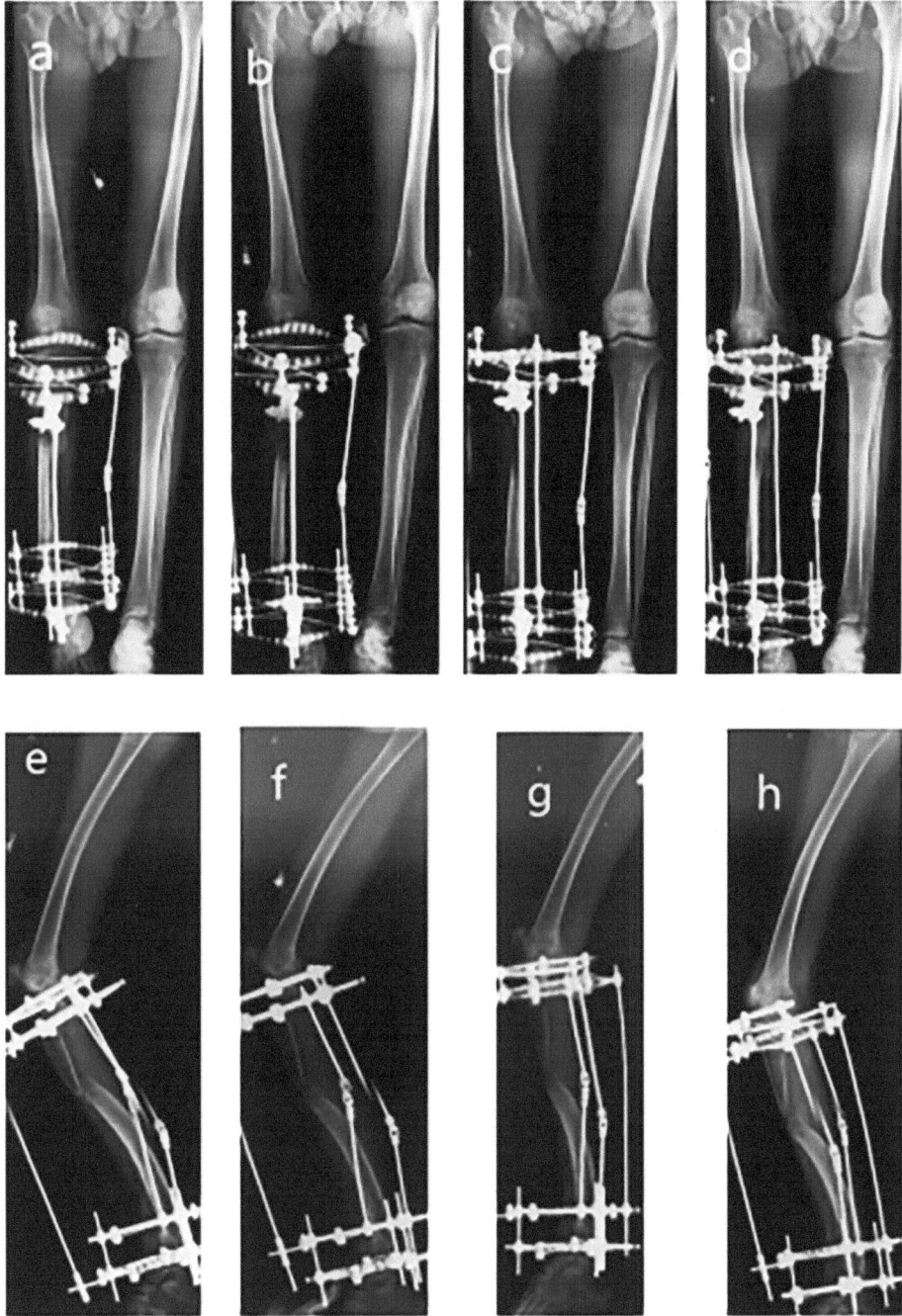

Figure 2. Series radiographs of the lower extremity after Ilizarov apparatus instalment. (**a**) AP view radiograph of 5th-month follow-up; (**b**) AP view radiograph of 8th-month follow-up; (**c**) AP view radiograph of 9th-month follow-up; (**d**) Lateral view radiograph of 10th-month follow-up; (**e**) Lateral view radiograph of 5th-month follow-up; (**f**) Lateral view radiograph of 8th-month follow-up; (**g**) Lateral view radiograph of 9th-month follow-up; (**h**) Lateral view radiograph of 10th-month follow-up.

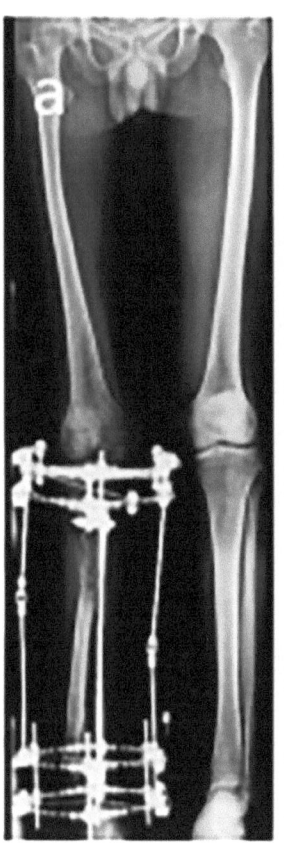 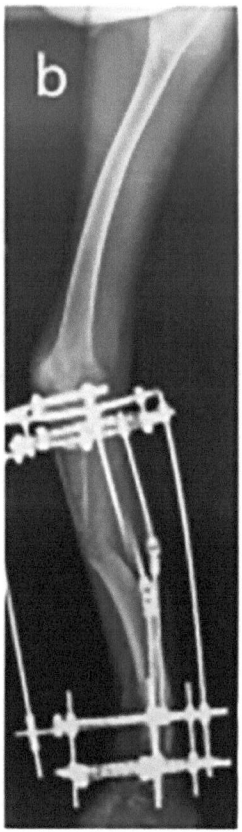 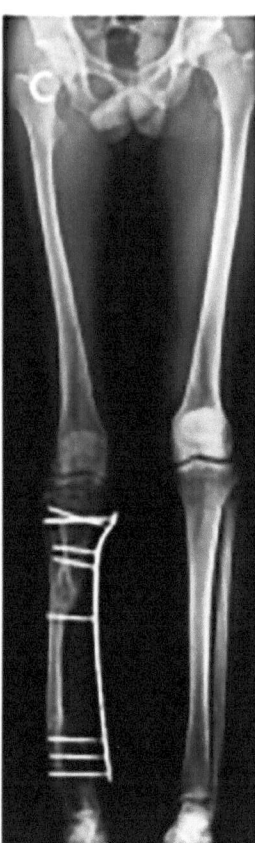 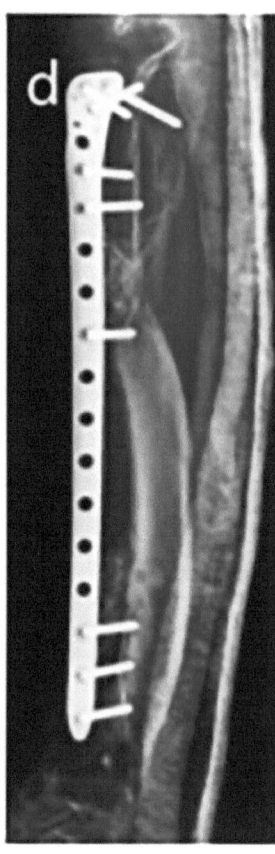

Figure 3. Removal of Ilizarov apparatus and externalized LCP. (**a**) AP view radiograph before removal of Ilizarov apparatus; (**b**) Lateral view radiograph before removal of Ilizarov apparatus; (**c**) AP view radiograph of externalized LCP fixation; (**d**) Lateral view radiograph of externalized LCP fixation.

Stage 3. Removal of the externalized locking plate: The patient was encouraged to walk with the support of two canes for three months after placing the locking plate. After that, the patient was able to walk freely with the externalized locking plate. Follow-up was carried out at regular intervals (once a month for the first three months and once every three months subsequently) on an outpatient basis. The locking plate was removed after 15 months (in January 2019), and the leg was immobilized in a slab for one month before full weight bearing (see Figure 4).

At stage 1, the necrotic and fibrous tissue was sent for pathohistological examination, and chronic osteomyelitis was confirmed. Intravenous empiric antibiotic treatment was continued for two weeks after the first surgery. Routine blood tests, including complete blood count (CBC), erythrocyte sedimentation rate (ESR) and C-reactive protein (CRP) were tested every two weeks to monitor the possible relapse of the infection. Bacterial culture from necrotic tissue reported negative for infection.

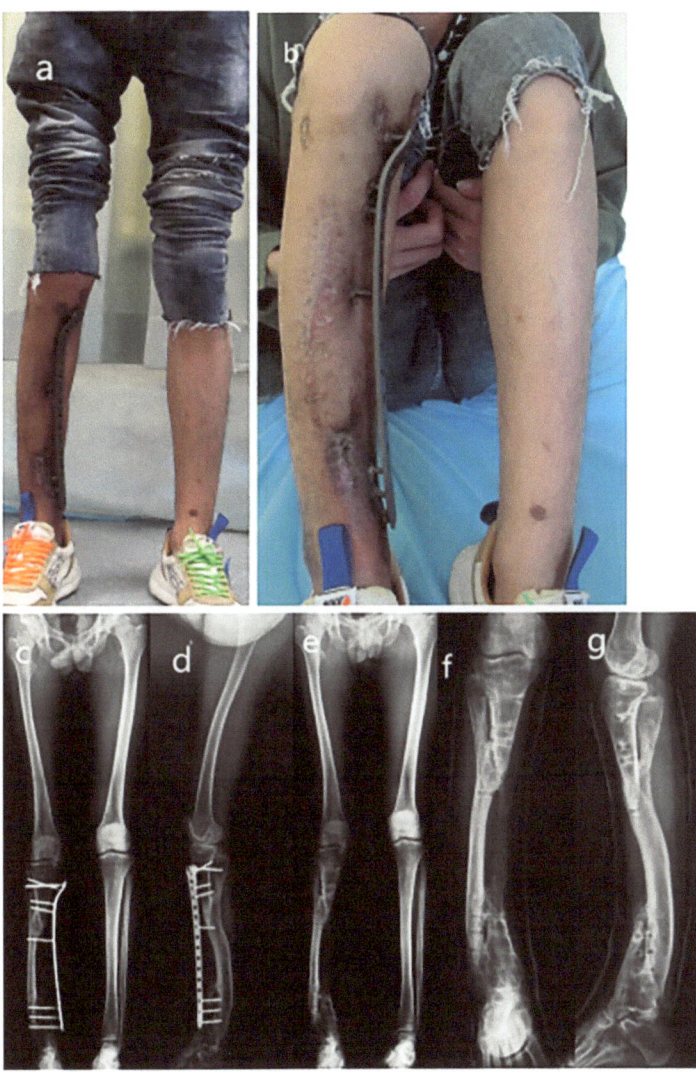

Figure 4. The appearance of the lower extremity and removal of the plate. (**a**) The appearance of the lower extremities; (**b**) Flexion of the knee joint; (**c**) AP view full-length radiograph of lower extremities before plate removal; (**d**) Lateral view full-length radiograph of lower extremities before plate removal; (**e**) AP view full-length radiograph of lower extremities after plate removal; (**f**) AP view radiograph of tibia–fibula after plate removal; (**g**) Lateral view radiograph of tibia–fibula after plate removal.

4. Results

The patient recovered uneventfully in the early stage of reconstructive surgery of lengthening and varus correction. The shin had been lengthened by 14 cm by the help of Ilizarov frame without knee or ankle spanning. In the later follow-up, the patient was able to walk with the Ilizarov apparatus, but it was quite inconvenient for him to wear such a bulky device. At the 12th-month follow-up visit, the distraction site displayed normal bone regeneration without complete consolidation. Therefore, a 5 mm locking plate was used to replace the Ilizarov frame to stabilize the tibia. Bone grafting was performed at the proximal interface of the tibia and fibula. The patient was braced for one month before weight-bearing exercise. The patient could walk freely with the support of an externalized locking plate, and he was satisfied with the low-profile external fixator. No wound infection, fracture of the tibia and fibula, or implant failure occurred during the 15-month follow-up. At the last follow-up visit before removing the plate, the ROM of the knee joint was nearly normal (135 degrees of flexion and 5 degrees of extension), but the stiffness of the ankle joint was noticeable. Assessment of the AOFAS score resulted in a score of 85 points (pain: 35, function: 40, alignment: 10). The muscle strength of the ankle assessed by the Lovett scale was level IV. The remaining leg length discrepancy of 0.1 cm required no application of a shoe lift. In addition, after removing the plate, the patient could engage in daily activities without limping. Moreover, the patient received empiric oral antibiotic therapy twice due to pin tract infections (PTI). However, the pin was fixed firmly without loosening, and no bone destruction and osteomyelitis was demonstrated by X-ray. Therefore, the olive wire was retained, and the skin and pin disinfection were performed daily. Fortunately, the PTI was controlled uneventfully at both times. During the last outpatient visit, the patient demonstrated a full recovery. In the recent phone call follow-up, the patient reported no adverse event and was satisfied with the status quo. Quality of life was assessed by the SF-36 scale during clinical visits, and the patient demonstrated a satisfactory activity of daily living in the last phone call follow-up. No serious complications (severe contracture or dislocation, etc.) happened during the treatment.

5. Discussion

This is a case of a young patient with segmental tibial bone defect and significant varus deformity of the tibia caused by chronic osteomyelitis (no relapse over the last ten years). The key is the correction of bone defect with misalignment in the lower extremity.

For patients with large tibial defect, there are three available choices: (1) amputation followed by prosthetics: Amputation could avoid the relapse of chronic osteomyelitis. However, the stigma after amputation could be prominent, and the young adult rejected this treatment decidedly. (2) Limb salvage surgery with custom-made implants to reconstruct the joint: A custom-made prosthetic from 3-D printing technology is a feasible choice for patients with severely destructed anatomical structures [12], but the severe LLD of this patient makes a custom-made implant unsuitable. (3) Limb salvage surgery with bone lengthening and tibial bridging: Autograft is not a feasible choice when the bone defect is more than 6–8 cm. Various apparatuses have been reported for bone lengthening, including Ilizarov frame, Taylor spatial frame (TSF) or Hexapod, and PRECICE [6–9].

PRECICE is an intramedullary limb lengthening system approved by the FDA; excellent outcomes with less pain and lower complication rates have been reported in over 250 cases [7]. However, this technique is not feasible for patients with abnormal intramedullary canal, as in this case. Additionally, although TSF and Hexapod are powerful computer-assisted deformity corrective tools, TSF is expensive and Hexapod is not available in China [8,9]. Moreover, for significant varus deformity with severe LLD, acute correction of angular deformity requires secondary surgery for lengthening. Therefore, we adopted the Ilizarov frame with spatial corrective potential, which provides relatively satisfactory effects and lower financial burden.

When the desired length and alignment is achieved, the patient wanted the bulky Ilizarov apparatus removed. There were several choices after hardware removal: (1) plaster support or brace, (2) rigid tibial nail, (3) plating, (4) externalized plating. Casting or bracing would restrict the weight-bearing exercises and might result in joint stiffness. Nailing is not suitable since the hypertrophic fibula does not have a normal intramedullary canal. The skin coverage and pin tract make conventional plating not applicable. Therefore, externalized plating was adopted in our study.

There were several details for this patient: a unilateral external fixator was not applicable due to delayed weight bearing and limited angular correction potential. Schanz screws in a one-sided external fixator could not provide sufficient purchase and accomplish massive lengthening. Therefore, Ilizarov frame was adopted. Moreover, for this patient, the compensation mechanism resulted in the osseous union between the tibia and fibula at the proximal and distal junction, and the hypertrophy of the fibula was so strong that it could withstand the body weight. Therefore, the compensatory fibula could work as a *bridge* to connect the tibia at both ends. With regard to the possible residual inflammation in the shaft of the tibia, we chose to remove the necrotic section of the tibia and elongate the hypertrophied fibula to correct the significant bone defect. Moreover, since the proximal and distal junction between the tibia and fibula was fused before corrective surgery, centralization of the fibula was not performed for better axial alignment. However, without the end-to-end union, the patient in our study demonstrated a normal gait and satisfactory daily life quality with tibial bridging.

As for the lengthening process, the recommended lengthening magnitude was 5–8 cm in long bones [13]. When the bone defect is substantial, the time to achieve the desired length can be extremely long. The lengthening process could be fraught with complications, such as PTI, neurovascular injury, muscle weakness, axial malalignment and nonunion or delayed union. Fortunately, no major complications such as neurovascular injury, infection, muscular damage, deep venous thrombosis (DVT) and re-fractures occurred. Serious complications such as severe contracture or dislocation were avoided during the treatment. However, the patient complained of intermittent PTI as well as the inconvenience of the bulky device in daily activities. The lengthening process was uneventful, but the mineralization and consolidation were insufficient at the time of Ilizarov apparatus removal. Concerning biomechanics, the stability of traditional plate fixation was worse than the locking plate, and the locking plate provided good angle stability [14]. Therefore, a 5 mm externalized locking plate was adopted after removing the Ilizarov apparatus. One month of immobilization of the long leg slab was implemented after the removal of the Ilizarov apparatus. Partial weight bearing was allowed after the removal of the slab, and progression to full weight bearing was initiated with discretion. Three months after the removal of the Ilizarov apparatus, the patient was able to walk freely with the externalized locking compression plate (LCP).

Postoperative complications have also been taken into account. PTI is common, but it is controllable with timely administration of oral antibiotics [15]. Rogers et al. reported that PTI occurred in 10% to 20% of cases of Ilizarov external fixators [16]. Moreover, they demonstrated the application of gentle compression dressings and reducing hyperglycemia and tourniquet time could reduce the rate of PTI. In addition, the bulky apparatus reduces patients' compliance, and wearing this device may decrease the quality of life and psychological happiness, which has been observed in adolescents [17]. Therefore, we removed the Ilizarov frame and changed it into a low-profile externalized plate. However, neurovascular injury, muscle weakness, axial malalignment and nonunion or delayed union are still common complications in massive lengthening, and discretion is required for patients with this condition [18–21].

There have been multiple cases reporting the application of externalized LCP in various regions of the body [22]. It has been shown that the main factors affecting the stiffness of LCP include working length, number of screws, distance from the plate to the bone and length of the plates [23]. Thirty millimeters is the upper bound of bone–plate distance to keep fixation stable in distal tibia fractures [24,25]. The increased diameters of the screws and the dimensions of the plate significantly enhance torsional rigidity but contribute little to compression stiffness. It is reported that externalized LCP could bear three times the body weight of an average 70 kg adult on axial loading only [26]. Thus, a 5.0 mm distal femoral locking plate was used in this patient.

Similarly, multiple cases have been reported regarding the Ilizarov frame on massive tibia lengthening. Kawoosa et al. reported a case of performing 20 cm lengthening and complex deformity correction on a centralized fibula using the Ilizarov technique with an excellent result [27]. They spent 17 months to complete the process of lengthening and consolidation at a healing index of 0.85 months/cm. Alkenani et al. also reported a case of right Gustilo IIIA segmental open tibia fracture with bone loss and other severe injuries [28]. Although the tibial defect was 14.5 cm, the patient was then admitted for Ilizarov application six months after the accident, and full limb length was restored. These cases corroborated that the Ilizarov frame was a positive alternative for patients with massive tibia lengthening.

To the best of our knowledge, no similar case with massive tibial defect and severe varus deformity due to chronic osteomyelitis was treated with Ilizarov frame, externalized plating and tibial bridging has been reported. Staged surgery is safe and relatively low-cost. The merits of our choices have been elucidated in the aforementioned context. Tibial bridging with successful fusion should be the touchstone for our staged treatment.

There also existed several limitations in our study. Firstly, meticulous care of a professional team with profound experience is usually required during the lengthening process. Moreover, our study was a case report rather than a cohort study, and externalized locking plate was unconventional. Moreover, the TSF frame might have demonstrated better outcomes than the Ilizarov frame, but TSF is more expensive than the Ilizarov frame. In addition, centralized fibula might be a better choice than tibial bridging.

6. Conclusions

Our study focuses on a patient with severe lower extremity deformity from chronic osteomyelitis in childhood. The Ilizarov apparatus was a powerful tool to lengthen the shortened long bone and adjust the deformity of the limbs in distraction–compression osteogenesis. Externalized locking plate provides an alternative to a traditional bulky external fixator because its low profile makes it more acceptable to patients without compromising axial and torsional stiffness. Moreover, in patients with static chronic osteomyelitis, a one-stage operation of necrotic bone resection and distraction osteogenesis is a feasible choice. In all, a combination of Ilizarov frame, externalized locking plate and tibia bridging is an alternative for patients in similar conditions.

Author Contributions: All authors contributed to the study conception and design. J.L. is in charge of the main idea and is the guarantor of integrity of the entire study; P.H. and R.L. are in charge of the study concepts, design, manuscript preparation and editing. Material preparation, analysis and editing were performed by R.X. and Y.D. The first draft of the manuscript was written by P.H. and Y.D.; S.R. and R.L. are in the charge of the language polish and the grammar revision. All authors commented on previous versions of the manuscript. All authors declare that the details of any images, videos, recordings, etc., can be published. All authors have read and agreed to the published version of the manuscript.

Funding: This research received no external funding.

Institutional Review Board Statement: The Ethics Committee of Tongji Medical College, Huazhong University of Science and Technology (IORG No: IORG0003571) gave a final APPROVAL on 20/11/2019 for the study, which was conducted by Xin Tang at Department of Orthopaedic Surgery, Union Hospital of Tongji Medical College, Huazhong University of Science and Technology.

Informed Consent Statement: Written informed consent was obtained from the patient for publication of this paper.

Data Availability Statement: Data sharing is not applicable to this article as no datasets were generated or analyzed during the current study.

Conflicts of Interest: The authors declare no conflict of interest.

Abbreviations

ROM = range of motion; LLD = leg length discrepancy; AOFAS = American Orthopedics Foot and Ankle Score; CBC = complete blood count; ESR = erythrocyte sedimentation rate; CRP = C-Reactive protein; PTI = pin tract infections; TSF = Taylor spatial frame; DVT = deep venous thrombosis; LCP = locking compression plate.

References

1. Ikpeme, I.; Ngim, N.; Ikpeme, A. Diagnosis and treatment of pyogenic bone infections. *Afr. Health Sci.* **2010**, *10*, 82–88.
2. Wirbel, R.; Hermans, K. Surgical treatment of chronic osteomyelitis in children admitted from developing countries. *Afr. J. Paediatr. Surg.* **2014**, *11*, 297. [CrossRef] [PubMed]
3. Koryllou, A.; Mejbri, M.; Theodoropoulou, K.; Hofer, M.; Carlomagno, R. Chronic Nonbacterial Osteomyelitis in Children. *Children* **2021**, *8*, 551. [CrossRef] [PubMed]
4. Schmitt, S.K. Osteomyelitis. *Infect. Dis. Clin. N. Am.* **2017**, *31*, 325–338. [CrossRef]
5. García-Gareta, E.; Coathup, M.J.; Blunn, G.W. Osteoinduction of bone grafting materials for bone repair and regeneration. *Bone* **2015**, *81*, 112–121. [CrossRef]
6. Aktuglu, K.; Erol, K.; Vahabi, A. Ilizarov bone transport and treatment of critical-sized tibial bone defects: A narrative review. *J. Orthop. Traumatol.* **2019**, *20*, 22. [CrossRef]
7. Paley, D. PRECICE intramedullary limb lengthening system. *Expert Rev. Med. Devices* **2015**, *12*, 231–249. [CrossRef]
8. Fenton, C.; Henderson, D.; Samchukov, M.; Cherkashin, A.; Sharma, H. Comparative Stiffness Characteristics of Ilizarov- and Hexapod-type External Frame Constructs. *Strateg. Trauma Limb Reconstr.* **2021**, *16*, 138–143.
9. Henderson, D.J.; Rushbrook, J.L.; Harwood, P.J.; Stewart, T.D. What Are the Biomechanical Properties of the Taylor Spatial Frame™? *Clin. Orthop. Relat. Res.* **2017**, *475*, 1472–1482. [CrossRef]
10. Alford, A.I.; Nicolaou, D.; Hake, M.; McBride-Gagyi, S. Masquelet's induced membrane technique: Review of current concepts and future directions. *J. Orthop. Res.* **2021**, *39*, 707–718. [CrossRef]
11. Alhadhoud, M.; Alsiri, N.; Alsaffar, M.; Glazebrook, M. Cross-cultural adaptation and validation of an Arabic version of the American Orthopedics Foot and Ankle Score (AOFAS). *Foot Ankle Surg.* **2020**, *26*, 876–882. [CrossRef] [PubMed]
12. Caravelli, S.; Ambrosino, G.; Vocale, E.; Di Ponte, M.; Puccetti, G.; Perisano, C. Custom-Made Implants in Ankle Bone Loss: A Retrospective Assessment of Reconstruction/Arthrodesis in Sequelae of Septic Non-Union of the Tibial Pilon. *Medicina* **2022**, *58*, 1641. [CrossRef] [PubMed]
13. Sailhan, F. Bone lengthening (distraction osteogenesis): A literature review. *Osteoporos. Int.* **2011**, *22*, 2011–2015. [CrossRef] [PubMed]
14. Aiyer, A.A.; Zachwieja, E.C.; Lawrie, C.M.; Kaplan, J.R.M. Management of Isolated Lateral Malleolus Fractures. *J. Am. Acad. Orthop. Surg.* **2019**, *27*, 50–59. [CrossRef] [PubMed]
15. Liu, K.; Abulaiti, A.; Liu, Y.; Cai, F.; Ren, P.; Yusufu, A. Risk factors of pin tract infection during bone transport using unilateral external fixator in the treatment of bone defects. *BMC Surg.* **2021**, *21*, 377. [CrossRef] [PubMed]
16. Rogers, L.C.; Bevilacqua, N.J.; Frykberg, R.G.; Armstrong, D.G. Predictors of postoperative complications of Ilizarov external ring fixators in the foot and ankle. *J. Foot Ankle Surg.* **2007**, *46*, 372–375. [CrossRef]
17. Sen, C.; Kocaoglu, M.; Eralp, L.; Gulsen, M.; Cinar, M. Bifocal compression–distraction in the acute treatment of grade III open tibia fractures with bone and soft-tissue loss: A report of 24 cases. *J. Orthop. Trauma* **2004**, *18*, 150–157. [CrossRef]
18. Xu, J.; Zhong, W.R.; Cheng, L.; Wang, C.Y.; Wen, G.; Han, P.; Chai, Y.M. The Combined Use of a Neurocutaneous Flap and the Ilizarov Technique for Reconstruction of Large Soft Tissue Defects and Bone Loss in the Tibia. *Ann. Plast. Surg.* **2017**, *78*, 543–548. [CrossRef] [PubMed]
19. Sella, E.J. Prevention and management of complications of the Ilizarov treatment method. *Foot Ankle Spec.* **2008**, *1*, 105–107. [CrossRef] [PubMed]
20. Donnan, L.T.; Gomes, B.; Donnan, A.; Harris, C.; Torode, I.; Heidt, C. Ilizarov tibial lengthening in the skeletally immature patient. *Bone Jt. J.* **2016**, *98*, 1276–1282. [CrossRef]
21. Hosny, G.A. Limb lengthening history, evolution, complications and current concepts. *J. Orthop. Traumatol.* **2020**, *21*, 3. [CrossRef] [PubMed]
22. Ebraheim, N.A.; Carroll, T.; Hanna, M.; Zhang, J.; Liu, J. Staged treatment of proximal tibial fracture using external locking compression plate. *Orthop. Surg.* **2014**, *6*, 154–157. [CrossRef] [PubMed]
23. Stoffel, K.; Dieter, U.; Stachowiak, G.; Gächter, A.; Kuster, M.S. Biomechanical testing of the LCP—How can stability in locked internal fixators be controlled? *Injury* **2003**, *34*, 11–19. [CrossRef] [PubMed]
24. Ahmad, M.; Nanda, R.; Bajwa, A.S.; Candal-Couto, J.; Green, S.; Hui, A.C. Biomechanical testing of the locking compression plate: When does the distance between bone and implant significantly reduce construct stability? *Injury* **2007**, *38*, 358–364. [CrossRef] [PubMed]
25. Kanchanomai, C.; Phiphobmongkol, V. Biomechanical evaluation of fractured tibia externally fixed with an LCP. *J. Appl. Biomech.* **2012**, *28*, 587–592. [CrossRef] [PubMed]
26. Ang, B.F.H.; Chen, J.Y.; Yew, A.K.S.; Chua, S.K.; Chou, S.M.; Chia, S.L.; Koh, J.S.B.; Howe, T.S. How externalised locking compression plate as an alternative to the unilateral external fixator: A biomechanical comparative study of axial and torsional stiffness. *Bone Jt. Res.* **2017**, *6*, 216–223. [CrossRef] [PubMed]

27. Kawoosa, A.A.; Butt, M.F.; Halwai, M.A. Deformity correction and massive lengthening on a centralized fibula with the Ilizarov technique. *Acta Orthop. Belg.* **2008**, *74*, 704–708.
28. Alkenani, N.S.; Alosfoor, M.A.; Al-Araifi, A.K.; Alnuaim, H.A. Ilizarov bone transport after massive tibial trauma: Case report. *Int. J. Surg. Case Rep.* **2016**, *28*, 101–106. [CrossRef]

Disclaimer/Publisher's Note: The statements, opinions and data contained in all publications are solely those of the individual author(s) and contributor(s) and not of MDPI and/or the editor(s). MDPI and/or the editor(s) disclaim responsibility for any injury to people or property resulting from any ideas, methods, instructions or products referred to in the content.

MDPI AG
Grosspeteranlage 5
4052 Basel
Switzerland
Tel.: +41 61 683 77 34

Medicina Editorial Office
E-mail: medicina@mdpi.com
www.mdpi.com/journal/medicina

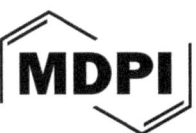

Disclaimer/Publisher's Note: The statements, opinions and data contained in all publications are solely those of the individual author(s) and contributor(s) and not of MDPI and/or the editor(s). MDPI and/or the editor(s) disclaim responsibility for any injury to people or property resulting from any ideas, methods, instructions or products referred to in the content.

www.ingramcontent.com/pod-product-compliance
Lightning Source LLC
LaVergne TN
LVHW072359090526
838202LV00019B/2586